Plant Energ

"I have not read or heard more in-dep physical features and natural history of o to enlarge our perception—this book is valuable. The foundation of this book is the interweaving of plant life stories and physical characteristics with the life lessons they incarnate for us. Above all, there is the wisdom distilled from the 'plant experience.' This book is an important contribution to the literature of plant wisdom."

MATTHEW WOOD, HERBALIST AND AUTHOR OF
A SHAMANIC HERBAL AND HOLISTIC MEDICINE
AND THE EXTRACELLULAR MATRIX

"*Plant Energy Medicine* is a tender and sensitive collection of writings that reveal the personalities of many common plants in a delightful and insightful way. The authors' deep connection and familiarity with plants shines as they guide us through exercises that are sure to deepen your understanding as you work with these gentle spirits. Treat yourself to a stroll through the spiritual garden of our plant brethren."

JILLIAN STANSBURY, ND, AUTHOR OF THE
HERBAL FORMULARIES FOR HEALTH PROFESSIONALS SERIES

"*Plant Energy Medicine* is riveting and a must-have for all students of plant science and for those who want to explore deeper into the plant world and the healing gifts that plants offer."

PHYLLIS HOGAN, SOUTHWESTERN HERBALIST
AND OWNER OF THE WINTER SUN TRADING CO.

"*Plant Energy Medicine* provides an in-depth understanding of the beneficial offerings of specific plants. The visual descriptions and the insights and energy impacts (chakra correspondences) the flowers provide are presented in a clear and easy-to-understand manner, backed by the authors' extensive knowledge and years of experience with flowers, trees, and flower essences. Through the book's guidance you are offered a way to explore the pathway plants provide to self-exploration, healing, and renewal."

ANNIE CHRISTOPHER, CO-OWNER OF FOSTER FARM BOTANICALS
AND FOUNDER OF ANNIE'S NATURALS

"This delightful, inspiring herbal brings readers the opportunity to enrich their self-awareness, growth, and healing through deepening their connection to plant wisdom. The authors share valuable insights gathered from their own personal experience, offering the reader practical hints, tools, and encouraging guidance for exploring their own personal plant journey. I really loved hearing the flowers' voices as they shared their wisdom and personalities. The photos are lovely, with so much information. Truly, a unique treasure of an herbal."

MARY BOVE, ND, AUTHOR OF *AN ENCYCLOPEDIA OF NATURAL HEALING FOR CHILDREN AND INFANTS*

"Rhonda PallasDowney and Sandi O'Connor have created a beautiful gift for all by creating this book. They introduce us to another way of connecting with the plant world that surrounds us. Through poetic descriptions, each plant leads us to a different and deeper understanding of ourselves. *Plant Energy Medicine* provides a means to gain insight and perspective into our current situations and to catalyze personal transformation."

KENNETH PROEFROCK, NMD, OWNER OF TOTAL WELLNESS MEDICAL CENTER

"This book is an amazing treasure chest about flowers and plants and how they help us. They can touch us physically, mentally, emotionally, and spiritually. When a flower or plant touches us spiritually, it is because the plant and the person are heart-to-heart. It is about love, and love is our greatest healing energy on every level of our being. Rhonda and Sandi are deeply in touch on this divine spiritual level with every plant they work with, which in turn transfers to the person who needs it."

EILEEN NAUMAN, AUTHOR OF *WALKING THE LAND*

"As our intelligent sisters of the green, the authors understand the power of the potential for our healing earth journey. I recommend this work so that we may find the reward of illumination within ourselves that the living green shows us through Rhonda and Sandi's work. The authors share with us their keen association—the relationship they have earned with the plants."

JOANNA CASTIGLIEGO SÁNCHEZ, RH(AHG), OWNER OF BOTANICA HERB SCHOOL IN ASSOCIATION WITH SOUTHWEST INSTITUTE OF HEALING ARTS

Plant Energy Medicine

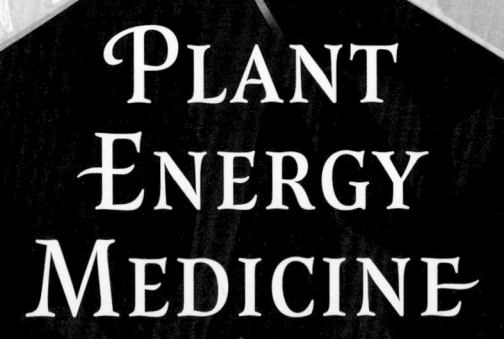

The Guiding Voice and Healing Vibration of 58 Plants

A Sacred Planet Book

Rhonda PallasDowney
and Sandi O'Connor

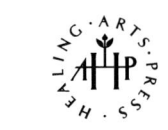

Healing Arts Press
Rochester, Vermont

Healing Arts Press
One Park Street
Rochester, Vermont 05767
www.HealingArtsPress.com

Healing Arts Press is a division of Inner Traditions International

Sacred Planet Books are curated by Richard Grossinger, Inner Traditions editorial board member and cofounder and former publisher of North Atlantic Books. The Sacred Planet collection, published under the umbrella of the Inner Traditions family of imprints, includes works on the themes of consciousness, cosmology, alternative medicine, dreams, climate, permaculture, alchemy, shamanic studies, oracles, astrology, crystals, hyperobjects, locutions, and subtle bodies.

Copyright © 2025 by Rhonda PallasDowney and Sandi O'Connor

Portions of this book were previously published in 2006 by Weiser Books in Rhonda PallasDowney's *Voices of Flowers: Learning to Use the Essence of Flowers to Heal Ourselves.*

All photos in this book are by Rhonda PallasDowney except where indicated.

All rights reserved. No part of this book may be reproduced or utilized in any form or by any means, electronic or mechanical, including photocopying, recording, or any information storage and retrieval system, without permission in writing from the publisher. No part of this book may be used or reproduced to train artificial intelligence technologies or systems.

Note to the reader: *This book is intended to be an informational guide. The remedies, approaches, and techniques described herein are meant to supplement, and not to be a substitute for, professional medical care or treatment. They should not be used to treat a serious ailment without prior consultation with a qualified health care professional.*

Cataloging-in-Publication Data for this title is available from the Library of Congress

ISBN 979-8-88850-175-7 (print)
ISBN 979-8-88850-176-4 (ebook)

Printed and bound in China by Guangzhou New Color Printing Co., Ltd.

10 9 8 7 6 5 4 3 2 1

Text design by Virginia Scott Bowman and layout by Kenleigh Manseau
This book was typeset in Garamond Premier Pro with Angie Pro, Myriad Pro, and Wedding Gothic ATF Wideused as display typefaces

To send correspondence to the authors of this book, mail a first-class letter to the author c/o Inner Traditions • Bear & Company, One Park Street, Rochester, VT 05767, and we will forward the communication, or contact the authors directly at **centerforplantstudies.com**.

Scan the QR code and save 25% at InnerTraditions.com. Browse over 2,000 titles on spirituality, the occult, ancient mysteries, new science, holistic health, and natural medicine.

To all the wisdom that has been passed down to us from our elders and ancestors, and in honor of the language of flowers and plants, and the green world that illuminates our path of healing.

We Are the Seeds

Through the long, cold winter
waiting out the dark
trying to beat the odds of survival
while hope grows in the heart

Dreaming beneath the snow
Awaiting the moment to grow
Gathering purpose and power
To finally become a flower

Imagine the stories
passing hand to hand
traveling the ocean in pockets
with memories of the land

The future is unknown
Can we learn to thrive?
Remember all the ancient wisdom
is held safe deep inside

You and me
we are the seeds
Let's grow a world
we want to see

You and me
we are the seeds
Let's grow a world
we want to see

Just like trees
our roots run deep
Our branches dance
in the mystery

Just like trees
our roots run deep
Our branches dance
in the mystery

SONG BY KATE WATTERS

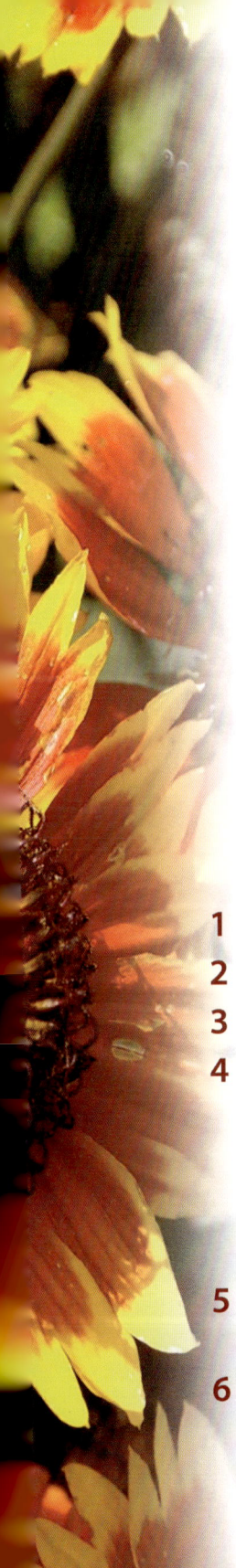

Contents

Foreword by Rosemary Gladstar ... ix
Acknowledgments ... xiii
Introduction: Synchronicity and Interconnectedness ... 1

PART ONE
Connecting Energetically with Plants

1 The Language of Plant Energy ... 14
2 Plants' Sensory Input ... 25
3 Dynamics of the Biofield ... 31
4 Flower Essences ... 38
   Unseen Gifts of Nature

PART TWO
The Wisdom in Plant Readings

5 Pathways Uniting Body, Mind, and Spirit ... 50
   The Chakras
6 How to Do Plant Readings ... 66
   Daily Insights and Plant Medicine Readings

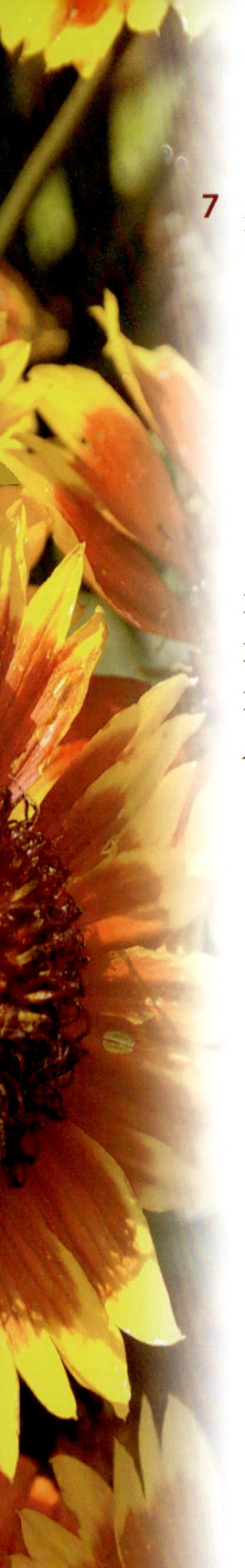

7   An Invitation to a Plant Journey   85
Welcome a New Doorway into Your Life

PART THREE
THE GUIDING VOICE OF FLOWERS, TREES, AND PLANTS

Aspen to Yucca   97

Notes   285
Bibliography   288
Index   294
About the Authors   302

Foreword

Rosemary Gladstar

Flowers adorn the face of the world and brighten every corner of the globe. In fact, humans couldn't exist without flowers or flowering plants. They are a part of every facet of our lives and every human celebration and ceremony, from birth to death. Flowers appear at weddings, as declarations of love; at religious ceremonies and pagan festivals, to mark the cycles of life; at births, to welcome the newest members of the family; and at funerals, to honor those who have passed over and to comfort those left behind. They adorn our art, our clothing, our gardens and landscapes, our homes, and our hearts. It's quite impossible to imagine life without flowers and plants, and thankfully we don't have to.

There are so many ways we can experience the exquisite nature of flowers: their often heady scents; their luxurious textures and colors; their radiant beauty that brightens everything around them; their enduring tenacity that allows them to just keep growing, surviving despite Earth's upheavals; their colorful and clever ability to lure and seduce the perfect pollinators; and their sensuous heart centers. There are also the inner teachings that flowers offer us when we learn to listen to them. By their very nature, flowers, and plants in general, teach us how to live a more joyful, harmonious, happier, healthier, and more balanced life. In fact, perhaps this is their greatest gift to us. But to hear their inner teachings requires attentive listening.

Foreword

In their beautiful book *Plant Energy Medicine: The Guiding Voice and Healing Vibration of 58 Plants*, Rhonda and Sandi generously and heartfully share with us the teachings they've received through years of attentive listening to these exquisite beings. Having cultivated a lifelong relationship with plants, and as practicing herbalists and flower essence practitioners, they have spent decades listening to and learning from plants, and they are thus skillful guides into the world of sacred plant medicine. Their work is both inspired and inspiring, and is imprinted with the beauty of the flowers and lessons they've learned from them. Reflected also in their teachings and life work are the multitextured experiences they've garnered working in the field of social services, along with their many years of studying plants, homeopathy, herbalism, flower essences, and other healing modalities. Through this lovely book that Sandi and Rhonda have co-created, these two friends bring a deep spiritual connection to their work.

Plant Energy Medicine: The Guiding Voice and Healing Vibration of 58 Plants was created as a tool to explore and deepen one's personal experience with the world of plants. In simple yet elegant language, the authors offer the wisdom and insights they've received from plants to assist us on our life journeys. More than merely reading about the messages of the plants, they invite us to put them into practice to help us gain a higher perspective on whatever life situation confronts us.

As the authors say, "Prepare for an extraordinary journey, a journey that calls forth the innate wisdom and power of the sacred medicine of the flowers, trees, and plants." This book is Sandi and Rhonda's gift to us—and such a wondrous gift it is!

ROSEMARY GLADSTAR,
FROM HER HOME AT MISTY BAY, VERMONT

ROSEMARY GLADSTAR is well-known as a leading practitioner and luminary in the modern herbalism movement. Her knowledge, expertise, love, and guardianship of the green world have made her legendary in the world of plant medicine. Rosemary has written and taught herbalism for more than forty years, is the author of eleven books (including the compendious *Herbal Recipes for Vibrant Health*), and is the founding president of United Plant Savers and past director of the International Herb Symposium.

Acknowledgments

The promise of friendship unfolds beautifully in a garden of joy.
ALDA ELLIS

Throughout our travels and life experiences we have known many people from all walks of life who have inspired us to trust our inner journeys and wisdom. With deep gratitude we extend our heartfelt thanks to the many Indigenous elders and herbal folk practitioners and teachers of the healing arts for sharing their profound relationship with plants and nature with us. We especially want to thank and acknowledge Rhonda's teacher, Matthew Wood, for his brilliance and wisdom in imparting his knowledge of the plant world. The wisdom of Matthew Wood has been passed down to many of us, as have the insights and experiences of many other great herbal teachers and elders.

We honor all those who have supported us in this work, for the gifts they offer to the world and for their efforts and authenticity in their review of this book. We are grateful for the opportunities to attend the many botanical medicine conferences that have flourished in recent years, which have led to longlasting friendships. Our hearts are filled with gratitude to Rosemary Gladstar for her foreword to this book and for the richness she brings to the plant world in so many ways. We also give thanks to our dear friend, songwriter and plant sister Kate Watters, of Wild Heart Farm in Rimrock, Arizona, for sharing her beautiful song "We Are The Seeds." And we give special thanks to our dear friend JoAnna Castigliego

Sánchez, director of the herbalist training program at Southwest Institute of Healing Arts (SWIHA), in Scottsdale, Arizona, for her profound knowledge of herbalism and for sharing her wisdom.

We want to thank a few more very special people in our lives. Rhonda's loving husband, Curt PallasDowney, has spent countless hours with her exploring earth medicine in the forms of flora and fauna. As a Western mystic, Curt has supported Rhonda in her many endeavors throughout the years. His love of nature and the human experience strongly encourages people to deepen their awareness, so it is with sincere gratitude that we acknowledge Curt's gifts and his immeasurable support and wisdom, including his contributions to this book.

As well, Rhonda offers her gratitude to her longtime friend Robbie Nelson, with whom she explored the healing energies of the plant world in the late 1980s and early '90s and, in later years, blended heart connection work with the Wisdom of Horses and Flowers retreats at Robbie's ranch in Dove Creek, Colorado.

Sandi's friend and loving brother, Gary ("Bear") Palisch, has encouraged her to open to exploring life in many different ways. Gary's support and commitment to human evolution has meant a lot to Sandi. Through his own explorations, Gary has inspired others to live life at its fullest.

These and other friendships have created the deep bonds of trust and integrity that have supported our work over the years, and for this we are eternally grateful. We thank Rosemarie Brown for her intuitive guidance and support, which have been immeasurable to the birthing of this book. We are grateful for Miss VJL and Kevin Chapman's expertise and assistance with some graphic formatting, and for Sarah PallasDowney's sharing of her heart-filled culinary nourishment during our work on this book. We are also deeply grateful to Renick Turley for sharing his love of the plant world and the many ways he expresses it; to Cody Lyon for sharing her love of flowers and horses and providing the photo of Angel; to Rene Ragan for opening a wider doorway into the bioenergetic life force field; to Pamela Becker of Big Vision Arts in Sedona, Arizona, for her beautiful illustrations of the chakras and the *Voices of Flowers* CD art; and to Joy Capp for her helpfulness and for all the ways she has shown up for us. And with deep gratitude we thank our friend and author Dawn Silver, D.N., for her exquisite timing and support to move forward in publishing our book.

We also want to give thanks to our family members and friends who offered support and permission to use their photos in our book. These include Tanya Downey, Adam Downey, Jennifer Downey, Sarah PallasDowney, Curt PallasDowney, Kylee Koepnick, and JoAnna Castigliego Sánchez.

In addition, with great respect and gratitude we thank Richard Grossinger for finding and connecting with us, and we are grateful for the expertise provided to us by our copy editor Margaret Jones and our project editor Lyz Perry. We are also grateful for all the beautiful efforts and energies put into the book by Virginia Scott Bowman, Kenleigh Manseau, and our ITI team.

Finally, we thank all of you dear readers who want to explore life and your inner journey in the company of flowers, trees, and plants.

INTRODUCTION

Synchronicity and Interconnectedness

If you want a child's mind to grow, you must first plant a seed.
AUTHOR UNKNOWN

Many of us experience those times in our lives when somehow, somewhere, and out of nowhere momentous happenstances occur when we least expect it. Events like this can coincide that seem on the surface to have no practical connection and yet are significantly related. Carl Jung, the Swiss psychologist, psychiatrist, psychoanalyst, and dream interpreter well-known for his exploration of how the unconscious mind communicates with the conscious mind, called this *synchronicity*.

Synchronicity and the interconnection of the unconscious and the conscious demonstrate the relationship with all things that come into our minds, feelings, and images as archetypes or symbols. This is an example of the archetypal design of the universe.

Many spiritual traditions—such as Western mysticism, Buddhism, Sufism, Greek traditions, Kabbalah, Indigenous cultures of the world including Native American peoples, and others—believe in naturally unfolding events, signs, and impulses that impact humanity's experience as it is exposed through mind, body, and spirit awareness to the unlimited potential of the universal energy of creation and searching for meaning.

Through this deeper universal connection, human beings experience their birthright, stepping into unity and harmony with themselves, each other, the ecosystem, and a way of life that nurtures sustainability—a way of life that offers interconnection and synchronicity in the both visible and invisible ways that human beings sense, understand, thrive in, and perceive their world and the universe.

Bernard Beitman, M.D., author of *Connecting with Coincidence: The New Science for Using Synchronicity and Serendipity in Your Life*, hosted a 2021 YouTube interview with author and publisher Richard Grossinger titled "Thoughtforms and Synchronicity—Assume the Impossible." With references to various scientists and psychologists, they discussed interconnection and synchronicity; in Dr. Beitman's words: "we human beings are like the dying caterpillar. We are eating up our habitat, our earth. We need imaginable individuals to begin vibrating at similar frequencies to recognize each other and come together as One to create a beautiful creature like that butterfly that lives lightly on the earth. A new science of synchronicity will help imaginable people recognize each other."

As these two thought leaders shared their synchronicity stories, they showed how our interconnectedness provides "markers for the cartography of the psychosphere," a term that refers to "a kind of mental atmosphere where a person's need defines and clarifies an intention, so that the mind can arrive at the needed information in extraordinary and wonderful ways."

> We live in that psychosphere and we take it for granted in a sense, as remarkable as it is and as inexplicable as it is by conventional logic. All the synchronicities cut across other kinds of paranormal aspects of reality. . . . In the psychosphere, we each have a higher Self communicating to us, and [we] see things more broadly than we can see right down here on earth.

Together they concluded that there is an inner guidance system within us, a higher energy at work, and they emphasized this power within. Beyond conscious knowing, Richard stated that synchronicity is not just chance. It doesn't fall under the algorithm that rules all thinking today. Scientists apply algorithms to explain how things happen. . . . There's more about this universe that we don't know than we do. . . . these lives we live are better lived when we take on the creative possibility of our own being and assume the impossible.[1]

RHONDA PALLASDOWNEY ON THE TEACHINGS OF BLACK COHOSH (*ACTAEA RACEMOSA*)

In 1980, while in my late twenties and facing a major life transition, my interest in natural medicine and healing remedies led me in a new direction. My inner voice guided me to go on a personal retreat. I set up camp in a remote area on some property owned by friends that was nestled in the lush, green, rolling foothills of the Appalachian Mountains of southeastern Ohio. My camp was situated in a forest of spruce and fir trees, sugar maples, white ash and beech trees, and red oaks. The trees became my friends of the forest as I studied their individual characters, the ways they shifted in the winds, and the sunlight that shone on their branches and leaves. I felt they were communicating their innermost natures to me. I gave names to each member of my forest family and certain plant relatives of the most prominent trees around my camp, feeling that they were my guardians and protectors. Many wild plants grew in my forest—wild ginger, spotted joe-pye weed, sassafras, wild grapevines, wild berries, goldenrod, wild asparagus, amaranth, black cohosh, blue cohosh, goldenseal, and American ginseng, to name but a few.

The camp was located near the small rural town of Ray, Ohio (then population 200), about forty miles from Rutland, Ohio, where the United Plant Savers Sanctuary now lives. I was often seen walking around with my plant book, asking questions about local plants and herbs. Two middle-aged mountain men who were brothers offered to take me into the denser parts of the forest to collect plants, especially American ginseng and goldenseal. These two men were my first plant teachers. They taught me how to identify, collect, and cultivate their Appalachian plants.

Many a night I slept with burlap bags filled with roots with plant parts surrounding me in my small tent. I felt a surge of energy while lying in my sleeping bag snuggled against the sacred gunnysacks that held my cherished findings. I traveled from one rich dream journey to another.

Throughout the summer I collected plants. The plant that called to me the most, however, was black cohosh. Black cohosh, also known as black snakeroot, thrives in soils rich in base elements. As I dug to get at the plant's root system, I found it to be extremely tangled and challenging to dig up. This brought up all the feelings I had buried inside myself. At that time in my life I was experiencing trapped feelings over my life's circumstances—frustration, anger, fear, and depression. Digging up the entangled black cohosh roots brought the dark force of my drama out in the open. I realized that all my fears seemed to hold me bondage, and I felt overpowered. I would dig up the roots and toss them, shouting out words I didn't even know were in me. Then I would take the shovel and heave it as far as I could as I reached deep into my inner battles. Following these acting-out episodes, I felt sad and remorseful for my actions. I would stand up in the digging area, walk over to the roots, gently pick them up, and return to the hole where I had been digging. Brushing off the clumped dirt clinging to the roots, I held them in my hands and apologized to them, letting my tears flow as I sucked on a root. This became my ritual for many days. The roots exuded a slightly smokey, earthy, mushroomy odor, and when I sucked on them they seemed to cool me off internally. I instantly felt relaxed, grounded, and at ease.

Black cohosh helped me to step outside of myself, to be an observer to my reactions and my feelings. It helped me confront my fears and the neglected parts of myself in a way that I had never experienced before. I let go of a lot of built-up anxiety and began sleeping better at night. In this way over the summer I established an intimate relationship with black cohosh as well as a new relationship with myself. Often at night I would gaze at the stars from the safety of my camp, where I followed the light of the moon in the trees, the shadows, and the many forms of nature that surrounded me. In the stillness of complete darkness I would travel to another realm apart from this earthly world and see myself as a pure light being—secure, unscathed, playful, and illuminated.

Six years later, in 1986, while living in Sedona, Arizona, I was once again feeling trapped by my life circumstances. I was involved in a manipulative and abusive relationship, feeling hopeless and stuck, struggling with my fears in a kind of inner darkness where I questioned my own self-worth. I was invited to attend an herb workshop in Flagstaff, Arizona, presented by Dave Milgram and Matthew Wood. There were about twenty of us in a comfortably sized room. At some point during his talk, Matt, who was sitting directly across from me, looked straight into my eyes. He picked up an old wooden medicine box filled with brown bottles and walked across the room and squatted down in front of me. He gazed into my eyes, reached into his medicine box, picked up a small bottle, and said "Ah-ha!" I wasn't exactly sure what that meant, but I could feel he was confident that he had found what he was looking for. He asked me to open my mouth. I did so, and naturally closed my eyes. The sensation of liquid drops dissolved under my tongue, trickled slowly down my throat, and landed in my stomach. I felt an overwhelmingly familiar energy move through me.

Matt then shared with me and the others that it was a flower essence. I sensed an immediate, subtle connection with this essence. It was as if the frequency of the plant was aligning my body, soul, and spirit with all of nature. Memories of my experiences in the Appalachian Mountains and my personal relationship with black cohosh came rushing back to me as I recalled how I had struggled with the entangled roots, pulling and digging them out of the earth and furiously tossing them as far as I could. I felt myself leaning into the healing energy of Matt's plant essence, being embraced by its nurturing presence. I felt grounded and peaceful. In a matter of seconds, a sense of relief and freedom swept through me. An awakening to my own personal patterns and behaviors, my emotions and thoughts, entered me all within the snap of a finger. In that moment I felt an inner shift, a drive and a determination to face my fears and gather my strength to move beyond all entanglements.

Opening my eyes, I gazed into Matt's eyes and asked, "Is this black cohosh?" He nodded his head and smiled, though little did he know my story behind it. His comment about the black cohosh flower essence was that it is "for those who feel entangled and hopeless." Matt also gave me *Mimulus guttatus*, yellow monkeyflower, a snapdragon-shaped flower with spotted red on its lower lobes. This flower essence, he said, was for "letting go of fear and for sticky relationships." *How fitting is that*, I thought. I couldn't help but inquire within myself how the physical properties of black cohosh's root emitted a similar response, as subtle as a flower essence. I was intrigued by the energy exchange within the plant's own makeup.

This experience of meaningful coincidence and the insights I gained from Matt were the start of a fruitful journey of teacher and student as I began my relationship with plants, trees, and flowers. Matt became a friend and mentor. He led me in my study of herbs as I researched plants and their characteristics and learned about the healing power of vibrational essences and importantly, the doctrine of signatures, the ancient idea that the physical characteristics of plants provide clues as to how they might be used—that plants have a "signature," that is, a color, texture, shape, scent, even the environment in which they grow, that resembles the body parts and diseases they heal. For example, Matthew's 1987 book *Seven Herbs: Plants as Teachers* has a fitting description of how the doctrine of signatures works with regard to black cohosh: "The dark, gnarled root indicates both a dark property and a bristling, contending nature. Black cohosh is a remedy for those who are caught in a state of brooding, dark hopelessness."[2] Wood continues: "The healer who masters this lesson [in plant-human correspondences] accumulates what [Native people] call 'monitou' or 'medicine-power'" . . . "a true remedy is an act of courage and insight, as much as the feat of a warrior or artist."[3] Reflecting on the healing power of black cohosh, how relevant it is that black cohosh showed up twice in my life for much-needed change.

Following the workshop, Matt spent a few days with me at my house in Back O' Beyond, near Cathedral Rock in Sedona. We explored the surrounding plant world and discovered a grove of yerba santa (*Eriodictyon californicum*) plants nearby. We studied yerba santa's doctrine of signatures, journeyed and meditated with the plant, and made a flower essence. The entire experience led me to a visceral understanding of the profound healing offered by yerba santa at all levels, and how its energetic gifts touched my innermost being. How amazingly enlightening this experience was for me when Matt said about yerba santa, "It teaches us to learn how to move with ease in the inner world and to know how to survive there." From there I developed a plant format and guide to support me in my plant studies. My yerba santa case study was included in Matt's first book, *Seven Herbs: Plants as Teachers*. This inspired me to further my study of the plant kingdom, for which I feel ever so grateful.

SANDI O'CONNOR ON THE MYSTERY OF WONDERWORKING

I grew up in a college town on the Mississippi River in midwestern Minnesota. As I grew older I lived in both the lakeside and farmland areas of Minnesota. Because I lived in the country, I developed a love of flowers, trees, plants, and various forms of natural healing. I connected with them on such a deep level that I could feel their unique vibrations. I wanted to learn more, and so I began reading books and magazines on plants and their healing properties. I was enamored of the excitement of learning about plants, and this eventually led me to renowned herbalist Rosemary Gladstar.

After delving into Rosemary's beautiful writing and the wealth of information she provided, I started searching for others who were into natural healing. I signed up for a newsletter published by Present Moment Bookstore in Minneapolis, and that's how I discovered Matthew Wood, the store's owner. One weekend I took a drive to Minneapolis. As a lover of books, walking into that bookstore made me feel as though I had walked into heaven. In the process of exploring the store, I saw Matthew Wood's office. I picked up information about him and vowed to return to meet him.

Because of my work hours, the only time I could visit the store was on weekends. Needless to say, Matthew wasn't there on the days that I was there. I was seeking books that would allow me to build my knowledge of the green world and holistic healing, and because my life was so full then I didn't make the connection with Matthew in person at that time.

As time passed, I had a few opportunities to travel around Europe. Following my last trip to Italy, I came back home and felt called to move to Arizona. One night, a close friend of a friend came through to me in a dream. She lived outside of Sedona, in Cottonwood, Arizona, and in the dream she encouraged me to move to Cottonwood. I packed up, sold my farm, and off I went to Arizona.

Landing in Clarkdale, Arizona, I found the perfect place to live. Through some sense of magic, I drove to nearby Jerome. There I heard some beautiful music coming out of a shop that pulled me in, where I met the shop owner. We had a beautiful exchange, and as a result she gave me a lead for a job that involved working with developmentally disabled adults with extreme behaviors, which was my area of expertise. Three weeks later, I had a job at Yes the Arc, an adult day program for people with developmental disabilities, located in Cottonwood. One day I met Rhonda, with whom we shared a client. At the time, Rhonda was a case worker for the State of Arizona. Little did we know that we were about to embark on a remarkable adventure together.

Because of our attraction to understanding human nature, each of our chosen professions had brought us to the same field, that of human services and special education, a field in which we each had over twenty-five years' experience. We both came from the Midwest, and we both had a connection to plants and wildlife that had been inspired as a result of growing up in the country, close to nature. And we both recognized certain patterns of the mind and their resulting behaviors. Our common experience of patterns and behaviors, along with our awareness of emotional structures, carried over into our understanding the integration process that leads to wholeness. Our intuition and conscious awareness of these patterns had deepened through our relationship with nature, especially plants.

It was through this connection that our paths met. There was an instant familiarity between us. During a break from the meeting we were in, this unspoken energy that we each recognized pulled at us to explore further. I subsequently participated in Rhonda's seventy-five-hour experiential flower essence program. Our connection continued to grow as we parlayed our experiences in the healing world of human nature with the vast world of nature itself.

I finally met Matthew Wood at Rhonda's house for an herbal consultation soon after that. I was struck by the profundity of Matt's healing insights into my condition. I had developed a deep pain to the left side of my groin which led to a visit to the ER. It was diagnosed as a kidney stone and I was referred to a specialist. In the meantime, before going to the specialist, Matthew came into town and I met with him. Right away he knew what herbal remedies I needed to take. Rhonda, being present with me in the consultation, jumped enthusiastically from her chair, rushed to her apothecary, and showed up proudly with all three remedy tinctures that she had recently made. They were agrimony, burdock root, and gravel root. Matt smiled and told me to take the doses right away. Within thirty minutes, the pain was gone. I stayed on Matt's program for months until the stones disappeared, and the doctor who had suggested surgery was in total amazement. I didn't need to have the surgery! This story confirmed my belief in the healing power of plants. In addition, we three shared our roots and a Midwestern comradery. Rhonda and I subsequently attended Matthew's herb class in Sedona during a fall weekend in 2010.

A BLOSSOMING CONNECTION

It is our hope and intention that in this book readers will recognize that we are all connected in our human journeys, and that everything in life is connected to nature. There's a message from all of these profound green beings around us, our plant teachers. They reflect back to us all the wonderful things that exist within each one of us. There is one thread of sweetness that runs through all living things, which we all share. This sweetness of life often gets buried by life's circumstances, such that we forget that it's there.

Most of us have been conditioned to think that we have to earn love. Awakening to this journey of life helps us to understand that love is already present within each of us. We don't have to earn love. Love is our birthright, something we are born with and that never leaves us, even when certain situations challenge us to love.

We can untangle our root system that has been knotted up from old patterns, old stories, old behaviors. These gnarly roots were entwined around the heaviness of our pain, like a rock that causes a plant's roots to grow around it. The rock is our old vibrational energy that causes us to see things with old eyes. Once we remove the rock, like the gardener who works the soil and removes all the rocks that interfere with the growth of the garden, our roots will spread out and go deeper, allowing us to take root in more meaningful and insightful ways as we acknowledge who we truly are.

The power that we have realized within ourselves is about speaking our truths and sharing. We have learned that we would rather not be seen as teachers or healers, but as instruments for helping others learn to heal themselves as we model life lived from a place of wholeness.

We want to lovingly share with our readers all that we've offered of ourselves from our own journeys—amazing journeys that all came about as if perfectly timed, and we are simply following the steps.

As you step deeper into the powerful, light-filled energy of your soul, may this connection infuse you with love and courage to be the highest version of yourself.

All of us are on this journey together, constantly fertilizing new growth and leading it to harvest. May you hear the flowers, trees, and plants whisper their voices to you and inspire you to thrive and blossom in unconditional love as you plant your seeds of inspiration and awakening.

This book takes off from Rhonda's 2006 book *Voices of Flowers*, which highlights forty-eight flowers and plants. We have added ten more plants, including trees, to this book. We also have gone deeper into the vibrational energy of each of these plants. As the journey evolves for us, so does the wisdom that we have gained from our plant teachers over the years.

We invite you to personalize your journey and awaken to your inner wisdom. We joyfully share our bouquets of inner wisdom that have awakened in us on our individual life journeys and on our journey together as friends and colleagues. As you read, allow yourself to open to this great mystery of life that is held by the plant kingdom. Prepare for an extraordinary journey, a journey that calls forth the innate wisdom and power of the sacred medicine of the flowers, trees, and plants. Hear their voices, feel their energy, sing their songs, speak their truths, and live as one with all creation.

Rhonda

Sandi

PART ONE

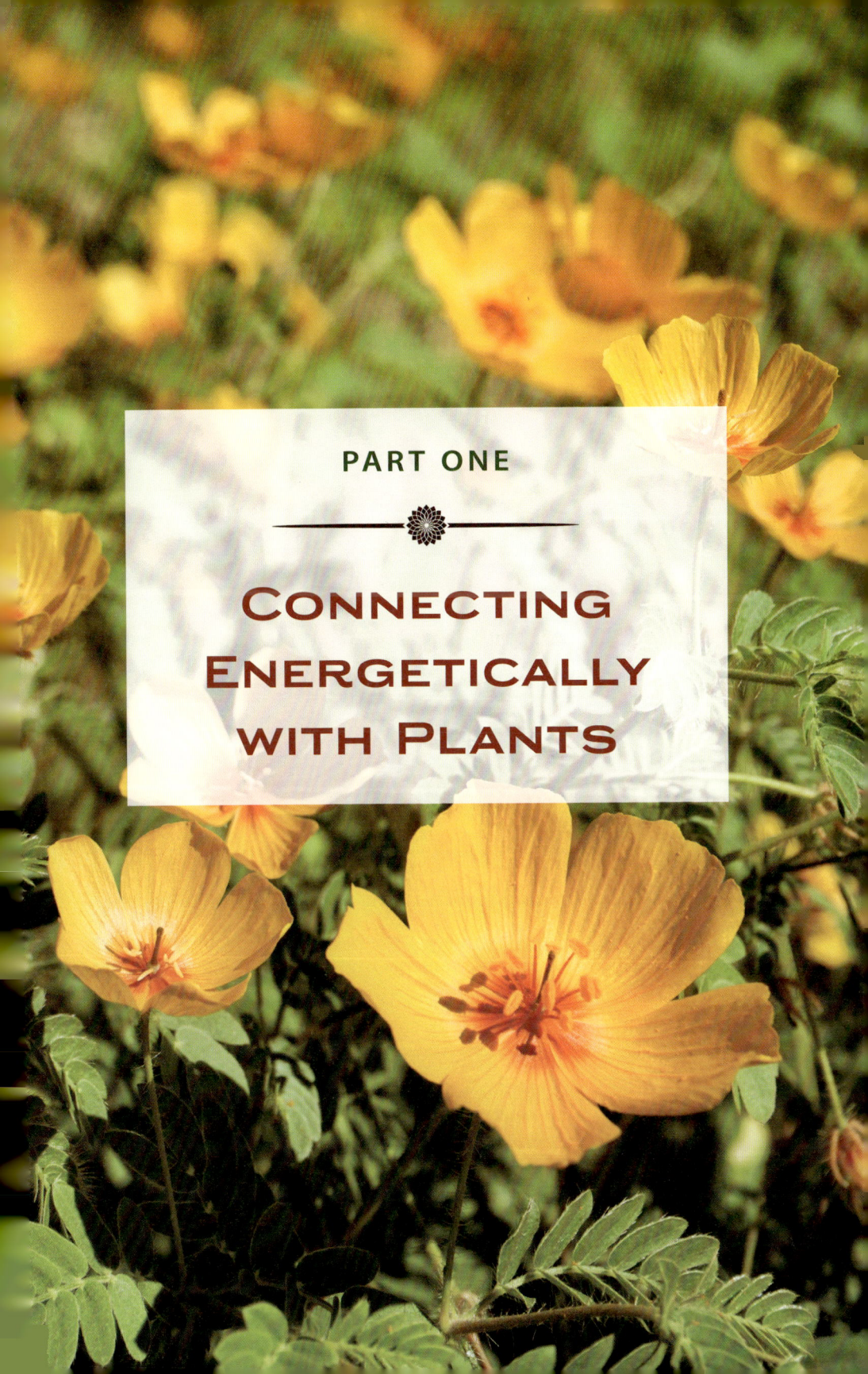

Connecting Energetically with Plants

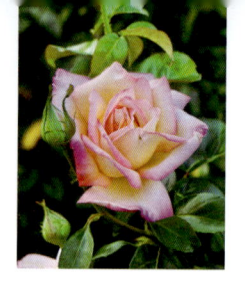

1
The Language of Plant Energy

The natural healing force within each of us is the greatest force in getting well.

HIPPOCRATES

HUMAN BEINGS—INDEED, all animals—are naturally interdependent with the plant kingdom. Plants offer us many gifts. Certain plants are believed to contain sacred and magical powers as well as natural medicinal properties. Plants have served as a primary source of nourishment and have also been used for heat, shelter, clothing, protection, and medicine.

Our relationship with plants goes back to earliest recorded history. There is a longheld tradition of relating to plants, talking to them and being with them, that is not well-understood by modern science. However, traditional and Indigenous cultures all over the world, going back thousands of years, have developed a sophisticated body of medicine that integrates knowledge of the language of plants to bring about healing, and this knowledge has been passed down to us through countless generations of medicine men and women. Today's herbal wisdom derives from the practices of these ancient and traditional cultures, which acknowledge the role of plant consciousness as an energy used in healing.

Plant energy medicine gently inspires change in the basic essence of our being, our energy, through a process of resonance. As is now confirmed by quantum physics, before we come into physical form we are first and foremost energy and vibration. Plant energy medicine seeks to

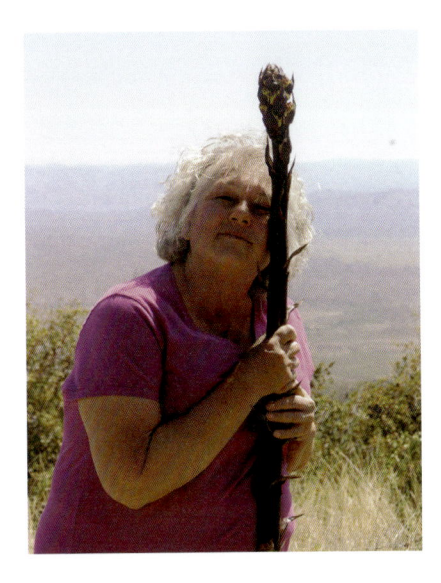

Sandi O'Connor being one with the century plant

encourage the healthy flow of energy throughout the body by employing the subtle vibrations of healing plants. Plant energy medicine offers a blueprint of any given plant that includes all the medicinal values that the plant carries. This blueprint identifies the signature and design of a plant. The signature of a plant refers to its characteristics and may include its unique form of root, stalk or stem, leaves, bark, blossoms, or medicinal properties. A plant's signature shows us how to gain access to the spirit of the plant.

The design of a plant supports its growth as well as the impact of that growth in its development from seed to fruit. Our awareness and experience of the natural evolution of plants draws attention to both the visible and invisible intelligence of the plant kingdom. By experiencing the intelligent nature and pure beingness of plants through our body, mind, and spirit, we go deeper into the human-plant connection. Doesn't it make sense, then, that the development of higher consciousness in human beings runs parallel to the same development of higher consciousness in the plant kingdom?

Human language is a living, changing phenomenon, as seen in the earliest pictographs of Stone Age humans, the petroglyphs of Indigenous peoples, the hieroglyphs of ancient Egyptians, and the digital bits and bites of computer age humans. So it is true for plants, whose language has evolved

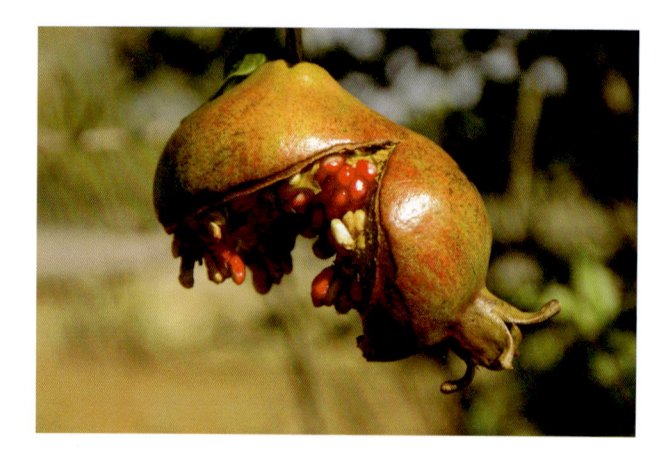

Pomegranate breaking ground

along pathways parallel to ours. Learning the language of plants is like learning the language of different peoples and cultures. It allows us to connect with a plant and that plant's biological family on much more intimate terms.

Just as human language is expressed in symbols, signs, letters, and pictures that represent an idea, word, or phrase, the language of plants is expressed by the plant's roots, vascular system, structure, stalk or stem, leaf patterns, veins, petals, blossoms, seeds and seed pods, as well as its cellular makeup. Learning the language of plants can help us connect to all levels of our being—physical, emotional, mental, and spiritual. By becoming aware of the energy that a plant carries, both in seen and unseen ways, we have an opportunity to become more mindful and step into a deeper state of self-awareness. This in turn supports a state of inner and outer balance, or homeostasis, as we become wise energetic beings with the support of plant energy medicine.

THE VITAL LIFE FORCE ENERGY

To become aware of the energy of a plant, one must first understand what the vital life force is.

Herbalist JoAnna Castigliego Sánchez writes the following in her curriculum *Breaking Ground*:

> Rooted in natural laws, herbalism captures our hearts and spirits and guides us along towards many wisdoms and knowings. Through

direct experiential association with the natural world of creation, herbalism is both an intuitive art and exact science. We best learn of nature with curious exploration, keen observation and eyes of wonder, with sensitive hearts filled with awe, with patience and deliberate awareness as well as deep contemplation and introspective thought. Through research and study, we blend experience with knowledge, and then learning is an appropriate context. There are fundamental concepts, groundwork that is required and mandatory as requisite foundational study for the newcomer to the herbal profession.[1]

Let's take a moment to understand the plant mind, not in the sense that a plant has a "mind" as we humans understand it, but referring to how a plant navigates its existence. In many ways, how a plant lives is instinctual. When you stop and think about it, it's the same as when a baby is born. The newborn is instinct and feeling first, and then sometime later, experience and training are added to that instinctive drive. We are all born with the instinct to survive, the same as any living organism that has taken on a physical existence.

Just as a fetus lives in its mother's womb and a seed lives in the soil, both fetus and seed naturally find their way forward through feeling and sensory perception. With further nurturing and environmental support, both the fetus and the seed naturally begin to develop a vital, energetic life force field. In a fetus, some heart rates are stronger and some are

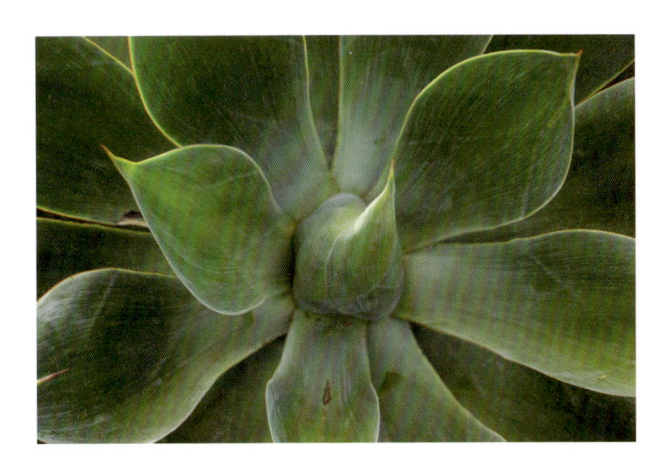

Emergence of a blue agave plant

weaker. Infants born with a physical disability generally have a lower life force energy and require more medical attention to build up their life force. The same is true of seeds. If a seed, which is an embryo, is undeveloped or lies dormant and is delayed in germination, the seed is put on hold. Often this is related to too much or too little water content and lack of oxygen.

All living things possess the vital life force energy, and they all have ways of processing sensory input. They possess what American herbalist Stephen Harrod Buhner calls "sensory gating channels . . . tiny apertures or gates or doors in specific sections of the nervous system's neural network."[2] The quaking aspen tree, *Populus tremuloides*, offers an example of how a plant's nervous system works via its signature of quaking or trembling in even the slightest breeze. Sunflower's flower head is radiant and bright, tilting toward the sun all day long, triggered by the intensity of the sun, which energizes its sensory input and neural network and sustains its life force. Yuccas are night-blooming plants, its blossoms opening to their fullest under a full moon—yet another example of how a plant connects with its life force and sensory system, as yuccas emit a sweet aroma that attract the plant's sole pollinator, the yucca moth, which flies only at night.

Known by a wide range of names in countless cultures—as *chi* in Chinese medicine, *prana* in Vedic medicine, and *Spirit* in traditional Indigenous medicine—the vital life force is a universal energy that flows through all living things, from the celestial to the molecular. It is essentially spiritual in nature. As herbalist, alchemist, and medical astrologer Sajah Popham says, "It's the animating factor that gives all forms their unique expression of life. It is invisible, but it can be seen through its effects upon a physical organism."[3]

The concept of the vital force began with Hippocrates (460–350 BC), the Greek physician known as the "Father of Medicine," who referred to it as a healing power in nature. Swiss physician and alchemist Paracelsus (1493–1541) called the vital force "*archeus*, an arch-principle dominating life processes in a biological entity . . . It was all-pervading and powerful within that milieu, yet invisible to the material eye. Only through its effects could the existence of the archeus be known. Through these, the

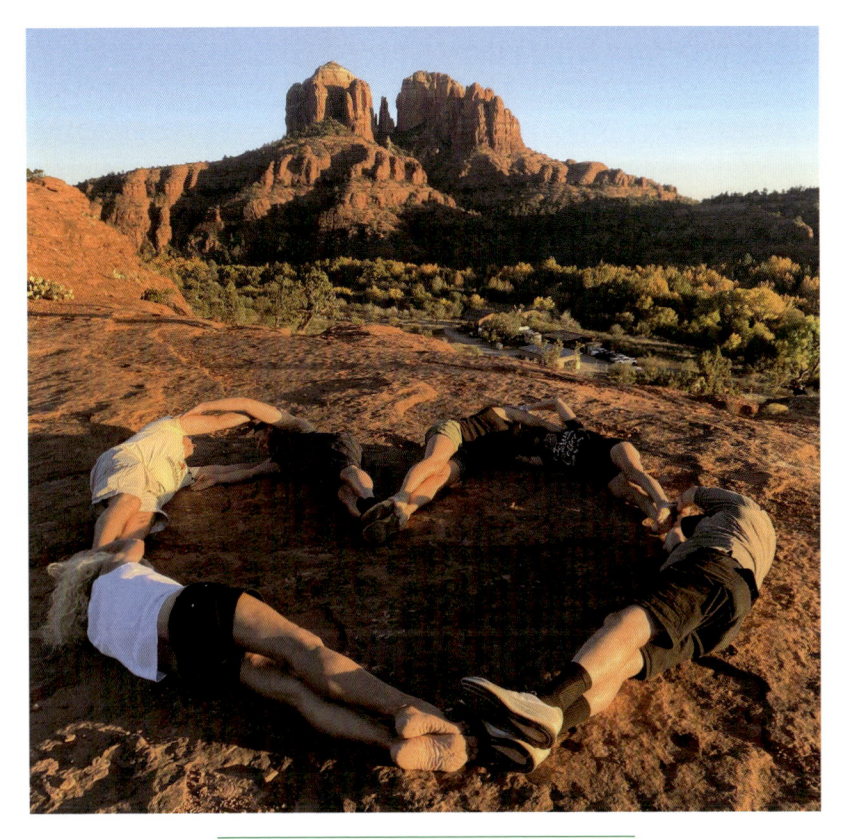

Living, breathing, human hearts as one

realization was possible that life was governed by a self-regulating and self-healing intelligence."[4]

Dr. Samuel Hahnemann (1755–1843), founder of the science of homeopathy, referred to the life force as the *dynamis*:

> [The] spiritual vital force (autocracy), the *dymanis* that animates the material body (organism), rules in unbounded sway and retains all the parts of the organism in admirable, harmonious, vital operation as regards both to sensations and functions, so that our indwelling, reason-gifted mind can freely employ this living, healthy instrument for the higher purposes of our existence . . . The material organism, without the vital force, is capable of no sensation, no function, no self-preservation.[5]

FEELING SENSATIONS THROUGH THE HEART

If we are first and foremost energy, vibration, then it is the heart that is the first physical organ to develop in a human being. It starts beating in a fetus before the brain is even formed. As everyone knows, it's the muscle at the center of our circulatory system that pumps blood throughout the body; in doing so it circulates the life force energy throughout the body. The heart is the sensory organ that gives us feelings, in that the real experience of the heart is connecting with what you feel. It's the feeling sense that we first develop while in the mother's womb. As Rosemary Gladstar points out, "What makes us human isn't all the information or knowledge . . . it's really our connection to the Earth and our Heart."[6]

As many ancient cultures have known, the heart is a source of intelligence, a kind of brain. Imagine that "in a period of seventy years in your lifetime, your heart beats one thousand times a day, approximately forty million times a year—nearly three billion pulsations all told. It pumps two gallons of blood per minute—well over one hundred gallons per hour—through a vascular system about sixty thousand miles in length (over two times the circumference of the earth)."[7]

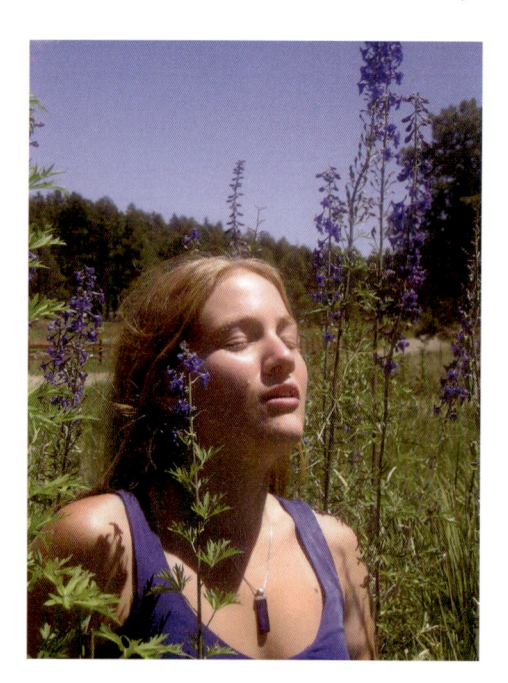

Jennifer Downey embodying the heart and breath connection

Much like the brain, the heart has approximately forty thousand neurons. This means that the heart has its own nervous system. Information from the heart, including all our feeling sensations, is sent to the brain. The heart's electrical impulses are approximately sixty times greater than the brain's, and its electromagnetic field is five thousand times greater; this affects the body at a cellular level. The rhythms of the brain, along with respiratory and blood pressure rhythms, attune with the rhythm of the heart, supporting the electromagnetic field produced by the heart.

Heart and Breath Connection

The heart is the keeper and the center of the true essence of who you are, the spirit of you. It is beyond space and time; it connects us to the infinite, which helps us connect to the core of our experiences as true human beings. Imagine the first breath you took as a newborn, leaving your mother's womb and entering the world for the first time. Bring that breath into your heart space, opening and feeling into the authentic person that you are—a breath of magic, of birth, of beauty and love that you came into this world from a place of innocence and trust.

Take a deep breath through your nostrils and down into your lungs, and further down into your belly. As you inhale, your belly should naturally expand and come outward as you breathe in. Feel your lungs open up. Allow air to enter and the oxygen from the air to move into your blood. Your heart and lungs work together to create oxygen-rich blood, strengthening your heart muscles as well as the very core of your being. As you exhale, relax your belly. Your chest cavity will become smaller and your lungs will depress. Breathing out releases any excess of electromagnetic energies such as incoherent thoughts and feelings, as well as unwanted carbon dioxide.

Breathing in deeply and exhaling fully revitalizes your entire being. Circulation, blood pressure, airways, bones, and even your psyche are strengthened as you become more conscious of your breath and the feeling in your lungs, diaphragm, and heart. Breath is the life force! It is the pure energy that feeds us, pumps us, and keeps us alive.

Come to realize the essence of your soul and the journey that your life has brought you to here and now. The heart is the bridge to the essence of your soul. It offers an expanded view of how you perceive the world. This world as we have known it is changing before our very eyes. Today, the collective consciousness is shifting to be more in alignment with the higher vibrations of the Earth and the cosmos, such that we are becoming more aware of a power or energy or source field much greater than us. We come together from a place of understanding to perceive the world through our hearts; this allows love to flow through us, just as this master pump circulates the blood throughout our body.

In the center of your heart space, imagine an opening, a doorway for you to feel, step into, and go beyond. Give yourself permission to love yourself no matter what, to feel what it is like to love yourself unconditionally. Here in this space we can begin to see, feel, and resonate with a reality that is beyond our past. We can create a design and the desire to be one consciousness by awakening to our own intrinsic divine nature, beyond expectations, moving into this moment as we become aware of the wisdom of the heart. We are given an opportunity to experience the magnitude of the universal electromagnetic field that is inclusive of all living organisms and that resonates with all living organisms. In the words of Stephen Buhner:

> All living organisms produce electromagnetic fields, all encode information, and all merged electromagnetic fields exchange information. The Earth itself is a living organism that produces electromagnetic fields filled with information. We are affected by the information encoded in these fields just by living on the Earth.[8]

When we as humans connect with plants in nature, in their natural habitats, we imbibe the electromagnetic energy field in which they live. We experience the views they live in, the kind of weather they thrive in, the soil that they emerge from, the sunlight they receive, the scents in the air, and the sounds of whispering winds moving through their plant bodies or the sounds of nearby calling birds.

These are examples of how we encode information from merely being in the presence of these green beings and imagining what it would be like to be them. And to take it a step further, we no longer have to imagine, we simply become one of them.

By connecting with the energy of your heart, you become more coherent and harmonious in every part of your body. Visualize your body as a vital, energetically flowing organism that is fueled by the light of the sun and the stars, and even beyond, to include the entire light-filled universe. See the light within you and expand it out to the light-filled universe, to every living thing. Imagine yourself merging and breathing with an invisible magnetic network of energy, the source of universal light that connects all things. What you feel, see, hear, and taste is an energetic channel to the light that permeates the cosmos.

Know that you are many notes in one note, many cells in one cell, one being of light in the universal light body. You have found your place, your belonging, your internal instrument in a cosmic symphony. This heart coherence, according to the HeartMath Institute, "is a synchronized and empowering state, physically, emotionally, mentally, and spiritually, allowing us to become our best selves."[9]

The exchange between humans and plants that occurs on a feeling and vibrational level becomes even more tangible when we get to know the true nature of the plant kingdom. Eileen McKusick, a pioneer in the field of bioenergetic healing, says,

> All energy is electromagnetic, its movement in our being. When we learn to flow with the movement of our emotions, to move with our natural inclinations toward what feels best and appropriate, then we learn to master conservation of energy, which enables us to keep our batteries high. This is not necessarily easy to do. Most of us have been taught to suppress rather than express our feelings and emotions, and there are limitless means of suppression that our culture provides.[10]

This is where plant energy intersects with the human energy field to effect healing. As Stephen Buhner says,

> Plants respond to the gesture of intimacy contained within the field projected by the heart. They respond, embedding new communications

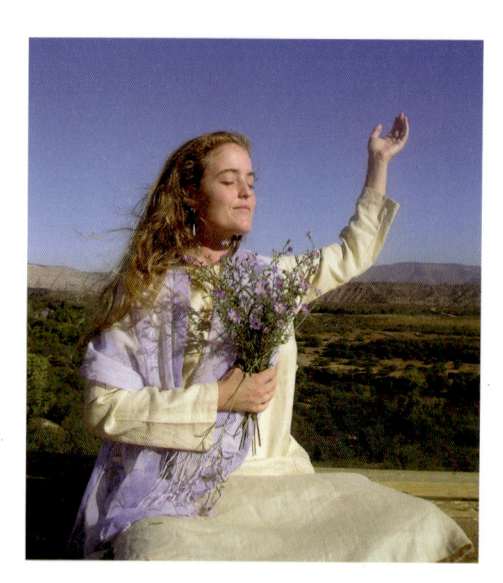

Tanya Downey in heart coherence with asters

within their electromagnetic fields, which your heart takes in, decodes, and uses to alter its own functioning once again. You and the living phenomenon with which you are making contact entrain, and a living dialogue begins to flow back and forth, extremely rapidly.[11]

Our experience has been that plants have their own natural state of coherence. They display not only their own individual electromagnetic field, but the electromagnetic field or life force energy of Gaia, to which they—and we—are all connected. Being with plants and resonating with plants helps us remember this. The innate, natural heart coherence of plants broadcasts this higher and more Earth-centered energetic frequency to we humans. An electrical exchange of energy occurs. The vibrations of plants influence the vibrations within us, and we in turn influence the vibrations of the universe.

2

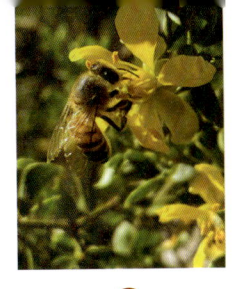

Plants' Sensory Input

How to think like nature... It's another dimension, a science from another world dimension. We have to lay down our logics, our science, and think of another science, a science into another dimension.

MATTHEW WOOD

IN HIS BOOK *What a Plant Knows*, Daniel Chamovitz, director of the Manna Center for Plant Biosciences at Tel Aviv University and visiting scientist at Yale University, gives a detailed scientific explanation for why plants have primary senses: in short, they are able to respond to their environment by following light: "The complex signals arising from multiple photoreceptors allow a plant to optimally modulate its growth in changing environments, just as our photoreceptors allow our brains to make pictures that enable us to interpret and respond to our changing environments."[1]

We know through simple observation that plants capture and use light by just watching them grow. They attune to both the condition and quantity of light. Through photosynthesis, they receive most of their energy through light. The quality of a plant's life and its behavior is directed by its searching for and ability to acquire light. As plants grow in the direction of light, they adjust their positions and move their leaves to sustain their life force.

Blue light receptors, called *cryptochromes*, are found in both plants and animals, including humans. Cryptochromes contain a circadian clock that follows the normal cycles of day and night. This internal clock synchronizes in people when we go to bed, when we're hungry, or when we're tired. In plants this internal clock influences leaf movements and photosynthesis. When the circadian clock's day/night cycle is artificially changed in a plant, the plant naturally experiences a form of jet lag, and it takes a few days for it to adapt to a new cycle. Thus both plants and humans are challenged to adapt to changing external conditions that affect their internal clocks.

For thousands of years, healers and herbalists have used fragrant, healing herbs, roots, stems, leaves, flowers, aromatic fumigations, gums, and resins in daily rituals and sacred ceremonies. Stories of the healing qualities of plants and their attributes, including their aromas, have been passed down from generation to generation and are documented in ancient texts from around the world, in China, Egypt, Rome, and Greece, in the Vedas, in both books of the Bible, and in the classic Taoist text known as *The Yellow Emperor's Classic of Internal Medicine*.

The oils and scents of myrrh, frankincense, and benzoin are derived from tree sap. The scents of bergamot, orange, lemon, mandarin, tangerine, and grapefruit come from fruit peels. The aromas of bay, cajuput, cypress, eucalyptus, lemongrass, myrtle, pine, and spruce are derived from leaves and twigs. Flowers such as rose, lavender, chamomile, rosemary, and neroli offer an abundance of fragrances. Scents from the leaves, stalks, and flowering tops are emitted from geraniums, basil, marjoram, oregano, peppermint, pulmarosa, thyme, chamomile, and clary sage. Barks from such trees as rosewood, cedar, spruce, cinnamon, mesquite, and pine all carry an earthy, delightful, individualistic smell. The roots of an array of plants such as black cohosh, sassafras, licorice, ginger, ginseng, yerba mansa, and many more produce unique odors and carry their own fragrances.

Plants emanate a tremendous variety of odors, which play a major role in their personalities. You may feel a sense of peace or love when you smell a rose; a feeling of being refreshed and cleansed when imbibing the scent of pine needles; or a tender-hearted moment of taking in honeysuckle's sweet fragrance and sucking on its honeyed nectar.

Not only do plants contain and send out their own odors, they can also pick up smells. This capability is much different from our advanced human olfactory system. Unlike humans, plants lack a central nervous system, and in the sense of smell for a plant, it is noseless. In addition to smell, plants can also sense, feel, and perceive their own odors as well as the odors of those plants that grow near them in their landscape. A tomato plant or a citrus tree can know, smell, feel, and sense when their fruit is ripe. A plant may know when there are invasive insects in their neighborhood, and they respond by releasing a combination of complex airborne chemicals and sensory information from one plant to another. Daniel Chamovitz describes this olfactory action in plants as "the ability to perceive odor or scent through stimuli."[2]

Olfactory communication between plants and animals is in fact multifaceted. Pollinators are attracted to certain flowers, fruits appeal to seed spreaders, and predators are repelled by certain plant odors. Plants respond to pheromones as chemical messengers that are triggered from one plant to another. They are able to somehow translate these signals into a physiological response that is linked to a plant's ability to smell.

Plants' nutritional source comes primarily from the soil they live in. The quality of the soil strongly influences the quality of a plant as a vital being. Plants can show us by where they live the kind of soil that feeds their appetites. The condition of the soil in turn affects how a plant tastes. In fact, smells and tastes are directly related in both plants and animals. In their book, *Brilliant Green: The Surprising History and Science of Plant Intelligence*, Stefano Mancuso, a leading scientist and founder of the field of plant neurobiology, and Alessandra Viola, a scientific journalist, describe how "the organs responsible for plants' sense of taste are certain receptors for the chemical substances they use as food, substances for which they probe the soil through the exploratory movements of their roots. The 'palate' of the plant world proves in this search to be as refined as that of the best gourmets!"[3]

Unlike humans, who use air as a pathway for sound waves in order to hear, plants, like snakes and worms, are without physical ears, yet they hear through the sound vibrations of the Earth as a natural composer, attracting attention to the cells of plants through her vibrations. Due to the existence of "mechanosensitive channels,"[4] the sense of hearing in plants is dispersed throughout the plant, in contrast to the ears, a single organ in humans. Plants can hear both underground via their roots, and above ground, in response to their outer environment. Mechanosensitive

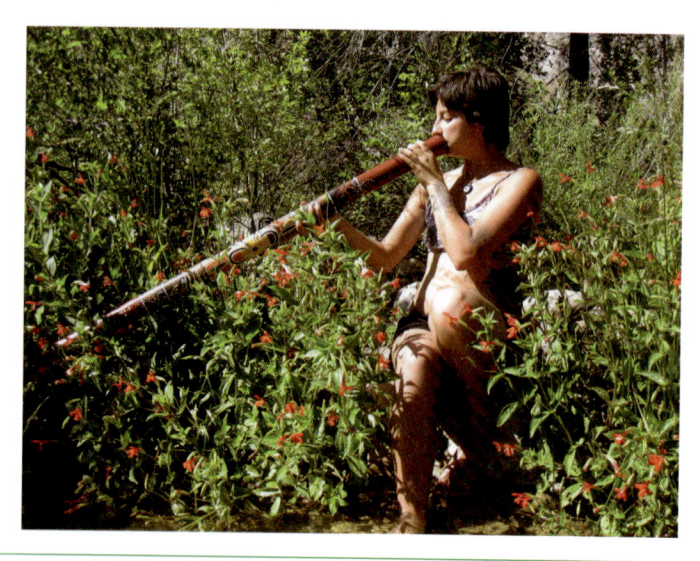

Kylee Koepnick, student, playing didgeridoo and offering sound healing for our class and the crimson monkeyflowers growing in a stream

channels in a plant are distinctive receptors that, when stimulated, enable a plant to feel or respond to the vibrations in their energy field.

There have been many studies showing how the sound frequencies of different kinds of music affect a plant's growth, from seed germination to roots (underground), to the aerial parts of plants (above ground). These studies show that the root system of plants carries a broader range of vibrational frequencies that guide the plant's growth. The plant's roots are drawn to certain frequencies and move toward them, or conversely, away from them. This is supported by a 2012 Italian study cited in *Brilliant Green*:

> The sounds made by the roots have been provisionally dubbed "clicking," because they characteristically sound like "clicks." In all probability, these tiny clicks result from the breaking of cell walls—made of cellulose and thus rather rigid—during the [plant] cells' growth. . . . The discovery opens up new scenarios in plant communication: the fact that roots emit and can perceive sounds would seem to imply the existence of a previously unknown underground communication pathway.[5]

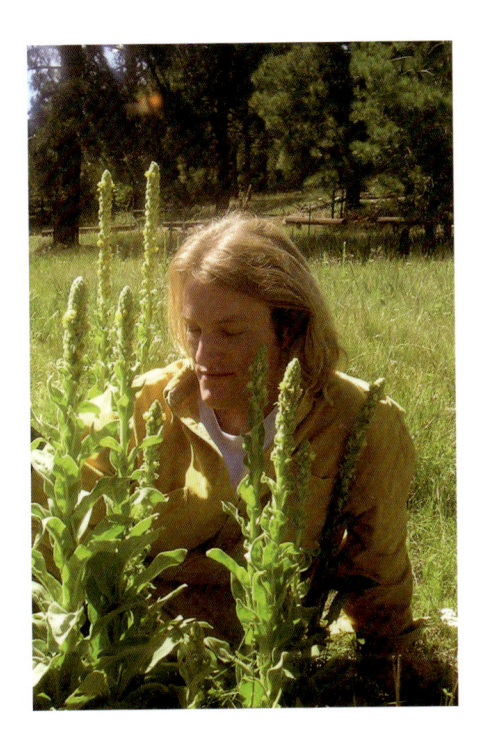

Adam Downey listening to what mullein has to say to him

Research by Israeli scientists also shows evidence of plants communicating via "clicklike sounds resembling the popping of popcorn"[6] at a similar volume as human sounds, but at higher frequencies, beyond the sound range of the human ear. A 2023 *National Geographic* article adds that "many different plant species make ultrasonic sounds to communicate stress."[7] And a 2017 article on the *National Geographic* Education Blog notes evidence that plants have the ability to detect water moving in pipes by sound alone.[8]

A March 2023 study at the Department of Molecular Biology and Ecology of Plants at Tel Aviv University discovered that certain plants such as evening primrose emitted more nectar when recordings of hawk moths flapping their wings or bees buzzing were played near them.[9] How do they hear? Motor proteins called *myosins* are stored in plants. These proteins are remarkably rich in their minuscule root hairs. Myosins can also be found in the delicate hairs in the human ear. In humans, vibrations in the ear canal cause these tiny hairs to detect sound. Plants have similar motor proteins that gather around these small root hairs that are able to perceive sound vibrations.

The mechanosensitive pathways related to a plant's sense of hearing are also associated with its sense of touch. These pathways or tiny receptors are everywhere on the plant, particularly on a plant's epidermal cells, those cells that are most affected by the plant's connection to its exterior environment. When a plant touches something, such as a sweet pea flower vining on a fence, the receptors are activated just as they are through sensing or feeling the vibrational frequencies of the Earth.

Pioneering naturalist Charles Darwin, in partnership with his son Francis, a botanist, conducted experiments on how plants move. In their 1880 book on phototropism, *The Power of Movement in Plants*, father and son expanded on their previous research on climbing plants. The Darwins were drawn to tropism, the involuntary, reflexive attraction of plants to stimuli, resulting in nutation, the spontaneous, usually spiral movement of a growing plant part. They were able to show that plants are sensitive to light, touch, and gravity, and that they move as a result. Since then, numerous studies have supported and expanded on these findings regarding the sensory system of plants, including their reaction to moisture, a physiochemical stimulus that can affect how a plant feels, tastes, hears, and smells.

Like the carnivorous Venus flytrap, plants can respond to being touched and injured. They can discriminate between the workings of insects and mammals and adjust the way they defend themselves. These stimuli, as well as the stimuli of wind, temperature, soil, moisture, exposure to cold and heat, light and dark, sounds and vibrations, all demonstrate that a plant has the ability to store biological information that allows it to feel, to sense, and to perceive both its internal and external environments and store this information as a kind of memory of its world.

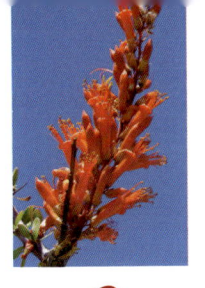

3
Dynamics of the Biofield

With energetic herbalism, as we tend our terrain, our ecology, and our spirit, we are, in essence, finding our way home. For me, the web that gathers together the multifaceted craft of herbalism is the equally ancient practice of honoring plant spirits.

KAT MAIER, CLINICAL HERBALIST

THE LONG HISTORY of documenting the relationship between plants and human beings shows there is a way to relate to plants—talking and being with them, feeling them—that may be different from what is currently understood by modern science.

Plants have wisdom to share. By creating a relationship with a plant and deepening that relationship, merging your spirit with the plant's spirit, feeling and imagining that your electromagnetic field is uniting with the plant's electromagnetic field, the strength of the plant's core essence is energetically transmitted to you.

Visualize the field of energy known as the biofield. In a human being this extends about eight feet out from your body, from below your feet to above your head, and from side to side. Although the biofield isn't visible to the human eye, it facilitates a subtle energetic exchange between you and another being who is in your biofield, or between you and your surrounding environment. Awareness of your biofield is a way of connecting with your own subtle energy, which is the higher frequency found in your electromagnetic energy field.

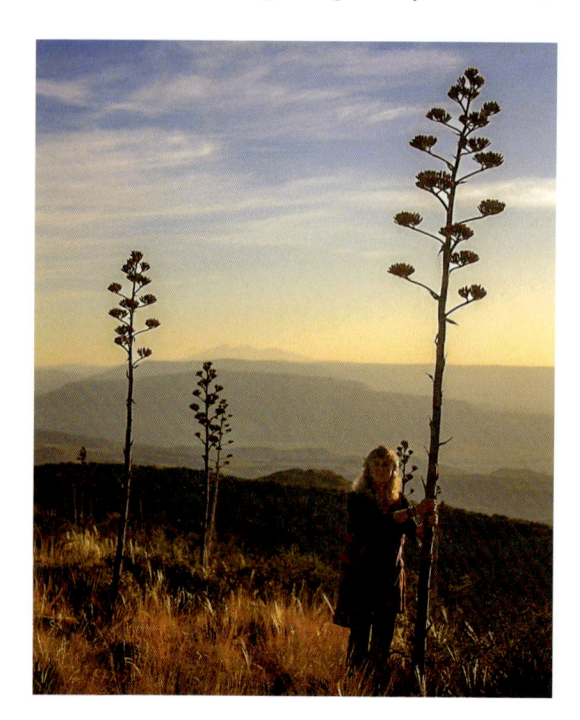

Rhonda PallasDowney in the biofield energy of a century plant tribe (photo by Renick Turley/Sedona Film)

A number of studies have confirmed that plants have a similar bioenergetic field.[1] This field of subtle energy extends all the way out from their surrounding habitat to below their root systems and above their crowns, and from side to side, similar to humans.

We believe that we humans can step into the bioenergetic field of a plant, which encompasses both the plant's electromagnetic field as well as our own. In other words, we can energetically merge with a plant's natural biofield. As a result, we experience an energetic exchange of some sort. What we do know, feel, and sense is that a charge takes place during that exchange with the plant. The charge may be deeply subtle or more tangible, and either way it is felt. Being in the presence of plants raises our voltage and deepens our perception.

Plants are like people. There are some plants that you are naturally drawn to, and others, not so much. The more you get to know a plant, spend time in nature with it, sit in silence with it, and even sleep with it, draw it, taste it, smell it, listen to it, breathe with it, observe its patterns, and notice what time of day or night the plant has reached its highest exaltation, you become intimate with the plant. You get to know it on a profound level.

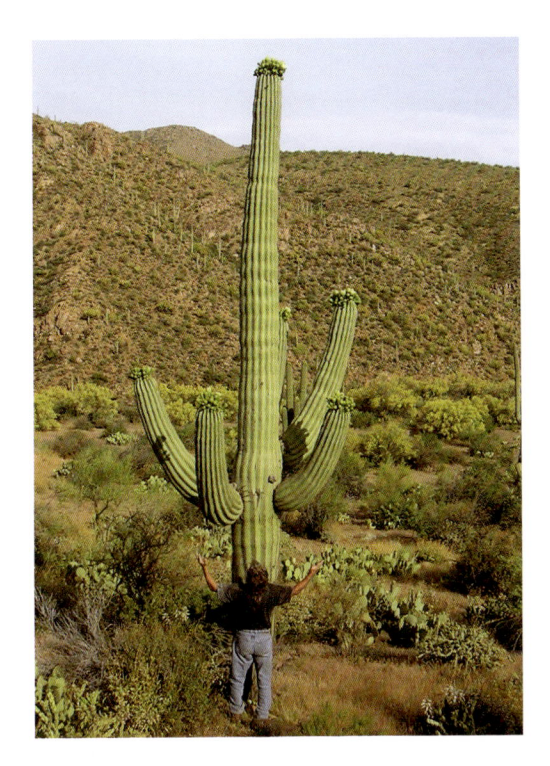

Curt PallasDowney and saguaro experiencing the biofield of the Sonoran Desert

Experiencing the biofield of a living plant and its environment can tell us more about the plant, how it survives and thrives, its condition of health and wellness, and perhaps what nutrients it needs for healing. The quantity and quality of a plant's biofield, including its relationship to moisture and light, soil and air, and oxygen and climate, indicate the plant's ability to adapt to its environment.

Just like humans and all living organisms, plants are challenged to adapt to the ecosystem, restore balance, transform energy, and adapt to the rhythm of the times. The awareness of our ecological interrelatedness as one system that comprises all living organisms widens our lens to restore and harmonize the vital force of every living thing as well as our awareness of the biofield of energy itself.

We learn to understand the synchronizing relationship of supporting the natural forces of nature. This relates to healthy conditions of life ranging from soil, organic farming, and the foods we eat to all the ways that naturally support our environment by reinforcing animal, plant, and human health and all the ways that we adapt with all living organisms.

When you shop for flowers or you grow flowers and plants, or you're out on the land wildcrafting, wouldn't you want to choose the plants that show their vibrancy and higher energetic frequency of life force? Do you stop and feel the energy of the plant? What a perfect example of your energetic biofield connecting with the plant's energetic biofield. Through that exchange, both seen and unseen, your connection with the plant deepens. It can't help but not.

For generations and generations, trees, for example, like animals, plants, human beings, and all of nature itself, have constantly been adapting both in morphological adaptations (physical changes that occur over generations based on environmental conditions) and in physiological adaptations (how the internal system thrives and responds to external stimuli) to gain or maintain homeostasis.

Learn to call on the nature spirit of a plant. When you do, most likely you will feel yourself merging with its energy, going deep by taking on how the plant feels, grows, moves, breathes, lives, touches, responds, communicates, gives, and receives. Becoming one with a plant's essence, its spirit, its intrinsic nature, you will hear and feel the plant's voice, song, and messages. As you experience the spirit of the plant, you may feel energetic vibrations, openings, releases, and teachings of the wisdom it holds. This exchange with the spirit of the plant will help you discover a profound, multidimensional relationship within yourself. Your relationship with the plant feels real, not something you are simply imagining. It becomes a shared experience. In this way you have encountered a true friend.

Feeling one with a plant is a sign that you have reached a deep-seated level of intimacy with plants that will only continue to grow. This kind of personal growth creates an inner opening that allows you to fully embrace and unite your own spirit with the nature spirit of the plant, tree, or flower. You have stepped into a mindfulness exercise of becoming one within yourself and one with the energy of the plant. Your awareness of this connection opens an inner doorway, awakening your awareness to the energy of the plant biofield.

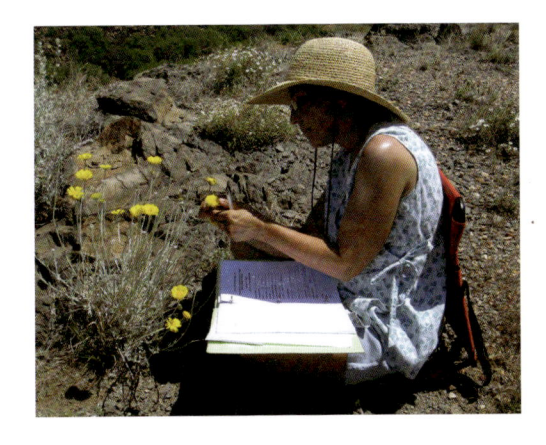

JoAnna Castigliego Sánchez, sister herbalist and friend, studying the doctrine of signatures of desert marigold

THE DOCTRINE OF SIGNATURES

Homeopaths and herbalists refer to the intrinsic qualities of plants in terms of the doctrine of signatures. The color, appearance, scent, shape, leaves, textures, roots, stems, flowers, and catkins, as well as the growth patterns and habitats of plants provide us with all the information we need to learn about the natural curative values of plant extracts, flower essences, and elixirs. It is believed that every plant, flower, and tree has its own signature, and that a remedy derived from a plant carries the signature of its natural source. Its medicinal profile is, at least in part, an expression of its place in the natural order of things. When we consider the doctrine of signatures, we open wide the doorway to the world of nature—its ecology and symbolism—and thereby gain a fresh, new insight into what it means for our healing journey. As Matthew Wood says,

> Although the doctrine of signatures depends upon a subjective examination of natural phenomena, this should not be seen as a flaw but as a strength. Through study of the natural history, environmental patterns, chemical properties, taste, smell, and appearance, a person can learn to see similarities between plants and people. Through experience, the interior eye is trained, and certainty in knowledge and practice is increased.[2]

Plant Examples of the Doctrine of Signatures

Chamomile (*Matricaria chamomilla*) has a creeping rootstalk that spreads, creating a carpet-like surface. The roots are delicate and easy to pull. The smooth, round, slender stems of chamomile bend and ease even in the slightest breeze. Its delicate bright green leaves have a lacey fern-like appearance with no stalk. They are light and airy and may alternate or grow in parallel on the stems.

Chamomile flowers appear as single, daisy-like flowers with white ray petals and fuzzy yellow centers that protrude toward the sun. Chamomile's soft fragrance offers a blend of honey and apple. Its touch is soft and delicate. The essence of the flower tastes fruity and mellow. Chamomiles exude a gentle presence of calm and harmony. You can feel the lightheartedness of this plant just by being with it. The plant contains a volatile blue oil (essential oil) that has a soothing, peaceful presence. Chamomile is used to treat irritability, nervousness, and tension, especially in children.

An herbalist may recommend drinking chamomile as a tea to relieve a headache or to settle the stomach. A homeopath will check the "keynotes," or primary traits, which indicate treatment using chamomile; in the case of children's conditions, one cheek may be hot and flushed and the other cheek pale and cold. Teething, peevishness, restlessness, sleeplessness, crying uncontrollably, and colic are crucial indications for treating with chamomile. Hot, green, watery stools are also an indication. A homeopath will also look for "modalities," such as the child improves in warm, wet weather and from being carried or rocked; the child's condition worsens in tantrums, anger, open air, and at night from 9:00 p.m. to midnight. A flower essence practitioner may give a chamomile flower essence to release emotional tension and to restore emotional balance and relaxation. Chamomile flower essence in adults creates a peaceful, balanced emotional relationship to illness through understanding and sympathizing with the underlying emotion that caused the illness.

Yarrow has leaves that are feathery, lacy, and saw-toothed. The signature of the leaves points to the plant's application as a wound remedy and for treating physical conditions associated to cuts, wounds, burns, and blood. The flowers have a lacy appearance and are bone-white with a little pink, signifying bones and blood. These signifying characteristics also show the plant's ability to thrive and heal. Yarrow can stop nosebleeds, is a natural emmenagogue (meaning it stimulates menstruation, and it also regulates menstrual cycles), and can break up stagnant blood. Its botanical name is *Achillea millefolium*, named after the Greek warrior Achilles who placed fresh yarrow leaves on the wounds of his soldiers on the battlefield to stop bleeding.

An herbalist uses yarrow to make a tea, tincture, poultice, salve, or ointment. A homeopath uses yarrow to treat hemorrhages indicated by bright red blood, bloody urine. A flower essence practitioner uses yarrow flower essence to treat those who feel "cut to the bone," exhausted, overwhelmed, vulnerable, like "the wounded warrior"—those who energetically need a shield of protection.

Onion is a bulb whose main signature is its odor and vapor that induce sneezing and cause the eyes and nose to water. Therefore, onion (*Allium cepa*) is a remedy given for head colds with symptoms of sneezing, watery nasal secretion, and mild tearing. An herbalist may recommend drinking cooked onion broth when these symptoms occur. A homeopath may recommend treating with onion to relieve the head cold and sneezing. A flower essence practitioner may recommend onion flower essence to help release suppressed feelings of grief and sadness by peeling off old emotional layers to get to the "heart" of the matter.

From seed to root to stem to leaf to blossom to pod and seed, we begin to understand the life of a plant that includes its entire energy system. Accessing a plant's underlying field of energy, we can connect with the healing vibrational energy medicine of plants, trees, and flowers to match or meet the healing energy of the whole person. We have explored deeper into the plant world—the signatures of plants, where they grow, the soil and environment they live in, who their neighbors are and who their tribe is—and in particular we have made space for the gifts of the healing and medicinal qualities that plants offer us as we dive deeper into our own energy systems—both the visible and the invisible, the essence of you and the essence of a plant.

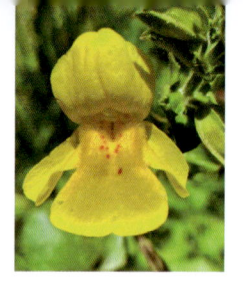

4
Flower Essences

Unseen Gifts of Nature

There is no true healing unless there is a change in outlook, peace of mind, and inner happiness.

EDWARD BACH

EDWARD BACH (1886–1936), a British medical doctor, homeopath, and spiritual healer best known for his development of the Bach Flower Essences, began his career in orthodox medicine, specializing in bacteriology, vaccination, and immunology. He was known for his discovery and treatment of seven different types of bacteria in the human body, which he referred to as "bowel nosodes." Yet Bach yearned to develop a natural approach to healing that was based in nature's plant kingdom, from which he believed all true medicines are derived. His approach involved identifying, understanding, and changing a disharmonious relationship with oneself and replacing the mental, emotional, and spiritual anguish that arises as a consequence of this imbalance with a balanced state of peace, belonging, and happiness. Bach's love of nature and the outdoors inspired him to seek plants with qualities that resemble human nature. Through his observation of people, he further identified certain human personality types and correlated them with particular plant expressions and personalities.

While walking through a field in the early morning dew, Bach had the sudden realization that each dewdrop embodied the properties of the

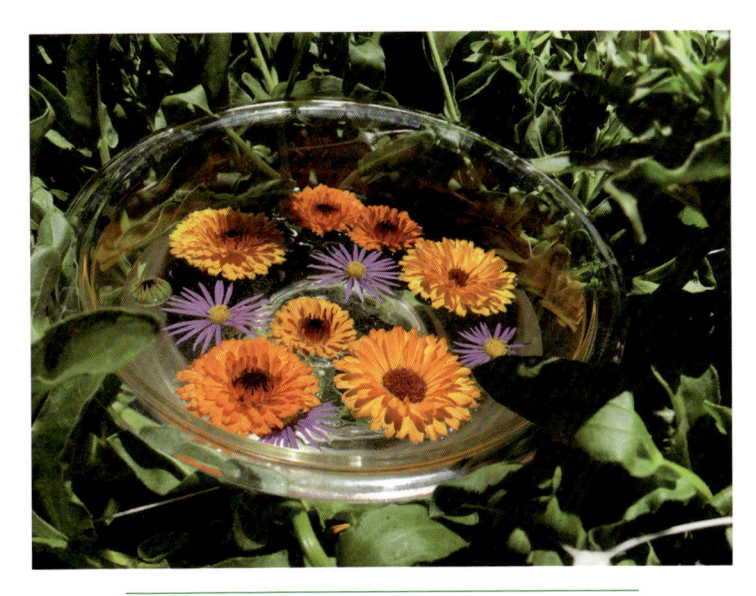

Flower essence infusion of calendulas and asters

plant on which it rested. The heat of the sun, energized through the fluid of the dewdrop, drew the plant's properties out into the dewdrop and exalted it with its power. Bach believed that this simple form of extracting the healing properties of the plant was a tangible experience. He began to collect dew from flowers, shake the dewdrops into bottles, take them back to his practice in London to prepare as remedies, and give those remedies to his patients.

Collecting dew from the flowers was a time-consuming process, so Bach sought a more direct method to extract a plant's qualities. He picked a few blossoms from several similar plants growing in the same area and filled a glass bowl with water from a clear stream. He covered the entire surface of the water with the petals he'd gathered and left them in full sunlight for several hours or until the flower petals faded slightly, to release the medicinal properties into the water, leaving the flower's imprint. He found the resulting flower essence water was energized by the power of the blossoms, creating a potent remedy. He then removed the petals from the glass bowl and preserved the liquid essence of the flower by adding some brandy to it as a preservative. He called the remedy a *flower essence*. In reference to Bach's groundbreaking flower essence method, Matthew Wood says, "Now we understand that these practices are significant in biological terms and not just odd, quaint, or 'mystical.'"[1]

Bach was satisfied that his simple, natural method was completely effective, as it contained the four natural elements of earth, air, fire (from the sun), and water, as well as the biological essence of the flower or plant. Interestingly, this essence had earlier been noted by the Pythagoreans and Paracelsians as the "quintessence" or "fifth essence," referring to the invisible, subtle, spiritual energy source that is experienced as an expression of the soul. As a whole, the four elements and the essence or "nature spirit" of the plant produce a powerful, effective means of healing.

Bach treated many patients with his new system of flower remedies. The most famous of them all, the Bach Flower Essence called Rescue Remedy, is used throughout the world as a first-aid treatment for such conditions as shock, trauma, terror, panic, and tension. Through his groundbreaking work with the plant kingdom, Bach believed that we can free ourselves from a disharmonious state, connect with our own divine power, and develop our unique energetic expression—our own energetic "signature," so to speak—with the help of flower essences.

THE VIBRATIONAL NATURE OF FLOWER ESSENCES

Flower essences carry subtle vibrational energies that realign disharmonies in human and animal bodies. Flower essence medicine works energetically in ways that capture the gifts of the whole plant's spirit, which is its medicine. This means imbibing the whole plant's properties, its life force and its electromagnetic energy, thereby connecting with its subtle vibrational energy.

At the core of the flower, tree, or plant's individual chemistry is a particular alchemical formula that includes its actual plant essence and the energy it produces. This alchemical formula, at the deepest level within us, offers us opportunities to develop new patterns of thinking and feeling. These new vibrational patterns in turn allow the budding of new energies that can further evolve us. This gift from the plant realm provides an opportunity to break through the illusion of separateness, that we are somehow separate from one another and from nature.

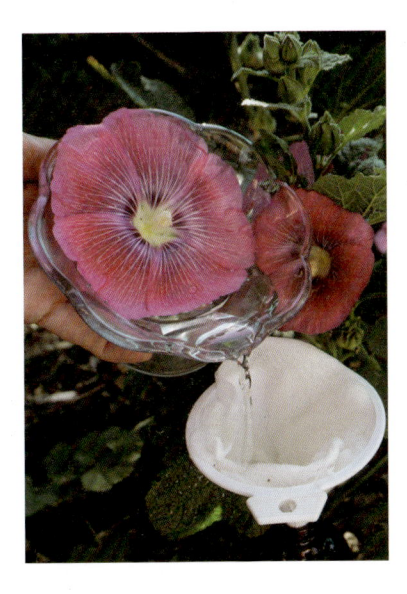

Hollyhock flower essence: there is no separation, trust the alchemy of a plant's energy

The power of plant essences is their ability to work with the human energy system to regenerate the chakras and endocrine glands. This interaction provides a path, an energetic vibratory frequency, for soul and spirit to unite. As this healing takes place, the resulting renewed mental and emotional balance provides physical healing and wellness for the whole person. As we begin to dissolve old patterns, the cosmic light body becomes anchored in our higher Self for longer and longer periods of

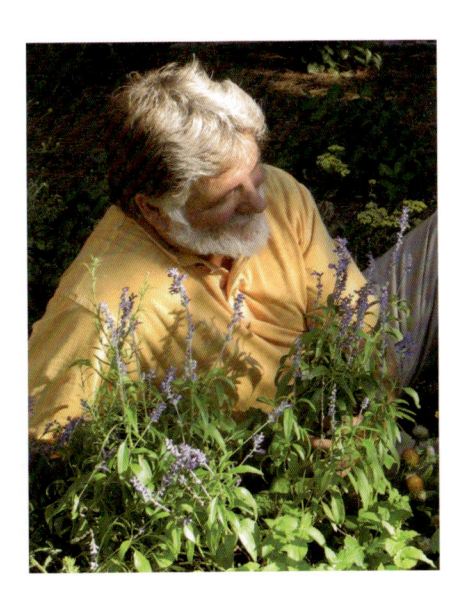

Curt PallasDowney taking in sage wisdom

time. Through this process, we're able to consciously plant the seeds of our inherent divinity in our energy field and in the vibrational frequencies we transmit to the world. Our subconscious mind in turn becomes fertile ground for eminent thoughts to arise. These higher vibrational thoughts and feelings shift our energetic frequencies and seed our body, mind, and spirit with fresh new perspectives. As we plant these seeds of cosmic consciousness, our cellular structure becomes lighter—more transmutable and fluid in relation to the environment. Becoming more aware of our own energy, we begin to live through these higher vibrational frequencies and learn that we are one with the Divine and all life forms.

As we work with flower essences and plants, we go deeper into the biofield's interconnected energetic awareness. This allows the feelings in our heart and our self-awareness to blossom. When we merge with whole plant medicine, we become resonators of higher energies and heighten the path of our personal transformation. Our vibrational resonance with plants allows us to attune to the electromagnetic field of light that is found within us and all around us. We establish a tighter bond with the electromagnetic vibrational influences and sensory input of plant energy medicine. By doing so, we broaden our awareness and increase the voltage of our energy field.

THE ART OF MAKING FLOWER ESSENCES

Flower essences, made from the blossoms of flowering plants as well as the catkins of trees, are charged with the subtle energetic life force and the unique signature of the flower or the catkin. The method is quite simple. Flowers or catkins are picked and placed in a clear glass bowl that's already been filled with purified water. The bowl is then placed in direct sunlight, or in some cases in moonlight if it is a night-blooming plant, until the flowers or catkins have faded into the water, leaving their energetic imprint in the water. The energy of sunlight (or moonlight) and water transfers the energy of the blossoms or catkins into the water, extracting a life force pattern that embodies the character of the plant. The result is called a *flower essence infusion*. The subtle energy pattern stored in the flower or catkin essence can be used for physical, emotional, mental, and spiritual healing.

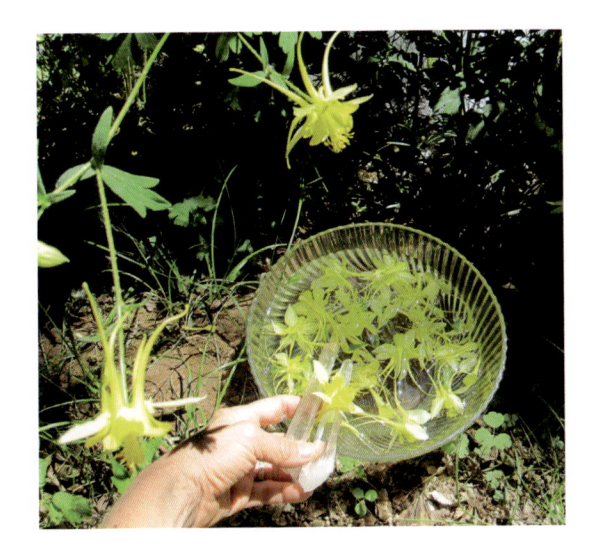

Infusing columbine flowers to make a flower essence

Plant substances are naturally adaptogenic. Flower and tree essences offer a subtle energetic influence on the ways we relate to ourself and how we adapt to stress and anxiety. These essences by nature embody a living energy. They help bring our awareness to how we can harmonize and calm, strengthen and restore, and normalize and reinforce a healthy and vital inner and outer environment.

Flower essences create a fertile garden within our own inner environment, which brings harmony to our natural landscape, which is our true Self. They offer an invitation to move beyond our limitations to open our inner doorways so that we can feel into and embrace living in a state of inner and outer harmony. They help us feel the world rather than trying to figure it out intellectually; they bring a sense of our interconnection with all living things; they help us let the timeless be in charge of time so that we can experience the mystery of our life's evolving journey.

That said, as each plant and tree has its roots, each of us comes into our own life journey with an innate primal force that expresses our individual spiritual and soul heritage, along with a DNA energy that affects where we have come from and how we can evolve into our authentic Self.*

---

*An in-depth description of how to make flower essences and journey with plants and flowers can also be found in Rhonda's book *The Healing Power of Flowers: Bridging Herbalism, Homeopathy, Flower Essences, and the Human Energy System*.

Are Flower Essences Safe?

We wildcraft many of our flower essences in remote areas where they grow in their natural habitats. Our flowers, trees, and plant essences are prepared on-site from natural resources in natural habitats or in organic gardens. Flower essences can also be prepared at home if preparing them in their natural setting is not practical.

We have many beautiful stories of finding the flowers, giving them our prayers, making their essences, and receiving their bounty. We honor the sacredness of this experience, and we bring this special energy all the way to the final product, the finished bottle of flower essence. Each flower essence bottle holds the richness and integrity of that particular flower. We formulate the intention that each unique flower essence will assist the person taking it on their personal journey.

Flower essences are nonaddictive and are generally very safe as long as the plant is safe! People with alcohol sensitivity should only use flower essences that are preserved with nonalcohol substances such as glycerin (however, note that flower essences preserved with glycerin have a shorter shelf life). Alternatively, one can place a few drops of a flower essence into a cup of boiled water; the heat will dissipate the alcohol preservative.

We have used flower essences with babies, young children, animals, and the elderly with no problems at all. Observe the effects and continue or discontinue use based on the response. Flower essences are very diluted and are widely considered completely safe.

The taste of our flower essences is delightful, refreshing, and mildly sweet. They are preserved with brandy or vegetable glycerine. We do not use grain alcohol as some flower essence manufacturers do. We add the plant's mother essence—that is, the direct essence from the mother plant without dilution—to purified water along with our preservative of choice.

If you have questions or concerns, please check with your health care professional before and during use.

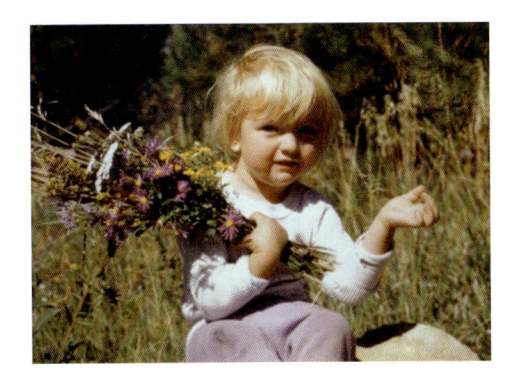

Sarah PallasDowney enjoying the comfort of nature with a bouquet of wildflowers

USING FLOWER ESSENCES

Flower essences help you gain a greater understanding of your innermost nature. They can work subtly or dramatically. Usually it takes some time to observe and feel the gifts of flower essences and how they make changes or cause shifts in your life.

Take three or four drops under your tongue two to four times daily according to your needs and level of sensitivity. You may decide to take a flower essence more frequently for the first few days—for example, six to eight times a day. This can heighten your sensitivity to the flower or plant, after which you can gradually reduce the dosage according to your own needs. Continue to take an essence as long as you wish.

You can also add flower essences to bathwater, spray bottles, the family water crock, or to your animal's water bowl.

Flower Essences for Children

We have found that by introducing children to the natural wonders of the plant kingdom, they become much more attuned to their surroundings and to the feelings of plants and the plant kingdom. Scents, colors, textures, shapes, and forms are exciting, fun, and appealing. The beauty and profundity of nature draws children into an imaginative, mystical world of beauty. As well, showing children photos of plants and letting them feel into the personality and nature of the plant, flower, or tree is like bringing them into the life force of the plant. This helps children identify and connect with the life force in themselves.

Telling children stories about plants and where they grow and asking a child what they see or feel when looking at a certain plant, taking time to stimulate the child's senses in this way, helps the child connect with their feelings and thoughts. A beautiful way to help a child change a thought form, mood, action, or feeling is to teach them a simple affirmation such as what is included for each plant in the compendium in part 3 of this book. Encourage the child to use their own words. Empowering a child with the energy of plants can help them grow deeper and wiser, which builds their self-confidence and helps them feel more connected with family and friends.

Add a few drops of essence water in a small glass of water or put drops directly in the child's mouth, depending on the child's desire for taste.

We have found that chamomile, calendula, and monkeyflower essences work well in treating restlessness, emotional upsets, fears, and nightmares. The beneficial effects come quite quickly. Sweet pea flower essence is rec-

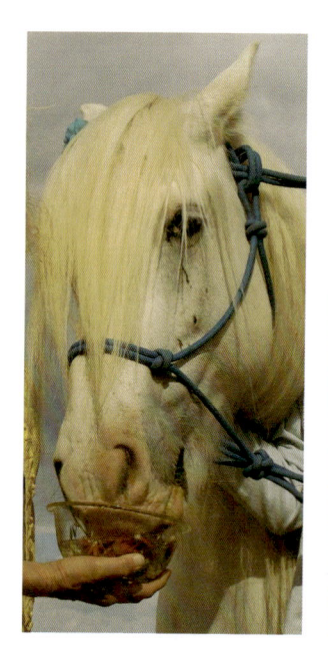

Angel breathing in the scent of flower essence water (photo by Cody Lyon/Rico Arts)

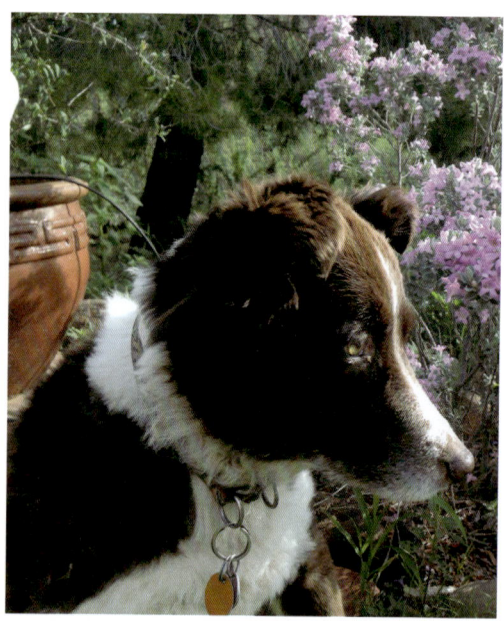

Nammuu focusing and feeling the moment

ommended for children who may feel left out or socially ill at ease. It helps them establish emotional security and social integration while fostering self-acceptance so they can connect with how they are really feeling.

Flower Essences for Animals

Flower and plant essences are very effective remedies for animals. When an animal is given a flower essence, either in a bowl of water or drops in its mouth, it can help the animal open a gateway into inner calmness and well-being. The plant's spirit can navigate along with the spirit of the animal to become a catalyst for healing.

Flower and plant essences for animals can be as powerful as flower and plant essences are for humans. They offer a place within the animal that reaches into emotional and physical discord to reestablish the link between body and soul, nature and spirit. Flower essences can also help an animal in unseen ways so they can live more comfortably.

Using flower and plant essences with animals is similar to how we use them with people. Generally, a few drops at a time throughout the day is sufficient. You may want to dilute the essence for tiny animals. With larger animals like horses, you can make your own essences for them to drink or add several drops to their water trough, or even put a few drops straight into their mouth. The principle "less is more" is a good one to follow with an animal, no matter the size.

Here's a heartwarming story about giving a wild rose flower essence to a dog with separation anxiety. I had given a wild rose flower essence to R.M., age forty-seven, to help her deal with her depression and apathy. Inspired by her good experience with the remedy, she told me a story about a situation she found herself in a few months later.

R.M. had offered to take care of someone's dog while the owner was out of town. The dog was high-strung and nervous. After five days of caring for the dog, it still hadn't eaten and had drunk hardly any water and rarely left its bed. R.M. worried that the dog could have kidney failure due to its listlessness, and she didn't know what to do.

Then she remembered her bottle of wild rose flower essence. She put four drops in a dropper bottle and filled it with water and put the drops down the dog's throat. Ten minutes later, the dog was up and drinking water. He started playing with a dog biscuit and proceeded to eat it. R.M. was relieved that the wild rose essence helped the dog, and the dog seemed happy to have regained its desire to live. R.M. had no more problems with the dog, and upon the owner's return she was happy that both R.M. and the dog were doing quite well.

PART TWO

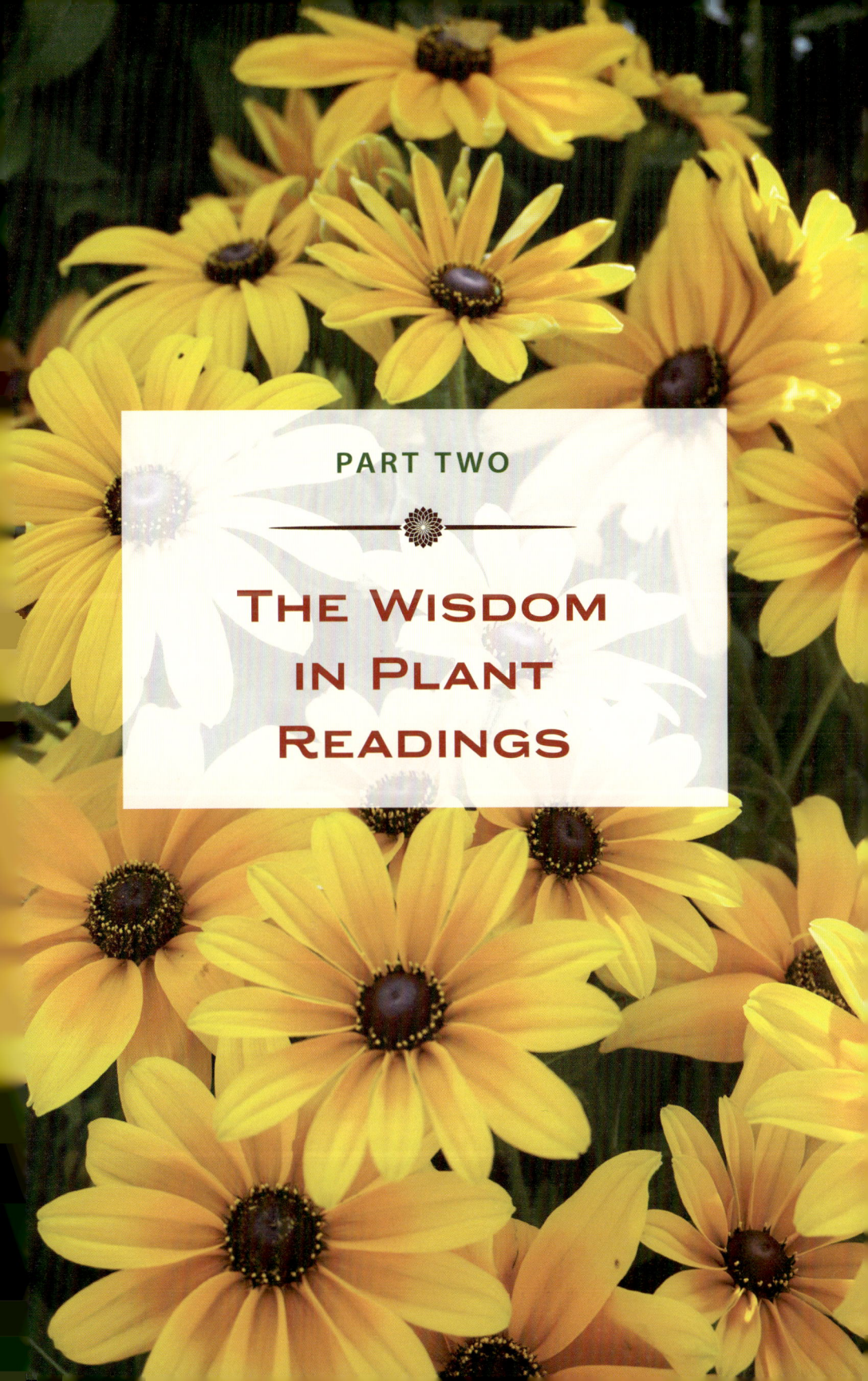

THE WISDOM IN PLANT READINGS

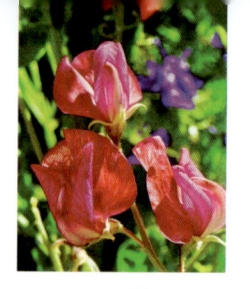

5
Pathways Uniting Body, Mind, and Spirit

The Chakras

And now here is my secret, a very simple secret: It is only with the heart that one can see rightly; what is essential is invisible to the eye.

ANTOINE DE SAINT-EXUPERY, *THE LITTLE PRINCE*

AS WE NOW KNOW, a plant is a complete energy system with a distinct vibration involving smell, sound, touch, and light. Plant spirits communicate to you through the color and sound vibrations specific to each of your energy centers, or chakras. We have learned over many years of working with plants that the colors of flowers as well as the whole plant's personality and electromagnetic field directly correlate with the chakra energy centers of the human body, including their colors and their corresponding glands.

Chakra is a Sanskrit word that means "wheel of light," which suggests something circular that moves. Working with our chakras as a system of subtle energy centers within the human body increases our awareness of our bodily functions; it helps us better understand ourselves, others, and the world. As you begin to form a relationship with the subtle intelligence of your own energy system, your chakras, then you will become more aware of your inner world and will know whether it is in harmony or out of balance.

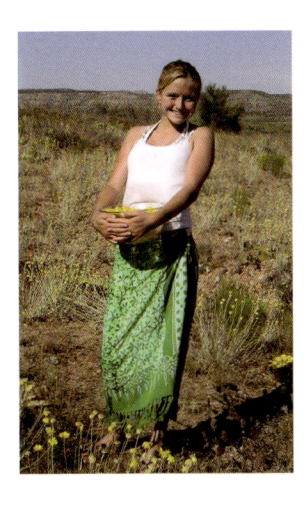

Sarah PallasDowney attuning with herself and plant energy

THE CHAKRAS AND THEIR COLORS

People have appreciated and responded to color and energy since earliest times. You choose certain colors for the clothes you wear, the paint on your walls, your furniture, and your living-room curtains, bath towels, kitchen wares, car, home, and even the foods you eat. We are surrounded by color. By becoming familiar with the colors of the rainbow and their correspondences to the energy centers of the human body, the chakras, you will begin to notice some very basic things about plants, nature, colors, and yourself.

For example, when we pay attention, it seems natural that plants and flowers in the red, orange, and yellow color range exude a warm, stimulating, vibrant energy. They generally appear to be more connected to the earth and to our personality self—to our roots, our emotions, and our thoughts. You can actually feel this resonance as you look at them.

Flowers in the blue and purple spectrum appear more connected to the sky. When you look at these flowers and notice their colors, they stimulate a sense of inspiration, insight, vision, and clarity. These colors are cooling, like a breath of fresh air. They take you into a deep place of self-reflection and insight.

The pink color associated with the heart rests between both the warm and the cool spectrum; it offers a mild sensation that is soothing to the heart.

The color white, associated with the crown chakra, the energy center at the top of the head, gives a sense of purity, oneness, sacredness, and connectedness.

Best of all, you don't have to be an expert at understanding the chakras when you work with plants. Simply imagine the energy centers in your body and the colors associated with them as reflected in the colors of flowers and plants. In this very natural way you will begin to experience the wisdom of the flowers, plants, and trees and what they have to offer. Let them deepen your own inner treasures as you receive these gifts from nature's bounty.

THE CHAKRAS, THE ENDROCRINE SYSTEM, AND THE VAGUS NERVE

If only for a moment, stop and connect with any of the sensations in your body—how you're feeling physically, emotionally, and mentally. What thoughts have been in your mind today or perhaps in the past few days. What shows up for you?

The chakras are associated with the sensations of their corresponding organs of the endocrine system, "the system composed of glands that release their hormones directly into the bloodstream for chemical signaling of target cells."[1] So, becoming aware of the chakras brings insight into the functioning of our glands and their locations within the endocrine system. This system is what's behind many of the functions of the body—sleep, heart rate, metabolism, immunity, hunger, thirst, body temperature, and so much more. When any of these functions are out of balance, the body's overall balance goes awry. Many illnesses are caused by stress that is the result of an imbalance between the endocrine system and the central nervous system.

Hormone secretions have their own language and unique interactions within the body as a whole. By becoming more aware of and adapting to our bodily functions, we enter into a new rhythm, a new dance, one that helps us become energetically stable. By understanding how stress affects our body-mind-spirit, we discover how to live artfully, in homeostasis, in a more peaceful state of being. The endocrine glands include the adrenal glands, which are governed by the root chakra and are associated with how we manage stress in our body. The gonads or reproductive glands are governed by the sacral chakra and are related to sexuality, water and emotions in general, creativity, and passion. The pancreas is governed by the solar plexus chakra and rules the digestive system and how it feels to be in our power. The thymus gland, at the center of our body, is governed by the heart chakra and relates to the ability to love ourselves and others from a place of unconditional love. The thyroid gland, governed by the throat chakra, relates to all the ways we communicate and express ourselves through voice, sound, and movement. The pituitary gland, governed by the third eye chakra, allows us to step outside our immediate circle to see the big picture, giving insight into who we are. And the pineal gland, governed by the crown chakra, offers the blissful understanding of oneness, that we are inseparable from the entire cosmos.

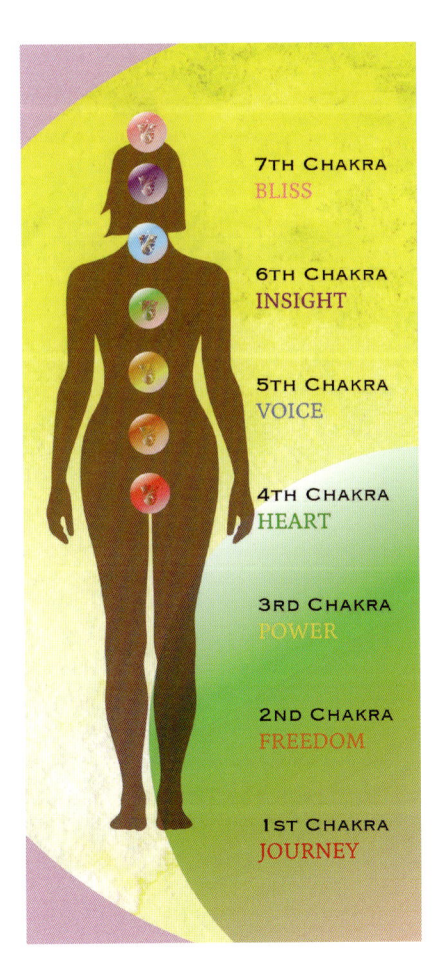

Chakra map (illustration by Pamela Becker, © 2022 Big Vision Arts)

Different philosophical systems, but especially those related to the practice of yoga, identify numerous minor chakras in the human body besides these seven major chakras. In this book we bring our attention to the seven major chakras, which are aligned from the root chakra to the crown chakra via the vagus nerve. The vagus nerve, also known as the tenth cranial nerve, runs throughout the body like a superhighway, connecting all the chakras and their associated endocrine glands. It is associated with the brain and the digestive, cardiovascular, and immune systems in particular. These functions of the human body are unconscious and involuntary.

By learning to access and understand the messages that your nervous system sends throughout your body via the vagus nerve, you may encounter various psychological and even physiological conditions that exist within you. The knowledge of where you hold energy in your body and any mental, emotional, or physical issues you may be feeling can be addressed as a result of your awareness of the endocrine system and study of the seven chakras. Such a discovery can lead you on the path of healing as you integrate plant energy medicine into your life. Experience guided chakra meditations through *Voices of Flowers: 7 Flowers & Chakra Meditation Sound Bath* (you can purchase the CD at centerforplantstudies.com).

FIRST CHAKRA: PHYSICAL, ROOT, OR BASE CHAKRA

My Journey

Element: earth

Focus: survival, physical security, foundation, boundless creativity

Color: red

Sounds/vibrations: tone of middle C, long *u* or long *o* vowel sounds, *lam* or *lang* (Vedic) sound; bass-toned and percussion instruments; didgeridoo

Endocrine gland: adrenals, located atop the kidneys. The adrenals produce steroid hormones, which regulate salt concentration in the blood; and hydrocortisone, which assists the body in its response to physical stress. The root or base chakra is located between the tailbone and the pubic bone.

Plant correspondences: Indian paintbrush, oak, paloverde

What is my relationship to my physical body?
How do I manage the stress in my body?

The root chakra has a grounding energy that connects us to the earth and establishes our foundation. This is an innate primal energy and the vital foundation of our spiritual and soul heritage—where we have come from and how we will proceed given who we are. It is about survival, power, and sensuality. It includes our physical needs such as food, shelter, clothing, exercise, and nutrition, yet it also includes a deeper awareness that takes us back to the roots from which we came. The earth takes us deep inside our darkness and helps us face our shadows, the unconscious forces that have driven us from the past to the present. Establishing an understanding of and a relationship with our root chakra initiates a deep internal journey into the discovery of our true self. It is the turning point for knowing who we really are; it gives us the strength to choose our direction in life in the context of this greater picture of ourselves and our origins. A strong and vigorous root chakra supports the performance of our vital life force energy.

SECOND CHAKRA: EMOTIONAL, SPLEEN, SACRUM

Emotional Freedom

Element: water
Focus: sexuality, procreation, passion
Color: orange
Sounds/vibrations: tone of D, next to middle C, *oo* vowel sound, *vam* or *vang* (Vedic) sound; bass-toned, percussion, brass, and woodwind instruments; didgeridoo
Endocrine gland: gonads, spleen. Located in the reproductive system, the ovaries and testes produce estrogen, progesterone, sperm, and testosterone, which affect the function of the

adrenal glands, the lymphatic glands, and the spleen, bladder, pancreas, and kidneys. The second chakra affects the process of elimination and the general detoxification of the body.

Plant correspondences: crimson monkeyflower, ocotillo, pomegranate

What am I feeling now?

The second chakra, or emotional center, is the driving force that gives us the incentive to get to where we want to go and helps us get in touch with how we feel about who we are. This chakra expresses what we choose to act out in our lives. Emotions give voice to our soul drama or soul pattern, which has developed over the course of our lifetime or even lifetimes. Feelings such as fear, anger, grief, and shame need to be understood and put in their proper perspective. Learning about how powerful our emotions are and their energetic impact on us and others can help us use our emotions as effective tools that can guide us to discover who we are or who we want to be. Our emotions can flow like a river, and their strength depends on the driving force of energy moving through us. We learn to yield and flow like a river, continually releasing, cleansing, changing, and evolving. We are constantly being pulled by two factors: releasing old feelings and emotions that limit us, prevent our personal growth, and possibly cause us to blame others for our suffering; and moving forward in new ways that free us from the bondage of old feelings and stuck patterns, in order to acquire a new identity.

The second chakra holds the key to our personal investment in ourselves, to our creativity and the birth of new emotional patterns, and to our ability to take care of and nurture ourself and others. By discovering who we are through our emotions, we can open to our own inner treasures of harmony, balance, and peace. Most importantly, we can feel a sense of trust in knowing who we are. We develop confidence, endurance, and emotional security.

The second chakra is the center of sexuality and sensation. As we come into a new identity, we experience the balancing of our sexuality. We learn new steps in the dance of life that stir our passion and excitement for living. We have accepted and embraced life's setbacks and we are creating a new way of living that supports who we are and what we've established in the foundation of our being. We create healthy relationships and navigate a creative emotional flow within.

THIRD CHAKRA:
PERSONAL POWER, SOLAR PLEXUS

Being in My Power

Element: fire

Focus: will, purpose, empowering radiance

Color: yellow

Sounds/vibrations: tone of E above middle C; *ah* sound; *ram* or *rang* (Vedic) sound; flutes, woodwinds, strings, and piano instruments; soft didgeridoo

Endocrine gland: pancreas/solar plexus. The third chakra rules the functions of the adrenals, pancreas, stomach, digestive system, liver, and gallbladder, some of whose functions are shared with the second chakra. The pancreas secretes insulin and glucagon to regulate blood sugar.

Plant correspondences: calendula, chaparral, sunflower

Am I ready to let go of my fears and step into trust?

The third chakra gives us our ability to think and reason, to find purpose and desire in life, and to empower ourselves to be who we need to be. It helps us understand our thoughts in relation to our feelings. It strengthens our mind to pursue a state of stability, courage, positive faith, hope, humor, and joy. This energy center brings about a balanced mental state

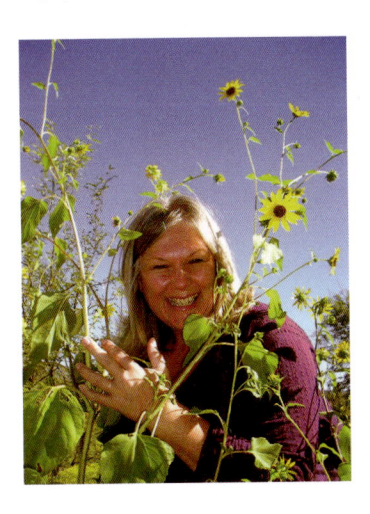

Sandi O'Connor being empowered with the radiance of sunflowers

of responsibility, mental objectivity, and wisdom. It teaches us to surrender the mind when we need to, and it's also the link between the rational mind and our psychic energies and enhanced intuition. It gives us the courage and faith to trust and act on our intuition.

The third chakra reveals a higher consciousness within the lower three chakras and helps us better understand ourself and others. It is the link between the lower chakras and the heart, uniting love and harmony to empower the process of dissolving or decrystalizing old patterns. By loving ourselves and taking personal risks to act in our own best interests, we develop honor, dignity, and self-esteem. In the third chakra we come to terms with who we are, why we are here, what we have learned, and what we desire. This journey with and as our true Self leads to dignity and self-empowerment.

By working with the third chakra we can dissolve our prejudices, judgments, and criticisms; learn how to effectively deal with anger; understand any hatred we may have and its roots; and dissolve and unplug from our fears, both rational and irrational. We become more assertive, advocating for ourself and capable of realizing our personal goals.

A conscious, healthy relationship with the solar plexus chakra helps us trust our intuition and the guidance transmitted from the higher chakras. The third chakra is complemented by the violet/purple ray of the sixth chakra, which indicates our ability to receive higher guidance and allow our spiritual aspirations and vision to move through us.

FOURTH CHAKRA: HEART CENTER

Opening to Love

Element: air

Focus: love, compassion, and forgiveness; heart awakening

Color: green or pink

Sounds/vibrations: tone of F above middle C, long *a* vowel sound, *ram* or *yang* (Vedic) sound; harp, organ, flute, wind chimes, and string instruments

Endocrine gland: thymus, located in front of and above the heart, beneath the breastbone. The thymus encompasses the functions of the immune and circulatory systems. It secretes thymosin and other hormones that regulate the immune system. It is associated with the right hemisphere of the brain and with tissue regeneration.

Plant correspondences: desert willow, manzanita, wild rose

Will I forgive myself? What nurtures my heart and excites my feelings?

The heart chakra is the link between the three upper and the three lower chakras. It is here, at the center, where spirit, vision, light, wisdom, and communication from above meet with matter, survival, procreation, knowledge, and personality from below. When the upper and lower chakras are balanced and their energy currents are flowing freely, the heart chakra radiates its creative energy and power. The merging of sexuality with the true expression of sexual love is generated, and passions of mystical awakening are stirred and experienced.

The heart center is the place within us where our personal development reaches a new level. This growth is demonstrated by our ability to let our heart dictate who we are and the choices we make. Our heart center awakens us to a higher expression of love, compassion, and will. We become open to unconditional love of self and others in a universal way that expands well beyond our families and friends. We begin to embody the balance between physical power and spiritual guidance and wisdom. Through this balance we become aware of what it means to invest in both spirit and matter. We develop a passion to live by a new honor system, trusting that Spirit, divine inspiration, and realizing the higher Self will lead us on our path. In turn, our journey becomes one of integrity, honesty, respect, forgiveness, compassion, and understanding. We learn to honor all things for who or what they are, without judgment or criticism.

The life aspect of the soul is rooted in the heart center. Here we can heal our heart wounds that may date back to our earliest memories and beyond, deep in our soul record. In our heart chakra we offer healing, forgiveness, and love of others. We come to realize that we no longer need to feed negative energies or limitations in relation to ourself or others, and that we can bless and love others while staying on our path. This awareness and growth enables us to decrystalize or dissolve the old patterns so we can follow our heart's desire and love freely.

FIFTH CHAKRA: THROAT CHAKRA

Voice

Element: ether

Focus: self-expression, communication, sound and vibration

Color: blue

Sound/vibrations: tone of G, above middle C, short vowels (*e, i, a, u*), *ham* or *hang* (Vedic) sounds; harp, organ, piano, and higher-pitched instruments such as flute, pennywhistle, and violin

Endocrine gland: thyroid. Located at the base of the throat, the thyroid wraps around the windpipe and secretes thyroxin, which regulates the body's metabolic rate. The thyroid is known as a lubricator of energy transformation. The throat chakra includes the throat, larynx, tongue, mouth, lips, teeth, esophagus, upper lungs, voice, bronchial tubes, and thyroid and parathyroid glands.

Plant correspondences: desert larkspur, juniper, Palmer's penstemon

Do I express myself from my heart?

The throat chakra is the link between the upper two chakras and the heart; it is where we receive the higher vibratory frequencies of the sixth and seventh chakras and connect those frequencies with the heart. The throat chakra is the chakra of creativity and spiritual willpower, as distinct from the power related to the emotions and the personality self. Having the willpower to face our fears, anger, barriers, or blockages means having the ability to call on Spirit to help us reach for and live in the light rather than the darkness. As we become more open to embracing the light and the higher energy currents within ourselves, we spontaneously bring spiritual guidance, creativity, and vision to our cognitive mind, and we are thus better able to bring in positive thought forms and attitudes. An opening or awakening of the throat chakra is indicated by our ability to speak our truth from an inner depth of awareness, creativity, spiritual guidance, and compassion. Communication takes place not only through vocal exchange, but through creative art forms such as dance, sculpture, painting, singing, chanting, and playing musical instruments.

True communication is the expression of our inner self (our voice, its sounds and vibrations, our thoughts, our inner truths and insights) to the outside world, and the responses that come back to us as a result. We become more self-aware of the ways we communicate and how others respond to us. We learn how to communicate clearly and honestly in order to be heard.

One form of communication that we don't always access is subliminal, that is, communication that goes beyond time and space. This type of communication, known as telepathy, involves exchanging nonphysical energy signals or information from the ethers, the rarefied element that traditionally is believed to fill the upper regions of space, or the heavens. Through inner listening and cultivating a calm mind, we gain the ability to channel communication from higher sources through a subtle vibratory exchange of energy. An example of telepathy is when we think about someone we haven't seen or talked to in years, and we subsequently receive a letter or phone call from that person. Another example is when we feel that someone close to us needs our help or is in danger. Most of us have experienced telepathy at some time in our lives. This is related to the fifth chakra.

SIXTH CHAKRA: THIRD EYE, EYE OF WISDOM, OR BROW CHAKRA

Insight

Element: radium

Focus: seeing, visualization, clairvoyance, intuition, and imagination

Color: violet/purple

Sound/vibrations: tone of A above middle C, long *e* vowel sound, *OM* (Vedic); harp, organ, piano, wind chimes, and high-pitched string instruments

Endocrine gland: pituitary. The pituitary gland is located slightly above the eyes, in the center of the forehead, in the area known as the third-eye chakra or the "eye of wisdom." The pituitary gland is a peanut-sized organ located at the base of the brain. It is known as the master gland because it secretes nine hormones that affect the function of the five lower endocrine glands, keeping them in balance and harmony with one another. The pituitary hormones serve many functions that relate to memory and sleep patterns. The hypothalamus is located directly above the pituitary gland and serves as a primary coordinator of the endocrine glands and the nervous system and much more.

Plant correspondences: aster, lupine, sage

Do I trust my intuition?

The third eye or brow chakra is the visionary chakra that gives us wisdom, balance, and spiritual insight. This is why it is referred to as the "eye of wisdom" or the "inner eye." The brow chakra teaches us about judgment, truth, honesty, harmony, and integrity, and shows us how our mind responds to the truths that we know. This center empowers us to acknowledge our wisdom and act according to the wisdom we receive. It releases stagnation and helps us define our purpose and refine our spiritual understanding. It enables us to allow light to come through our third eye and to receive the messages that light brings. The third eye is the vibrational point where the darkness from the center of the Earth and the light from the center of the sun merge as one. Light and darkness together create a balanced sixth chakra. This energy center works with the mental aspects of the third chakra and allows a higher vision and spiritual aspiration to guide our thought forms.

The third eye gives us the ability to see our memories, dreams, thought forms, and imagination. At this center we take in, hold, clarify, create, and manifest visual information. This chakra is a gateway that allows us to step beyond ourself and access the higher power that is already inherently within us. It opens us to clairvoyance and psychic awareness and the ability to see beyond time and space. It helps us access information that tells us about a person, place, or event from within our mind's eye. We may see lights, color, images, our own emotions, or the emotions or energy fields of others. Through the sixth chakra we gain access to long-distance vibrational healing by sending our prayers and healing to others without their being physically present.

This energy center awakens our intuition and our insights at a deep level. It gives us the power to tap into a higher vibrational frequency that links us with the collective unconscious, to lead us to a state of oneness. It is through this powerful connection with the collective unconscious that our energy is shared and united. Clear third-eye perception brings mental focus and acuity.

SEVENTH CHAKRA: CROWN CHAKRA

Bliss

Element: magentum
Focus: awareness, oneness with the unified field, peace and understanding
Color: white/gold
Sound/vibration: tone of B above middle C. There is no particular sound to chant except for the sound of the universe coming through us as the frequency of the sacred syllable *OM*; harp, organ, wind chimes, and high-pitched instruments.
Endocrine gland: pineal. The pineal gland is a small, ovoid body about the size of a pea, situated centrally in the brain and attached to the third ventricle of the brain. The biological role of the pineal gland is not well-understood. Its primary hormone is melatonin, which regulates the cerebrum, the hypothalamus, and the body's sleep/wake cycle. The crown chakra is located at the top of the head and is associated with the cerebral cortex, the central nervous systems, the pineal gland, and all the pathways of the nerves and electrical synapses within the body.
Plant correspondences: saguaro, yerba santa, yucca

What guides me to connect with my higher Self?

The seventh chakra is associated with both conscious and unconscious thoughts, including our beliefs, how we see ourself, how we see others, and how we view the events in our life. This energy center is associated with the strand of consciousness that is anchored near the pineal gland.

The actual passage into the seventh chakra occurs spontaneously and effortlessly, aligning us with our spiritual essence and an intrinsic knowing that is linked to our higher consciousness. Higher consciousness means a broader relationship with the Self and with the unified field of energy that is bigger than, yet inclusive of, the physical world and our experiences in it. Higher consciousness includes our ability to live in the here and now, to plant the seeds of our thoughts in a higher power, and to nurture these seeds so they will manifest. This consciousness comes from an inner place that allows us to reach for knowledge and obtain wisdom. Our brain, as a vehicle to the mind, is then infinite and unlimited.

As we gain access to the crown chakra we find we can be nowhere yet everywhere all at once. The crown chakra is where we explore, study, and experience the infinite reservoir of knowledge that influences the way we receive information, the way we interact with the world, our beliefs and values, the way we view ourself and our internal patterns, and the way we evolve in our spirituality. By working with the seventh chakra we become more aware of our relationship with a unified field of energy. We consciously begin to devote time each day to the sacred, which can include prayer, meditation, writing in dream journals, doing healing work, using flower essences, or other practices. We become the purpose of our life's work, and through our awareness the bond between the heart and the sixth chakra becomes more evident. We feel a vibrant energy flow through all the chakras and throughout our entire being. We become conscious of all the chakras and how they work together to create our biological existence. We learn to see ourselves as a system of energy, being mindful of every situation we find ourselves in and the way we hold or give away our power.

The chakras are traditionally symbolized by the lotus flower, the petals of which unfold as it emerges into full bloom. The lotus is a sacred and beautiful flower, precious in India. The transformation that lies at the heart of the flower's opening can be compared to the opening of a chakra. The lotus emerges from the mud, symbolizing our journey from the earth's darkness, and evolves into a thousand petals (the famous thousand-petaled lotus) that glows with radiant light out of the crown of our head. The lotus has completed its evolution and has now reached its highest peak of manifestation, that of infinite bliss, expanded consciousness, and divine communion.

Plants have a root system that grows out of the darkness of the earth. The developmental process of a plant is much like the evolution of a chakra.

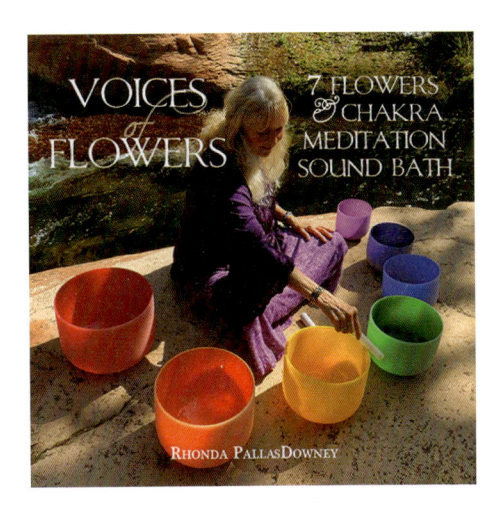

Experience guided chakra meditations through Voices of Flowers: 7 Flowers & Chakra Meditation Sound Bath *(purchase the CD at centerforplantstudies.com; CD cover art by Pamela Becker of Big Vision Art & Design, Sedona, AZ)*

The plant begins as a tiny seed in the earth, then forms a root to stabilize and grow. The plant requires earth, water, fire (sun or light), air, and sound vibrations to help it develop. It then forms a stem (a spine) and leaves as it emerges into the uniqueness of its own energetic vibration. Finally, the plant produces a beautiful flower at its crown, the top of its head. The flower expresses the plant's intrinsic identity when it reaches its peak of blossoming, merging its roots, anchored in the darkness of the earth, with the radiant light of consciousness. The flower evolves, completes its cycle, and surrenders to the infinite. Like we humans, plants have cycles of growth and development, closing or opening to expand into their fullest blossom as they experience the process of budding life followed by death.

By going deeper into your relationship between each organ of your endocrine system and its corresponding chakra, you will strengthen your ability to merge your personal energy with your higher consciousness. Experience the integration of each of these chakras and endocrine glands as a complete energy system in all the ways that you feel, think, and respond to yourself and to all of life.

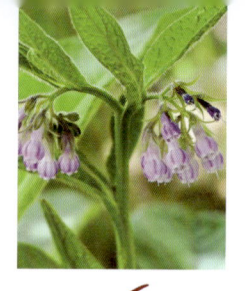

6
How to Do Plant Readings

Daily Insights and Plant Medicine Readings

There is no peace that cannot be found in the present moment.
                                                    TASHA TUDOR

BY DEVELOPING A relationship with the plants highlighted in this book, you will access their wisdom. The more you work with these plants, the more deeply you will come to understand how they connect to your own body and to your entire being, physical, mental, and spiritual.

The simplest practice of all is to use any one of the flowers, trees, and plants in this book as a focus for daily meditation. Find a solitary place where you can listen to your heart. What is it saying? Begin by choosing a plant that calls out to you or that you already have in mind. Review the compendium of flowers, trees, and plants in part 3 of this book to see if this plant has a particular quality that stands out for you. You can also look through the photos of plants in this section and randomly select a plant to be your guide for the day. Be with that plant and contemplate its qualities. Carefully look at the image of the plant, take in its primary quality, and read about it. If you have a flower or plant essence from that plant, take a few drops, then close your eyes and imagine the energy and color of the flower or plant embracing you. If you are focusing on healing a particular issue that relates to a certain chakra, visualize the energy and color of your chosen plant in that energy center in your body. Let yourself be imbued with the presence of the plant as fully as possible. Then open your eyes and remember this experience throughout the day, holding the plant's message in your heart.

DAILY PLANT ENERGY READINGS

Listening to the voices of our fellow green beings and their messages brings profound knowledge of both the plant realm and ourselves. Doing plant readings is one of the best ways to learn the language of plants and understand their messages. Similar to the way tarot cards can provide insights or answer questions, a plant reading can be a wonderful tool for self-reflection and self-discovery that can help you grow in your awareness and open new doorways that allow you to connect with your own divine nature as reflected in the plants. Working with plant energy in this way is relaxing and pleasant, as you free your mind of any lingering thoughts or emotions to focus only on the plants and their messages.

To begin, find a quiet place where you won't be interrupted. Set your intention to create a special space for the wisdom of the flowers, trees, and plants to speak to you. As well as an appropriate physical space, quiet your mind for visualization and imagination. Using a liquid flower or plant essence as you do your plant reading can enhance your experience of the vibrations of the flower, plant, or tree you have chosen.

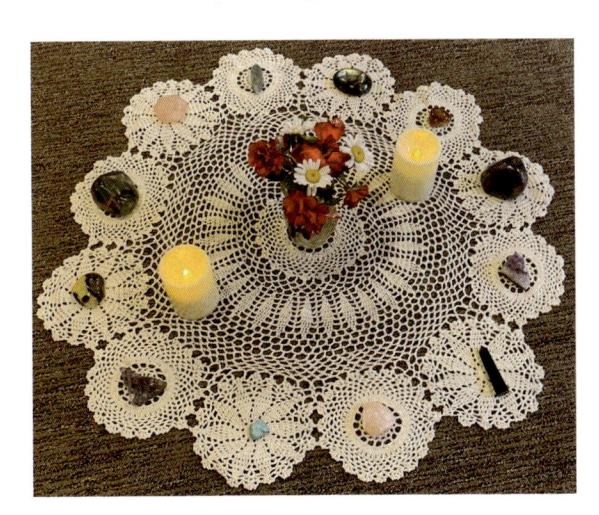

Creating space for a plant reading

To begin, simply choose a plant you're drawn to in this book, or close this book and then randomly open to one of the pages in the plant compendium in part 3 to see who shows up. We recommend you keep a plant journal to record your plant readings, along with any insights you may have regarding the relevance of a plant's message to your life or a particular situation in your life. Be assured that the magic of the plants will attract you to the exact message you need at the time. The act of writing down insights from a plant will increase your self-knowledge and strengthen your connection with the nature spirits of the plants. Using a plant journal can also be a helpful way to visualize the spreads we'll be discussing later in this chapter.

When you are ready to begin your plant reading, ask yourself, *What is my intention? What is my present issue? What message from this magical green being would serve me best now?* Take a moment to record your thoughts in your plant journal. If you don't have any special thoughts or concerns in the moment and you simply want to be open to receiving the plant's message, you can simply rest in the silence of your mind.

Once you've chosen your plant, look at its photo and read the description of its primary quality in the compendium in part 3 of this book, and allow yourself to imbibe that quality. Take that feeling deep inside yourself. Imagine the plant talking to you. Notice the plant's voice, its insight, its chakra correspondence, and its affirmation. What is it reflecting back to you? Take note of colors, its signature, its personality. Notice how the flower, tree, or plant expresses itself and why you are attracted to it. The colors, qualities, and messages of the plant will likely mirror something within you that already exists or that wants to be expressed. After contemplating this way for some time, write down your impressions in your plant journal.

If you are using a flower or plant essence, take three or four drops before you contemplate it. You may want to read about the plant out loud from this book so as to reinforce the description. After doing so, close your eyes and listen to the wisdom of the plant within your heart. Take some time to allow the plant's message to sink in. Pay attention to the subtle energy, senses, or emotions you may experience. If you wish, note your findings in your plant journal.

You may wish to work with one plant for several days or even longer. Remember, you are free to choose any plant, anytime. Follow your heart's desire. You may find there are certain similarities among the flowers, trees, and plants, and the affirmations offered by each plant in this book. Through conscious repetition of the affirmations, the power of words and thoughts will become seeded in your consciousness. This will allow you to create a healing field within your body that expands your biofield to ignite positive changes in your life. Plants, like all living beings, come from one source—the same source that all living beings share. Let go and trust the process.

Another wonderful approach is to share a single plant reading with a friend or friends. By pairing up with another person you can formulate a shared intention, or you can work together with separate but related intentions. You may be surprised by the field of energy that two or more of you can manifest. The resulting combined experience can create a synergy that raises your individual and combined energy fields and increases your voltage.

You can take your reading even further by contemplating the chakra correspondence for the plant you've choosen, which is listed in the plant compendium in part 3. Note which chakra energy centers are affected by the plant, then read the affirmation for the plant you've chosen. Repeat the affirmation out loud. Again, if you wish, you can write down the affirmation in your plant journal or you can create an affirmation in your own words. Consider placing the affirmation on the bathroom mirror so you can see it every morning, or in a special spot where you will see it throughout the day. Use the affirmation as often as you wish, especially before going to bed and when you wake up in the morning. If you are working with flower or plant essences, take a drop of the essence as you repeat the affirmation.

No matter how you work with plants, by doing so regularly you will soon discover that you've created a profound relationship with them, one that will take you on an incredible journey of self-exploration and discovery. Allow the plants to grace you with their beauty, wisdom, and power. Let them nurture and embrace you with their light-filled energies. Remember, just as all seeds grow with tender loving care and guidance, by allowing the flowers, trees, and plants to nourish and guide you, you too will blossom into the fullest expression of yourself.

PLANT ENERGY MEDICINE SPREADS

In the pages that follow you will find four different plant energy medicine spreads to choose from: the Flower Spread, the Seed Spread, the Five Elements Circle of Life Spread, and the Chakra Spread. You may want to familize yourself with each spread before you choose which one to use, so review them all and go with the one that calls to you. You will need to have your plant journal handy to record each plant in the diagram of the spread you've chosen, along with your observations and insights. Once you've determined which plant spread you are most drawn to, take some time to silence your mind. Follow the suggestions for establishing your intention. Remember, this is a process of joining with the spirits of the plants and calling on them for help.

A plant reading is a ceremonial process in itself. No matter which spread you choose, take a few moments to get comfortable and focus your mind. Once you've chosen which plant spread you are drawn to, write down the spread's diagram in your plant journal. Then begin by choosing a plant for each position in the spread. Choose whichever plant you are drawn to or one that chooses you, then write the plant's name down in the appropriate area in your diagram. As you choose a plant for each position in a particular layout, be aware of the position of the plant in the layout as you hold your intention in your mind. Continue with the spread, adding all the rest of the plants in the layout you've selected by jotting down their names in the diagram in your plant journal. Take a moment to look at each plant and its position. Then read about each plant one by one, starting with the first position. Go to the plant compendium in part 3 and look up each plant's voice, insight, chakra correspondence, and affirmation. Notice any feelings, thoughts, or images that come to you as you experience each plant or flower and its specific position in the spread.

After you've reviewed each plant in your spread, go back and try to gain a bigger perspective of the entire reading. Bring in the energy of all the plants in the layout and listen to what they say to you. Let yourself be guided intuitively to any place or position within the plant layout that calls to you. Let the plants tell your story by reflecting their wisdom back to you.

If you like, you can ask yourself questions such as: Which plant am I most drawn to? Where in the reading does the most energy show up for me? In what way has this plant reading opened my awareness about myself, my situation, or my intention?

Notice any overt or possibly hidden messages in the reading. Which particular plant message is the most meaningful to you? What have you gained from considering the big picture of your plant layout? What is the overall message given to you by all the plants in the layout?

As you come to completion with your chosen plant layout, give thanks to the flowers, trees, and plants and their messages. Let yourself absorb the reading and the magic of the green beings as your story unfolds.

The Flower Spread

This spread teaches you about your inherent connection with your roots (Mother Earth) and your awakened consciousness (star beings). It brings awareness and encourages you to tend to the blossoming of yourself. The messages that arise with this spread will strengthen your personal power and understanding of yourself. They provide guidance and support and help you achieve a higher perspective on your life situation, as well as give new meaning to your life choices.

For this plant medicine spread, the layout is shown on page 72.

Position One: Foundation (Root)

This position and the chosen plant represents the foundation of your present situation or your current relationship with yourself. Your foundation is associated with the root energy center that connects you to the earth and serves as your grounding energy. The foundation position takes you to the root of your question or to the foundation of your quest. It points you toward the strength of your foundation. It may indicate what is happening in your life on a deeper or unconscious level that has not yet been brought forth and is buried in your dreams and your deep-seated emotions, memories, desires, and thoughts. The root position helps you gain awareness of your relationship to the source of the situation.

```
                    ┌─────┐
                    │  7  │
                    └─────┘
            The Overview (Sun and Sky)

                    ┌─────┐
                    │  6  │
                    └─────┘
            The Outcome (Flower Head)

┌─────┐                                     ┌─────┐
│  4  │                                     │  5  │
└─────┘                                     └─────┘
Receiving (Left Leaf)                Giving (Right Leaf)

                    ┌─────┐
                    │  3  │
                    └─────┘
          Direction of Movement (Stem)

                    ┌─────┐
                    │  2  │
                    └─────┘
              Environment (Earth)

                    ┌─────┐
                    │  1  │
                    └─────┘
               Foundation (Root)
```

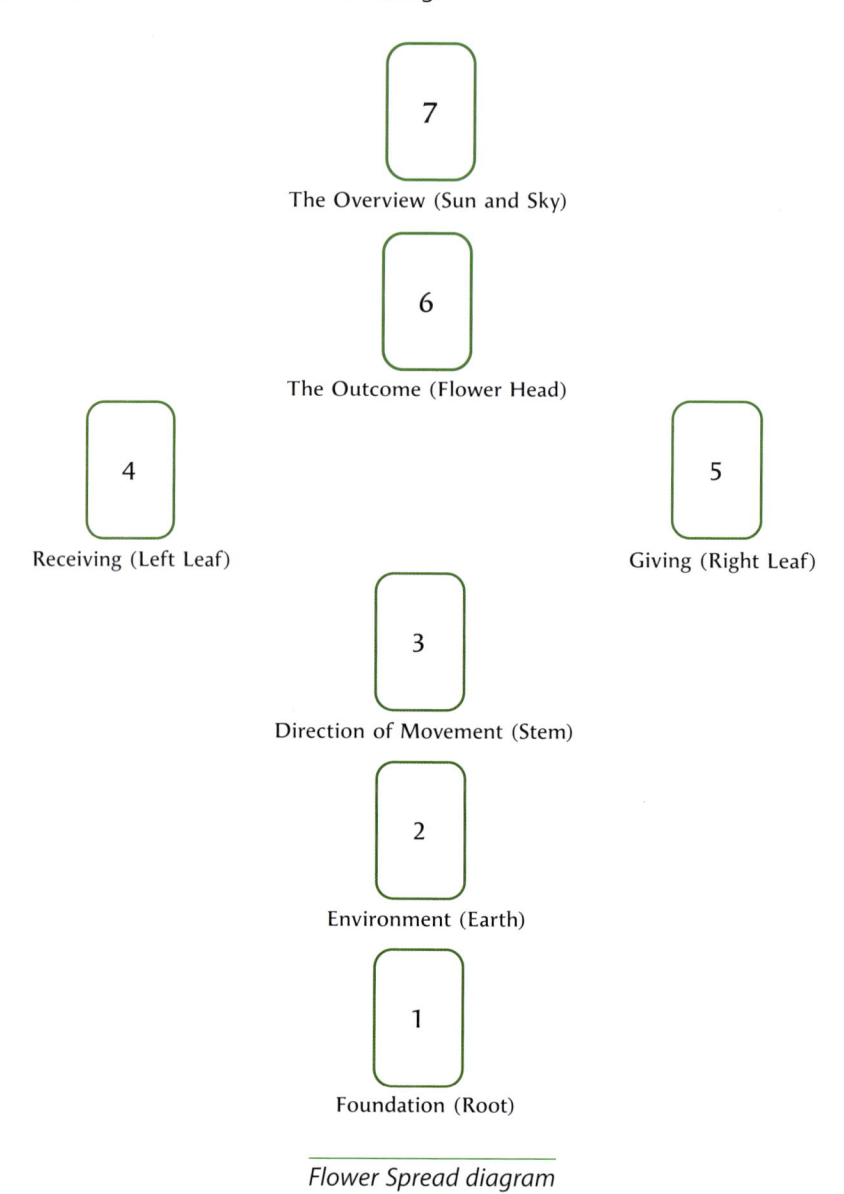

Flower Spread diagram

Position Two: Environment (Earth)

The second position and your chosen plant relates to the soil, which is a metaphor for the environment you are providing for yourself in which to grow. The message behind this position calls on you to get in touch with your lifestyle and your personality self to see how you care for your root energies. Are you providing a rich, nurturing environment, one that is well-watered and well-tended? Or have you neglected your environment? The plant you draw will reveal what is the most nurturing environment for your intention or desire. This message reveals a deeper understanding of how the environment of your thoughts, emotions, and attitudes affects your roots.

Position Three: Direction of Movement (Stem)

This position and the chosen plant speaks to you of the energies that move through you and motivate you. What inspires you to make choices and take new directions in life? What draws you to the actions you take? Do your choices reflect your inner environment and the root energies in which you reside? The message of this position tells you more about your process and how it is working for you. It offers insight into what direction your movement should take. This position offers insight into what will nurture your growth, how to make better choices, and how to find the next step on your path.

Position Four: Receiving (Left Leaf)

The left leaf indicates a receiving position, and the plant you have chosen for this location in the spread relates to circumstances both outside and within yourself. This plant indicates the energies you are taking in—what you are breathing into your being, how you are receiving these energies, and in what way you are internalizing them. What is in your psychic space and how is it feeding the situation? This plant speaks of being receptive to the higher wisdom that allows you to build on your roots, your environment, and the direction you choose to take. It is about receiving your gifts, talents, and abilities and nurturing them.

Position Five: Giving (Right Leaf)

The giving position and chosen plant relates to circumstances both outside and within yourself. This plant indicates the energies you are giving out, what you are exhaling and releasing. The giving plant speaks to you of the way you express and balance yourself in the world and points out what you need to let go of that holds you back. Your direction is becoming clearer, your creativity stronger, and by nourishing yourself, you will feel yourself growing in ways that not only feed you but also feed others.

Position Six: The Outcome (Flower Head)

The outcome position and chosen plant resembles the blossoming flower at its fullest. The message of this plant is the revelation of what you will achieve. It assures you that you have the freedom and innate capacity to reach your fullest exultation, to express your core essence. This card speaks to you of emergence. It offers a natural resolution, completion, and understanding of the outcome of the reading.

Position Seven: The Overview (Sun and Sky)

The overview position and selected plant is associated with higher consciousness and divine wisdom. It indicates how to align yourself with your spiritual essence and intrinsic knowing deep inside. The overview provides the perspective of wisdom and the healing power of grace to the outcome. The flower head blooms and fades, but the sun in the sky remains. This plant honors what is sacred in your heart, allowing it to connect with your higher wisdom. See, feel, and experience yourself as a vibrant, whole being.

The Seed Spread

You may have come to a time in your life when you realize how worn-out you feel, how tired you are of certain patterns in your life, and how much you are in need of a retreat or a change in your life. You may be looking forward to time out from your mundane responsibilities, or you may yearn to be in silence. If you are feeling these things, you may be in need of renewal, the focus of the Seed Spread. Renewal is a natural part of a continuous process of cleansing, building, and creating. Renewal is about taking time to consciously release old habits of mind and body that are no longer desired or needed. Take time to be with yourself. Let go and relax. The cards you choose in this Seed Spread can empower your process of renewal and rekindle your relationship with yourself.

In the Seed Spread you will choose four plants. The first position, "planting the seed," represents what you are sowing. The second position,

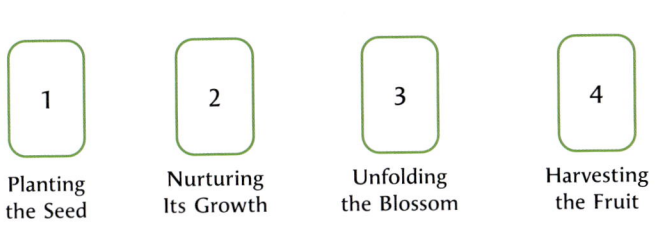

1	2	3	4
Planting the Seed	Nurturing Its Growth	Unfolding the Blossom	Harvesting the Fruit

Seed Spread diagram

"nurturing its growth," is the quality or direction of your growth. The third position, "unfolding the blossom," represents the fullness of what you have unfolded. The fourth position, "harvesting the fruit," represents what you will produce, or the fruit of your efforts. The four cards are laid out in a horizontal line, as shown above.

Position One: Planting the Seed

Before you choose your first plant for the Seed Spread, take a moment to reflect on how you've been feeling. Get in touch with ways you may feel you are not connected with yourself. The plant you choose for this position is about acknowledging your need for change and healing. Gently bring your focus to that silent, powerful place at the center of your being. Allow the silence in this sacred place to envelop you. When you feel ready, choose a plant. Let the plant bring to your awareness the energy that can help you with your renewal. Contemplate the image of the flower and its message, insight, and affirmation. Rest in the source of your renewal.

Position Two: Nurturing Its Growth

When you choose your second plant for the Seed Spread, ask for guidance from the flowers for the energy that will support, nurture, and give you life. Allow the plant to help you grow this renewing energy. Awaken the bud of new life within yourself. Let your thoughts and images of this plant share its qualities with you. Notice how this plant nurtures and supports you—listen to your inner voice. Let the soil in which you plant your seed—your inner environment—be tended and cared for as you experience an expansion in your awareness. As you nurture and renew yourself, the seed opens further and begins to grow.

Position Three: Unfolding the Blossom

When you choose a plant for the third position in the Seed Spread, you may already be feeling a sense of renewal dawning. This plant will guide you in the direction of your renewal. Choose a plant and notice how it helps you feel uplifted and reconnected within. Read the flower's voice and hear its words. Listen to its message and contemplate its energy. Let your inner being come forth. Embrace the feeling of freedom and renewal. Allow yourself to blossom to your fullest, feeling refreshed, whole, and at peace with yourself.

Position Four: Harvesting the Fruit

The final position in this spread indicates the fruition of your growth. The seed has opened and sprouted, the bud has formed, and it has blossomed. You are now ready for the harvest. Having been gifted with new awareness and understanding, welcome and honor your renewal by joyfully sharing the abundant harvest of your fruits.

The Five Elements Circle of Life Spread

For this spread, each of the four elements is placed in relation to its direction: earth in the north, fire in the south, air in the east, and water in the west. These four form a complete circle, as if you were looking at a map of

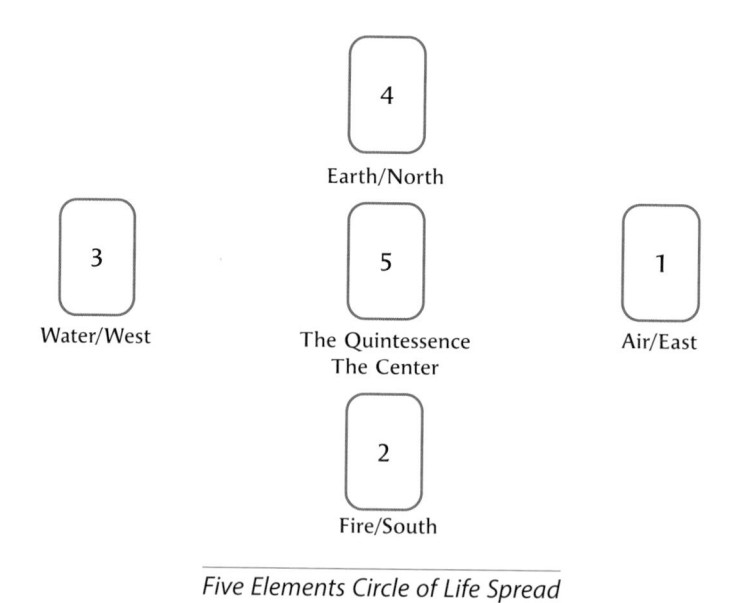

```
                    ┌───┐
                    │ 4 │
                    └───┘
                 Earth/North

  ┌───┐           ┌───┐            ┌───┐
  │ 3 │           │ 5 │            │ 1 │
  └───┘           └───┘            └───┘
Water/West    The Quintessence    Air/East
                 The Center

                    ┌───┐
                    │ 2 │
                    └───┘
                  Fire/South
```

Five Elements Circle of Life Spread

the world with the addition of the elements. Various cultures and people have different associations with the elements and the four directions. This plant spread is based more on European Celtic associations.

The center of the four elements is called the *quintessence*, which indicates the heart of the reading. This represents an invisible or unseen energy source that can be felt and experienced as an expression of the seed of the universe, the core essence and the divine presence of all living things. Overall, the four elements that surround the center plant, the quintessence or the fifth element, produce a powerful and effective means of healing. The five elements are used in making a flower essence. The core essence of the flower is considered its quintessence. The elements of air, fire, water, and earth are the living foods that sustain and nurture us. They support all of life and give us everything that we need.

This spread allows you to experience and understand your relationship to each of the elements, including your own quintessence, which is the essence of you in your highest form. It helps you to cultivate a higher perspective about your life situation. It takes you to a deeper connection with the very essence of your being.

Position One: Air/East

This position in the east represents the air in which we live and breathe. Just as the sun rises, bringing forth a new day of illumination and power, we are given new hope energized by the light, allowing us to proceed from a place that expands beyond our physical world. As the eagle soars, we can see far below us, yet be connected to our earthly ways. As spring emerges, new buds and plant growth bring freshness and beauty, adorning the earth with living colors and natural bounty. We are sustained by the oxygen provided by plants. Without them, we could not survive. The east represents new beginnings, new life budding, and inspiration. As you take in a breath of fresh air, imagine you are taking in the green bounty of plant energy deep inside your throat and lungs. Breathe in the wisdom of this plant's message and allow it to move through your entire being. This position represents clarity. You may have a fresh, new idea or want to tackle a new project. A doorway may open in some way that gives you a new insight about yourself or about the situation you are in. You may be guided to speak your truth, sing your songs, and listen to how your voice sounds and its vibrations.

Position Two: Fire/South

The south is the place of the element of fire, represented by the sun, the source of light and heat. It is sunlight that makes possible the process of photosynthesis, especially in plants, where the synthesis of complex organic materials such as carbohydrates from carbon dioxide, water, and inorganic salts, with the aid of a catalyst such as chlorophyll, provides the enrichment of vitamins and minerals. The selected south plant is associated with your personal growth and the fire or inner light within you. The message of this plant may call on you to get to know yourself better, to look at the ways you reason and think, to find your purpose and desires in life, and to empower yourself to be who you truly are. The power of the south and the sun gives you the courage and faith to trust your intuition and innocence and act on it. It strengthens you to live life in joy and humor, to trust your childlike self. By doing so and by loving yourself, you develop honor, dignity, and self-esteem. Choosing this plant gives you an opportunity to allow your creativity to come through, to develop your ideas, and to trust the power of your thoughts and intuition.

Position Three: Water/West

The west is represented by the element of water. The flowing action of water creates change on the Earth. Its movement changes the Earth's appearance. Water feeds the Earth, and without it Earth would become barren and unable to produce plants, trees, and flowers. Water sustains us by stabilizing our bodies internally, aiding us in the process of elimination and detoxification, managing blood pressure and preserving cellular efficiency. Water is related to our emotional center. It is the driving force that gives us the incentive and the creativity to get to where we want to go and to help us get in touch with how we feel. When our emotions become stagnant and there is no flow, we shut down. Our thoughts become dry and negative. The heart closes. A steady flow of water within the body can penetrate negativity, nourishing us, and fertilizing our thoughts with water's healing power. When we feel this loving flow, our heart opens and we are able to love others. The plant you choose for the west is here to offer insights into what you are feeling in the present. The west is also symbolic of taking time for retreat or going within. Taking time for yourself through introspection, especially before making decisions, allows you to be present, to feel from the inside before acting on the outside. A renewed self-expression and creativity keeps you flowing and moving, offering a rebirth in how you pursue your purpose.

Position Four: Earth/North

This northern position represents the element of earth, which provides all living things with sustenance and nourishment. The north represents a time of renewal, purity, and quickening of the spirit. Although the Earth appears dormant and barren in the cold and windy winters of northern climes, the seeds of inner reflection are still alive deep within the earth. A breath of spiritual renewal takes place in the midst of cooling winds. The north plant reflects a time of gathering strength, becoming clear with your intent, and finding earthly resources to bring into your life. The north is the place of the elders, who offer wisdom on how to live in harmony with the Earth through such activities as tool-making, building shelter, cultivating, and farming. The message of the element of earth deals with our relationship to the material world and our ability to survive. The plants and trees anchored in the Earth provide us with food, shelter, clothing, and medicine. Through natural laws we learn how to navigate the material world, grounding our energy in ways that connect us to the Earth, building a foundation for how we want to live our life. Our relationship to the material world impacts our life force and the ways in which we breathe and move. This plant reveals the wisdom, harmony, and support you need to create in the world. The Earth as your literal ground offers an abundance of resources, both inner and outer. As you honor and respect her, you come to honor and respect yourself and all of creation. The message here is to honor where you came from, who you are, what you are becoming, and to express gratitude for all living things.

Position Five: The Quintessence/Center

This card represents the core essence of your being, the divine presence that is already inherently within you. This is your sacred center, the heart of the matter, the place where you can always go for prayer, meditation, silence, and connection with your true Self. The quintessence shows you that you are an expression of the divine source that lives and breathes through you. This is the place that aligns you with your higher power, giving you wisdom and spiritual insight. The message of this plant is to remind you to go to a higher source, your sacred space, the place that gives you personal freedom and expression. In this place you may come to understand the truth that all living things are interdependent. You may soon discover how your own personal essence integrates, receives, and gives back to the seed essence of the universe. This plant teaches you your role in the circle of life. If you wander from this place, remember this is only an illusion, for wherever you are, whatever you're doing, the sacred center is only a breath away.

The Chakra Spread

Begin the Chakra Spread reading by establishing your intention for your path of healing. This spread is about listening to the voices and messages of the plants that connect with your energy centers or chakras. Remember that each chakra resonates with the others, integrating and mirroring who you are. You may wish to review chapter 5 "Pathways Uniting Body, Mind, and Spirit: The Chakras" before beginning this spread. For example, if your intent is to gain insight about a particular health issue and how that issue affects your whole being, begin by connecting with the plants in the book and choosing a plant one by one for each chakra, keeping your focus clear. Some plants may naturally be associated with the chakra energy center you are working with. Some may not. Don't be concerned about the color of the plant or that it needs to correspond with the color of the chakra. In this spread you are receiving insights from any of the plants in relation to any of the chakras. Let's say you choose the blue flag iris for the first chakra regarding a particular health issue. When you read about the blue flag iris you will find that its message is about perseverance and pacing yourself. Perhaps blue flag will give you inspirations or an insight into how you can better pace yourself and avoid burnout. Or maybe you will choose the black-eyed Susan to represent your fourth chakra. Although the colors of black-eyed Susan are not associated with the colors of the

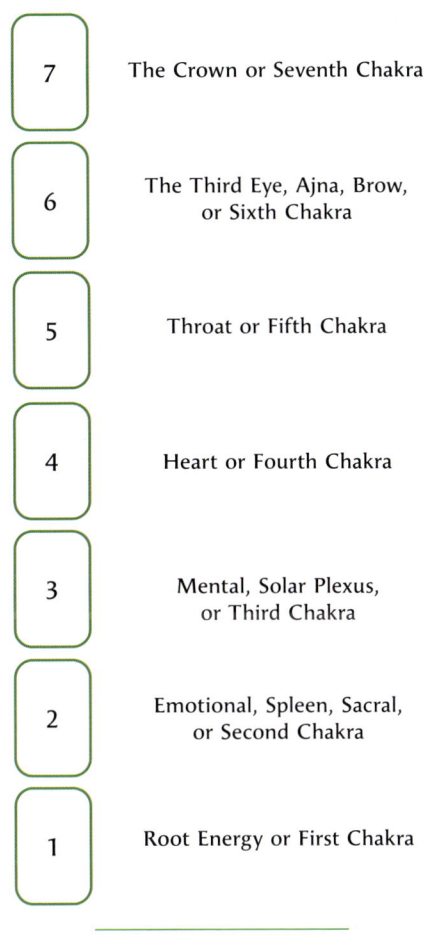

```
┌───┐
│ 7 │   The Crown or Seventh Chakra
└───┘

┌───┐
│ 6 │   The Third Eye, Ajna, Brow,
└───┘        or Sixth Chakra

┌───┐
│ 5 │   Throat or Fifth Chakra
└───┘

┌───┐
│ 4 │   Heart or Fourth Chakra
└───┘

┌───┐
│ 3 │   Mental, Solar Plexus,
└───┘      or Third Chakra

┌───┐
│ 2 │   Emotional, Spleen, Sacral,
└───┘      or Second Chakra

┌───┐
│ 1 │   Root Energy or First Chakra
└───┘
```

Chakra Spread diagram

fourth chakra, the message and the voice of black-eyed Susan may bring to your awareness the ways in which you shut down your heart and feel challenged to love.

The layout of the Chakra Spread is very straightforward. You'll simply create a vertical line, with the first position at the bottom and the seventh position at the top, as shown above.

Position One: Root Energy, or First Chakra

When you choose a plant that will reflect your relationship with your root chakra, focus on your physical connection with yourself and with the

Earth. The plant you choose may bring to you an awareness of the physical ways in which you survive, such as the food you eat, the amount of exercise you do, where you live, where you work, and the physical environment you choose to be in. The root chakra is also the center of primal energy. It reflects your spiritual and soul heritage—where you came from and how that has affected who you are now, and where you want to go. Whether your parents were poor, middle-class, or wealthy, the way in which you connected to your material survival as a child and now as an adult may not be the same. The root chakra points to survival in relationship to yourself, your life force, and the way you breathe and move with the earth.

Position Two: Emotional, Spleen, Sacral, or Second Chakra

When you choose a plant to give you insight into your relationship with your second chakra, your intent is related to your emotions, what you are feeling. You may want some deeper insight into how you flow with the emotional current within or how you express yourself creatively. You may also feel the flow of your expression as a sexual, sensual, and passionate being. Perhaps you will gain some insight into the deeper currents within that affect the flow of your overall emotional health. Drink plenty of water and eat good, nutritious food, letting the energy flow within you so you can come alive!

Position Three: Mental, Solar Plexus, or Third Chakra

When you choose a plant to reflect on your relationship with your third chakra, you invite introspection into the way that you think and view yourself. You begin to notice how your thoughts, positive or negative, feed your emotional body and how you walk on this Earth. You may learn to think and perceive in clearer ways, without judgment and criticism. The plant that you receive at this time may bring insight into your dignity, values, desires, thoughts, and higher will. Perhaps you will be guided to align with divine will, trusting your intuition and your knowledge.

Position Four: Heart, or Fourth Chakra

When you choose a plant for insight about your relationship with your fourth chakra, you may come to a deeper understanding of the value of forgiveness, letting go, and learning to live and feel what it is to love unconditionally. As your heart becomes more open, you may feel an extension of warmth radiating outward and find yourself becoming more tolerant and generous toward yourself and others. A doorway to your path of healing is opening wider. Allow yourself to let your heart guide you in the choices you make.

Position Five: Throat, or Fifth Chakra

When you choose a plant for insight into your relationship with your throat, as represented by the fifth chakra, bring your awareness to your throat area and feel the vibrations of the sounds you make. Your throat communicates your inner self to the outside world. Our inner self includes the sounds and vibrations of our voice, as well as our thoughts, inner truths, and insights. Notice the way you communicate with the words you choose and the tones you make. Are you listening to your heart when you speak to others? Are you listening to the ways that others communicate to you? Perhaps there are other creative forms of expression such as dance, sculpture, painting, singing, chanting, writing, or playing an instrument, which can fulfill your expression for life.

Position Six: The Third Eye, Ajna, Brow, or Sixth Chakra

When you choose a plant for insight into the sixth chakra, you may gain a deeper understanding of the importance of trusting your perceptions, intuition, and the way you view the world from a higher perspective. Form a new relationship with the higher power that is already within you. Feel an opening in your psychic awareness and the ability to see beyond your inner circle, beyond time and space. Receive a broader vision and an expanded view of your intent for this sage wisdom spread. Experience a deeper understanding of your intent. Allow the power of illumination to come forth.

Position Seven: The Crown, or Seventh Chakra

When you choose a plant for insight into your relationship with the seventh chakra, be comforted to know that you are connected with and part of an all-inclusive presence in which separation does not exist. Although at times you may feel alone in the circumstances that you face in life, know that on some level, someone else somewhere is experiencing something very similar. Come to realize that all of humankind and all life forms on this Earth are part of a bigger design, and that we are all in this together. As you gain access to the energy field of the crown chakra, you become aligned with a higher power that is linked to the collective higher consciousness. Your connection with the crown chakra opens a new way of viewing yourself—the intent of this reading—as well as the way you interact with the world. Feel a vibrant energy flowing throughout your body, emotions, mind, and heart. Open to see beyond your wildest imagination. Step into the portal of oneness and bliss!

7

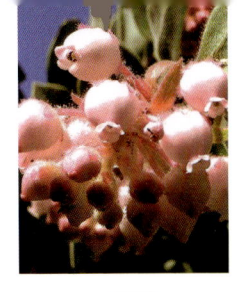

An Invitation to a Plant Journey

Welcome a New Doorway into Your Life

It is the marriage of the soul with Nature that makes the intellect fruitful, that gives birth to imagination.

HENRY DAVID THOREAU

STRAPPING ON MY backpack and adjusting the belt around my waist, I start walking, breathing in the fresh scents of spring all around me. I hear the crunching sound beneath my feet and observe the dried-out, curly, purplish-brown seed pods that fell on the ground last spring. I am on a journey to meet an old friend, Grandmother Manzanita. I take a moment to appreciate a locust tree a few yards away. Its bright green, lacey, pinnate leaves plummet to the ground, like grapes falling from long branches. Reflecting on its drooping racemes of softly scented white flowers that I observed last year, I recall how I took in the tree's distinctive fragrance while being mindful not to get too close to its twisted, branched thorns. I feel a quickening as I anticipate today's journey. I step around the cattle guard and begin the hike up the rocky dirt road that leads to Allen Springs, a road I have hiked many times, on many plant journeys.

I notice the town of Jerome sitting on Cleopatra Hill to the northwest of where I stand. Jerome is a old mining town situated on a cliffside,

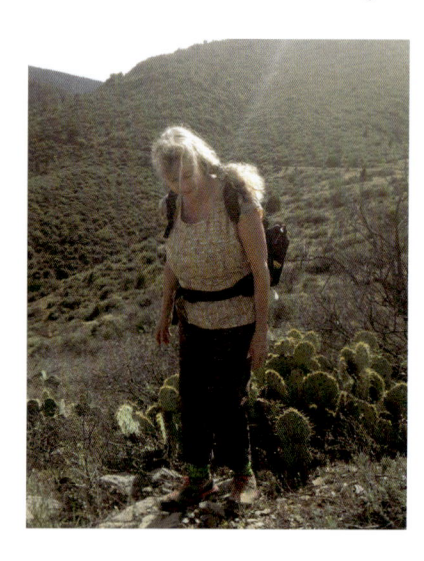

Rhonda on her plant journey (photo by Curt PallasDowney)

once famous for its deposits of copper. Houses of many colors and shapes cling to the hills. My attention, however, is fixed on the landscape before me as I walk around the large rocks, careful of my footing. As I approach the top of the hill, the vast, panoramic view pulls me in. My excitement builds. The San Francisco Peaks in nearby Flagstaff, Arizona, appear in all their glory to the north, their snow-laden crests brushing up against a clear blue sky. They are dormant volcanic peaks that rise above the flush sedimentary layer of the Colorado Plateau, reaching a height of 12,633 feet at Humphrey's Peak, the tallest summit in Arizona. These mountains are sacred to thirteen Native American tribes. For a moment I reflect on a powerful plant adventure I once experienced in that area with treasured herbalists Cascade Anderson Geller, Matthew Wood, and Phyliss Hogan.

To the east and centered below me is our beautiful Verde Valley, with its lush green grasses, junipers, shrubs of catclaw and red root, scrub oaks, yuccas, prickly pear cactus, and tall skeletons of century plants scattered on the hillsides. I face southeast and follow the dirt road until it branches off on the right, descending into one of my most special magical forests. Turning a corner, I sense the presence of my enchanting plant friends awaiting me, pulling me forward. The forest sounds reverberate in every cell of my being and awaken all my senses. My eyes are captivated by the beauty before me. I take a few more steps and then place my backpack next to an old oak stump shaded by a large gambel oak close by. Almost

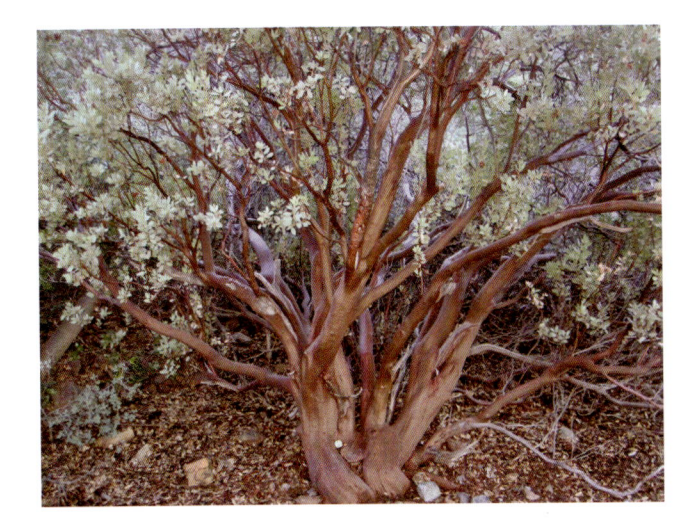

Grandmother Manzanita

directly across the path from me is my cherished tree friend whom I have named Grandmother Manzanita, one of the oldest and largest manzanitas I have ever seen. I have known her for nearly thirty-five years and have experienced her through all the seasons, as over the years her growth has reflected my own back to me.

She presents a rich reddish-brown presence. Her smooth and colorful branches reach out to me, beckoning me to come closer. Sliding my hand across one of her extended arms, my fingertips touching and exploring the firm bark, crevices, and bulges of the branch, I feel the strong yet sensual nature of this beloved tree. Touching my nose against her branch, I take in her earthy aromas of geranium, sandalwood, and patchouli, paired with her higher, citruslike notes. I press my lips against a flower's bud and taste its apple-honey, resinous liquid as it slowly moves into my throat and down into my heart, where I feel its subtle vibrational frequency.

Slowly, I step back and return to my backpack, which is jam-packed with all my tools for making an essence from the tree: my medicine bag packed with cornmeal blended with kinnikinnick, a traditional Native American smoking blend of mullein leaves and flowers, osha root, red willow bark, juniper berries, and yerba santa leaves; a large glass container filled three-quarters full with fresh spring water; two quartz crystal wands that I use for holding flowers I intend to create essences from (you can see the crystal wands in the photo on page 43 depicting making the columbine flower essence);

a small, unbleached cotton muslin cloth; a small and a large funnel; labels, pen, colored pencils, and notepad; and two eight-ounce brown glass bottles with about a quarter cup of E & J brandy in each, which I measured earlier at home. I find my altar cloth near the top of the bag and lay it on the ground. Then I meticulously place each item on the cloth and turn to Grandmother Manzanita with the medicine bag in my hand. I take a few moments to contemplate and feel our heart connection. Grandmother Manzanita's blessings have offered me a deep vibrational field of energy within me and all around me. My heart opens to receive her gifts.

Taking time to feel the warmth of the sun, I breathe deeply of the scented and fresh air of the forest, listening to nature's sounds and consciously releasing all my worldly and personal concerns. Being fully in the moment, I take a pinch of the kinnickinnik blend from my medicine bag, and with reverence to the four directions I offer this gift of herbs along with a prayer of gratitude:

> To the east, to the element of air that we breathe, sustained by oxygen provided by trees and plants, represented by new beginnings, new hope, and for allowing myself to perceive from a place beyond the physical world;
>
> To the south and the element of fire and the sun, the source of energy that provides light and heat, making possible the process of photosynthesis, where the synthesis of complex organic material with the support of chlorophyll gives us vitamins and minerals, the warmth in our bellies, the power and courage to trust and let go of fear, and to live life with strength and wisdom
>
> To the west and the element of water, and the flowing action of water creating movement and change to sustain the Earth, our bodies, our oceans, streams, and rivers, and all life forms; to trust the inner navigational flow within me, my own driving force, as it gives me the incentive to live my life's passion

> To the north and the element of earth, which provides all living organisms with sustenance and nourishment, silencing my mind for a time of renewal and a quickening of my spirit, honoring and respecting our Earth Mother and all that she provides for us.
>
> To the quintessence, the sacred center that aligns the core of the Earth with the center of the heavens and comes together as the heart of it all, the sacred place in me and in all life forms that connect me with my deepest sense of Self, trusting my role in the plant kingdom as our electromagnetic fields come together in the circle of life.

Then, as a gesture of respect and gratitude, I gently sprinkle the herbs from my medicine bag around the roots of the tree, its branches, and lightly toss a pinch in the air. As one of my students, an Alaskan Inuit taught me, I also remove a hair from my head and place it on the tree as a gift from me to the tree and to the entire plant kingdom.

I gaze into Grandmother Manzanita's flowers and then close my eyes. Feeling into the energy of the tree, I ask her permission to remove some of her flowers. Trusting my intuition and discerning our connection, I am aware that in this subtle field of energy that we share, I have been granted permission to gather the tree's flowers. Opening my eyes, I look around at the tree's flowers to see who may be noticing me. Several clusters of flowers stand out. I imagine their tiny ovoid flowers are bobbing their heads for attention. They seem to be calling me to notice them. They cheer me on to choose them and provide me with their sweet essence. Tenderly, with my two crystal wands, I remove a flower from its cluster and place it in the jug of water. Repeating this action, I continue to pluck a single flower or cluster of flowers one at a time using the crystals, placing the blossoms in the water.

The flowers are noticeably vibrant as they float to the top of the jug of water, which I've placed between the striking reddish-brown branches of the tree for security. Their essence will be heard, felt, tasted, touched, and connected to a secret inner world for all those who are ready to step into the heart of vibrational plant medicine.

I step back from Grandmother Manzanita and return to the old oak stump directly across the path to take a seat. Feeling the hard wood beneath me, I adjust my body to fit the contours of the stump so I can sit comfortably. With colored pencils and notepad at hand, I methodically begin to draw the tree. Its branches, stems, and flowers together offer a vivid impression of Grandmother Manzanita's features. I then close my eyes to begin a plant journey with Grandmother Manzanita. In this journey, I open my awareness to how she feels, grows, moves, breathes, lives, responds, communicates, gives, and receives. As I bring my attention to each part of her body, moving from her outstretched roots to her branches, stems, and flowers, I feel that I am one with Grandmother Manzanita. I sense her deep taproots searching for water, yet liking the hot climate of the upper Sonoran Desert. Visualizing my own roots descending from the soles of my feet, I feel my perineum touching and embracing the deep roots of Grandmother Manzanita. We become intertwined, pulsating as our taproots merge deeper into the ground below us, transporting feeder roots and fibers to receive and absorb nutrients and water.

Anchored in the earth, I find my way to where our below-ground roots meet our above-ground parts. The uppermost roots find their way to the trunk, which in turn supports the twisted yet smooth surfaces of the branches of the tree. We move together, my body and her eye-catching, reddish-brown branches. The bark of the branches has beautiful streaks, probably bleached by the sun shining through the tops of the forest, and I notice that in places the bark is shredding to reveal reddish wood underneath. I know that Grandmother's glandular secretions cause the bark to be slippery, and that's what creates the smoothness of the bark and the feeling of movement and grace she exudes. To my mind the branches seem to be arteries extending from her trunk, while the trunk is her heart, which pumps arboreal fluids throughout the branches and leaves.

Grandmother Manzanita's thick, leathery, ovoid, and dull blue-green leaves appear to me as a network of veins alternating along her branches. She reflects back to me the inner workings of the human body. It's no wonder, then, that manzanita can be used as a urinary tract astringent, for its doctrine of signatures consists of the way it can move fluids throughout the human body. Manzanita also acts as a mild vasoconstrictor for the uterus and can be helpful for painful and heavy menstruation.

I listen for Grandmother's messages, which generally come from her flowers, yet include her entire being. The flower of any plant, for me, is the highest splendor of the plant, although parts of most plants hold medicinal value. When I turn my attention to Grandmother Manzanita's flowers, her messages and teachings become even stronger and more powerful. I feel an inner shift, an intuition about what she is communicating to me.

Her urn-shaped pinkish-white flowers are vessels containing droplets of nectar, hanging elegantly from its slender stems. They emerge in terminal clusters that are sticky and hairy. Each of her flowers form a tear-shaped tubular bud with a yellow tip. Five flower petals form a circle at the tip of each flower, and five at the bottom. A flurry of tiny white stamens arise from the center. Like the bees and the hummingbirds, I am attracted to the flowers' apple-honey fragrance.

As I focus on the flowers, my breathing becomes deeper and calmer. I feel an opening in my heart, and my entire being blossoms into a gentle release. The authentic expression of Grandmother Manzanita in all of her beauty and grace connects my spirit with hers. We are one. I see and hear the deep humming sound of her voice as though it were my own. Embracing her spirit, her intrinsic essence, I experience energetic vibrations, openings, and releases. I listen to her wisdom teachings and her message:

> My love and radiance pour out to you. Trust what you feel in your heart. Connect with your natural flow. Live life from a place of loving yourself. Feel the sweetness of life's flow pulsating through your heart and your whole body. Give yourself permission to relax and experience joyful freedom. Blossom into a gentle release. Enter your heart-filled vessel.

By now, a few hours have passed, and the jug of water holding the blossoms has been thoroughly infused by the sunlight streaming through

Grandmother Manzanita. The flowers in the water have faded and show signs of wilting. Her essence is captured! Removing the flower water from the tree, I place a muslin cloth in the funnel to act as a strainer, then pour most of the water into one of the brown glass bottles I brought with me. The brandy acts as an immediate preservative. I have an additional clean cloth in a plastic bag, which I spread on the ground to place the funnel, muslin, and accessories on.

Next is labeling the bottle with the common name of the flower, its botanical name (if you know it), the date, and the location where the essence of the flower is made. I write "MT" for "mother tincture" on the label, clarifying that this is a concentrated form of the essence straight from the mother plant. This is a reminder to me to use the mother tincture as a reserve from which to make stock bottles, that is, a diluted form of the mother tincture. The mother tincture can have an indefinite shelf life if properly stored in a dark glass bottle in a cool, dark place.

Once I've filled the bottle and labeled it, I sit down to drink the remaining flower essence water from the water jug. Before tasting it I notice its creamy color with a slight hint of yellow. Usually it is clear, but in some cases it can be various shades of yellow and milky white. I raise the jug to my lips. To drink this unadulterated elixir, which I consider the champagne of the plant, straight from where I have just harvested and made it, is the pinnacle of this journey. I take this opportunity to toast Grandmother Manzanita, to thank her for her gifts, and to receive her blessing by drinking her essence. I close my eyes and take another sip or two, discerning the subtle honey-apple taste of the essence, and note the sensations arising from imbibing it. Grandmother Manzanita's essence is lukewarm, not just from the heat of the day, but from the flowers themselves. A tingling feeling arises in my throat, esophagus, and lungs, and lingers in my heart. This stirring energy seems to unite my heart with the essence of my soul.

I write down my experience of drinking this flower essence water in my plant medicine journal, and jot down the key rubrics for positive healing patterns, as well as for symptoms and patterns of imbalance. When I've finished documenting all that has guided me in this journey, I return the remaining essence water to the root crown of Grandmother Manzanita, pouring from the jug, giving a short prayer of thanks to the earth, air, sun, and water, and especially to Grandmother Manzanita, for sharing her gifts with me. I thank Spirit for receiving these blessed gifts, and ask her permission to carry them with me as I return to the world.

I walk across the path from Grandmother Manzanita and turn to face the great gambel oak tree (*Quercus gambelii*), Grandfather Oak, who has also been my friend of many years. Together this pair emanates a powerful life force to their surrounding plant offsprings.

Grandfather Oak sits on a thick hillside. Clustering shrubs of red root, *Ceanothus americanus*, grow beneath his thick, scrubby canopy, and today they are in full bloom, their snowball-shaped blossoms releasing a sweet mountain scent, freshening the air all around me. I take in several long, deep breaths, inhaling all of nature. I sense the profundity of what it must feel like to live here all day and all night, day after day, year after year. In this moment I feel the sprightly, multidimensional field of nature alive in me and outside of me, touching every part of my being.

At about thirty feet, Grandfather Oak, which is a gambel oak, stands much higher than other scrub oaks in his vicinity (see the photo of Grandfather Oak on page 203). His branches are irregular and crooked, making him impervious to heavy snow in the winter, and he has a thick trunk and rough, brownish-gray bark. I imagine a deep root system, though in reality the gambel oak's roots are only about fifteen to twenty inches below the ground—not a deep root system compared to larger oak trees, but still a strong system, well-anchored in its strength and fortitude.

I walk up to Grandfather Oak, wrap my arms around his broad trunk, and gently press my face against his coarse, scaly bark. As I breathe in his earthy, bittersweet scent, I visualize my breath flowing downward with the trunk of the tree. I imagine a powerful grounding aroma inside of me moving into the tree's roots, making him one with me. Could it be that my heart is connecting with the heart of Grandfather Oak? That's what it feels like! In my mind's eye I perceive two hearts beating as one, the heart of Grandfather Oak beating in sync with my own heart. I sense a powerful force that comes from within Grandfather's trunk, nourishing my own life force. I imagine the hum of Grandfather's presence vibrating through the heart of the tree and softly pulsating within me. I feel that Grandfather Oak and I are united as a single living wonder. I connect with a deep inner wisdom that gives me all that I need to survive in the world. My inner core feels strong and stable. I feel renewed on my life's journey.

Grandfather Oak's many gifts include its broad-lobed, reddish-orange and golden-yellow leaves in the fall, quite striking to the eye. In early spring, fuzzy male catkins droop like tassels hanging from the tree's branches. Female flowers grow in clusters with a ring of small leaves or bracts at the base, and eventually evolve into an acorn. The acorn holds its own force of life as an extension of the tree. For millennia the acorn has symbolized the boundless potential for new growth and development—fertility and strength at all levels of being for both the oaks and for all living organisms.

In his book *The White Goddess*, mythologist Robert Graves refers to the oak as "Düir," meaning "door" in various European languages. "When Gwion writes in the Cad Goddeu, 'Stout Guardian of the door' . . . he is saying that doors are customarily made of oak as the strongest and toughest wood."[1] Oak is a doorway between Heaven and Earth. The evolution of the catkin into an acorn is the ultimate embodiment of the power of all the natural elements that feed the oak. The catkin, as it becomes an acorn, is a doorway to the infinite, where we can plant new growth and new seeds of awareness. The branches of oak reach up to integrate the divine power of the universe, just as we humans assimilate the elements of earth, air, fire, and water in the energetic field that unites all living organisms on our cherished Earth Mother.

The grounding strength in me, captivated by the life force from and heart connection with both Grandmother Manzanita and Grandfather Oak, anchored my awareness to my energy field.

Before my journey, I had been feeling the loss of a dear friend. Grief, as I have come to understand it, is a tool for shifting energy from holding on to letting go by allowing myself to honor my vulnerability and to accept how I feel.

The experience of my connection with Grandmother Manzanita and Grandfather Oak gave me an opportunity to use the natural vibration of nature and the plant kingdom to support my healing journey to renewal.

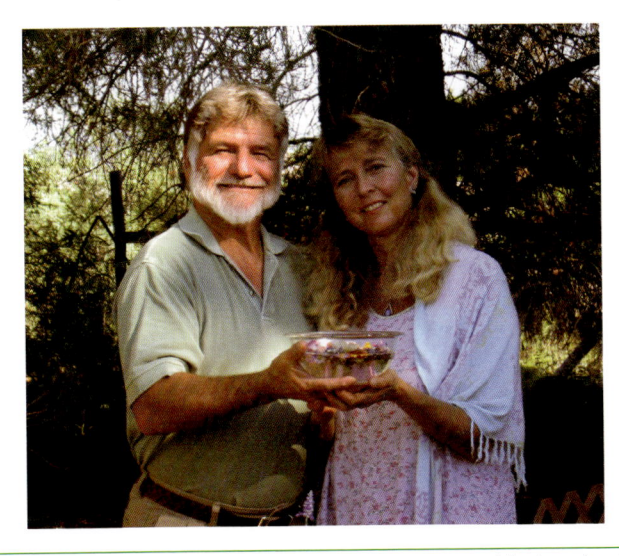

Curt and Rhonda offer a toast to your inner journeys with the plant kingdom
(photo by Renick Turley/Sedona Film)

On our human path, we encounter transformational events that lead us to stumbling at times, feeling insecure, hopeless, and fatigued, and that leave us wondering what this journey of life is really all about.

My connection with these two beautiful, wise, and wonderful beings stayed with me as I strolled upon the dirt path through the oaks, manzanitas, and red root bushes. Red root (*Ceanothus americanus*), to me, offers life-supporting energy and clarity about the ways we choose to create new patterns in our lives. For a moment, I stop near a red root bush to smell its blossoms and reflect on this.

Then, moving forward, I step into the opening of high desert flora alongside the majestic views that encapsulated me in the beginning of this plant journey. Now, with a nourishment of inner strength, feeling reconnected with my heart, breath, voice, and beingness, I feel strong again in who I am, happily reunited with myself, and ready to embrace my return home.

We invite you to explore the seen and unseen world of the plant kingdom. Discover deeper the kingdom within you. Illuminate your awareness and your relationship with all living things.

PART THREE

❖

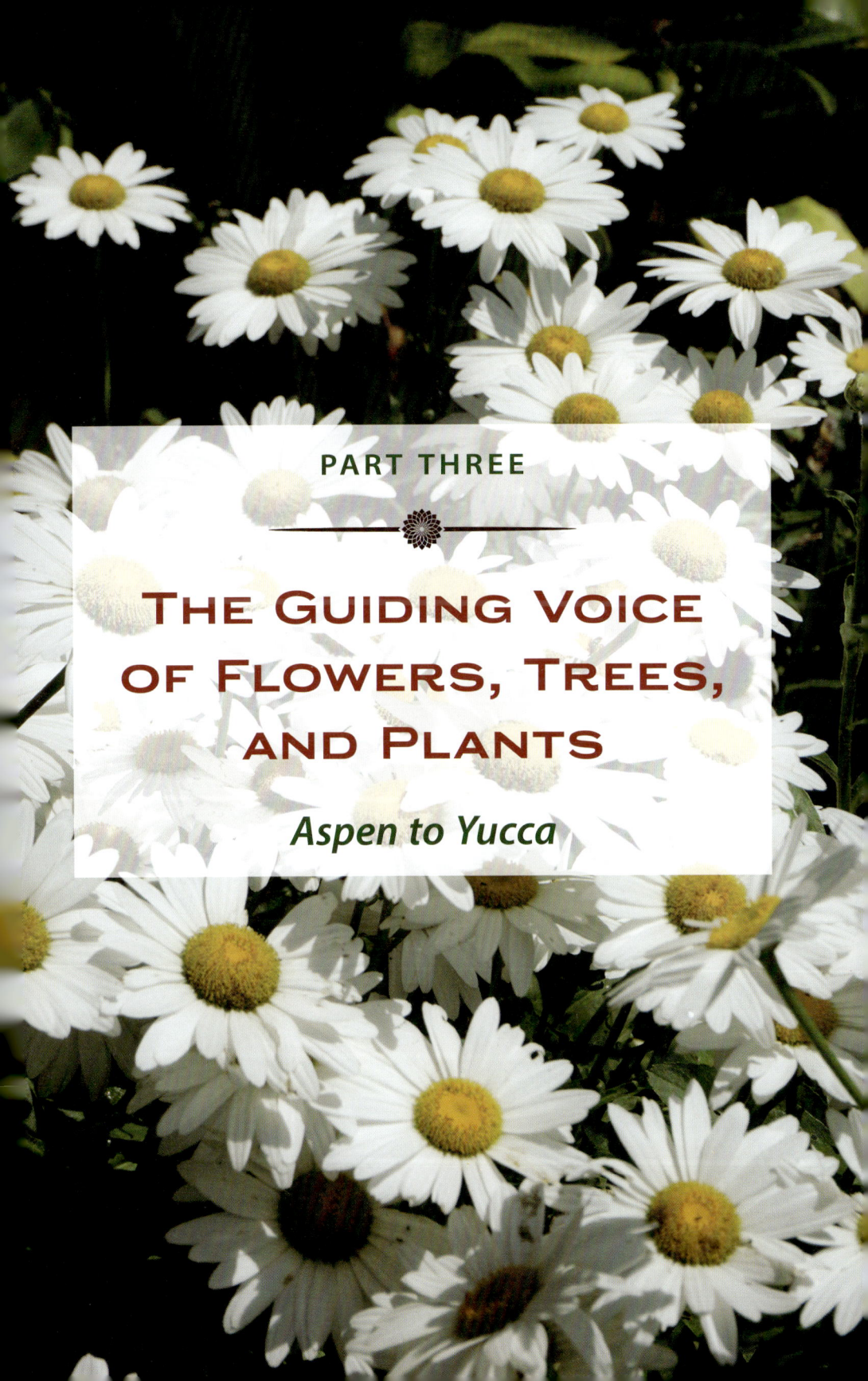

THE GUIDING VOICE OF FLOWERS, TREES, AND PLANTS

Aspen to Yucca

LIST OF THE FLOWERS, TREES, AND PLANTS AND THEIR PRIMARY QUALITIES

Aspen	Gentle Rhythms	101
Aster	Insight	104
Bells of Ireland	Healing Inner Child	107
Black-Eyed Susan	Authentic Self	110
Blanketflower	Enthusiasm	113
Blue Flag Iris	Perseverance	116
Bouncing Bet	Blissful Union	119
Calendula	Peacefulness	122
California Poppy	Emotional Clearing	125
Century Plant	Transformation	128
Chamomile	Emotional Harmony	131
Chaparral	Cleansing & Survival	134
Cliff Rose	Self-Acceptance	137
Columbine	Inner Beauty	140
Comfrey	Support	143
Crabapple	Open Heart	146
Crimson Monkeyflower	Emotional Power	150
Desert Larkspur	Self-Expression	153
Desert Marigold	Experience with Ease	156
Desert Willow	Nurturing Love	159
Echinacea	Vitality	162
Evening Primrose	Self-Worth	165
Hollyhock	Circle of Life	169
Honeysuckle	Balance	173
Indian Paintbrush	Boundless Creativity	176
Juniper	Deep Cleansing and Renewal	179
Lupine	Higher Purpose	183
Manzanita	Heart-Filled Vessel	186
Mesquite	Trusting the Invisible	190

LIST OF THE FLOWERS, TREES, AND PLANTS AND THEIR PRIMARY QUALITIES (CONT'D)

Mexican Hat	Freeing Pain	194
Morning Glory	New Beliefs	197
Mullein	Intimacy	200
Oak	Grounding Strength	203
Ocotillo	Creative Life Force	206
Onion	Healing From Grief	209
Ox-Eye Daisy	Inner Awareness	212
Palmer's Penstemon	Truthful Communication	215
Paloverde	Feeling Rooted	218
Peace Rose	Serene Peace	221
Pinyon	Trusting In Patience	224
Pomegranate	Passion	227
Prickly Pear Cactus	Strength To Be Me	230
Purple Robe	Awakening Vision	233
Sage	Inner Wisdom	236
Saguaro	Protector	239
Scarlet Penstemon	Self-Confidence	243
Strawberry Hedgehog	Sensual Pleasures	246
Sunflower	Empowering Radiance	249
Sweet Pea	Inner Security	253
Thistle	Feeling Centered	256
Vervain	Inspiring Direction	259
Walnut	New Beginnings	262
Wild Rose	Heart Awakening	266
Willow	Compassion	269
Yarrow	Energy Protection	273
Yellow Monkeyflower	Trust The Flow	276
Yerba Santa	Self-Discovery	279
Yucca	Focus	282

> *When the temple bell rings, I still hear the sound coming from the flowers.*
>
> UNKNOWN TIBETAN MONK

The wisdom contained in flowers, trees, and plants is subtly intelligent and ever-changing. There are specific qualities and energies that you will discover as you begin your study of plant energy medicine. Whether you choose a plant to imbibe as a medicinal elixir or use as a daily meditation tool, or if you try any of the various plant energy medicine spreads described in this book to gain insight, this section provides essential information about the plants you choose to work with. You can also randomly open the book to any page in this section and see who is drawn to you.

The flowers, trees, and plants in this section are listed in alphabetical order. For each listing you will find the plant's primary quality as well as its voice, insight, energy impact/chakra correspondence, and affirmation. Explore the plants and listen to their voices. Develop your own relationship with these vibrant living and life-giving green beings! Invite plant world into your life. Speak the affirmation of each flower, tree, or plant. Imbibe its essence. Imagine being in its presence. Let the spirit of the plants and flowers guide you and help you to discover the depths of your innermost mysteries.

> *Everything that is in the heavens, on earth, and under the earth is penetrated with connectedness, penetrated with relatedness.*
>
> HILDEGARD OF BINGEN

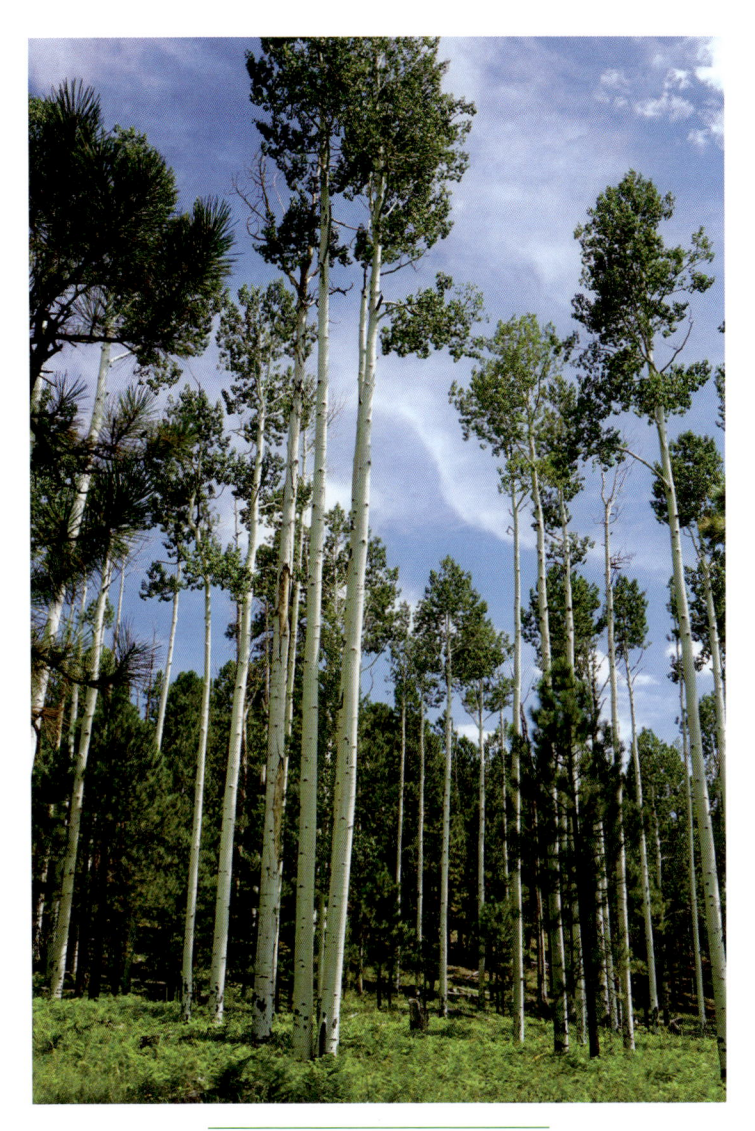

Aspen colony awakens to spring

ASPEN
(Populus tremuloides)

Primary quality: gentle rhythms
Energy impact/chakra correspondence: first, second, and third chakras

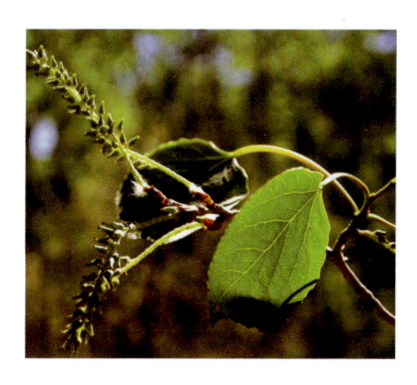

Aspen catkin budding

Voice of the Flower (Catkin)

Come sit with me in my aspen grove, close your eyes and listen.

Experience the sensation of the earth below you. Imagine my roots encircling you and connected as one big root system. They form an underground blanket of safety and protection.

Tiny, discreet flowers emerge from my amber buds and form into firm, bold catkins. My tiny cottony seeds are eventually lifted by the winds, enabling pollination. They are a reminder to let go and trust your own natural rhythm. Let the journey take you right to where you need to be.

My rounded, flat, delicate, shiny green leaves offer a lemonlike scent swooping before you as you inhale my uplifting presence. Hear the sound of the wind rustling through my leaves as they dance with the movement of the wind, quaking in even the slightest breeze. And when the winds are quiet, I appear still and centered, present, yet awaiting my next movement. I surround you with my gentle rhythms as I awaken the natural rhythm within you.

Feel my calmness washing over your body, mind, and spirit. Let the ebb and flow of your rhythm build as you deepen the awareness of your own inner pulse. Let it take you to where it wants to go.

Allow the support of my community to surround you. Take in the natural beauty of my whitish-gray bark and how I stand tall and determined to reach new heights in the mountain forest. Trust the energy of awareness that this brings you. Feel your natural rhythm move with the winds in your life as you adapt to a new shift in your awareness.

Insight

Aspen brings your awareness to your rhythm and movement, to your voice and to sound in general. From a place of trust, follow your inner guidance to express yourself in all the ways you move through life. Let your own natural rhythms guide you on your path.

Aspens propagate mostly through their root sprouts, which share a single root structure. Since multiple stems sprout from the same root system, they are replaced with new growth. This allows a colony of aspens a life span of thousands of years. Above ground, Aspen's colony may appear as separate trees, however, they are all genetically identical. The trees of a colony all come from the same source below ground, yet their individual identities are revealed above ground. We all come from the same form or substance as human beings, yet we develop our own unique sense of identity in who we are. Each of us has our own individual expression in how we adapt to and move in the world. We carry our own natural rhythm as we adjust to new ways of living and being.

The striking whitish-gray and smooth bark of the aspen contains salicin and populin, which are used to make aspirin to treat joint pain, back pain, nerve pain, and prostate discomfort. The healing properties of aspen are also used as an antiscorbutic, diaphoretic, diuretic, expectorant, and purgative.

Aspen's catkin essence is subtle and offers a gentle presence.

✦ Affirmation ✦

I trust that my life is unfolding with my own natural rhythms as I adapt to new ways of living and being.

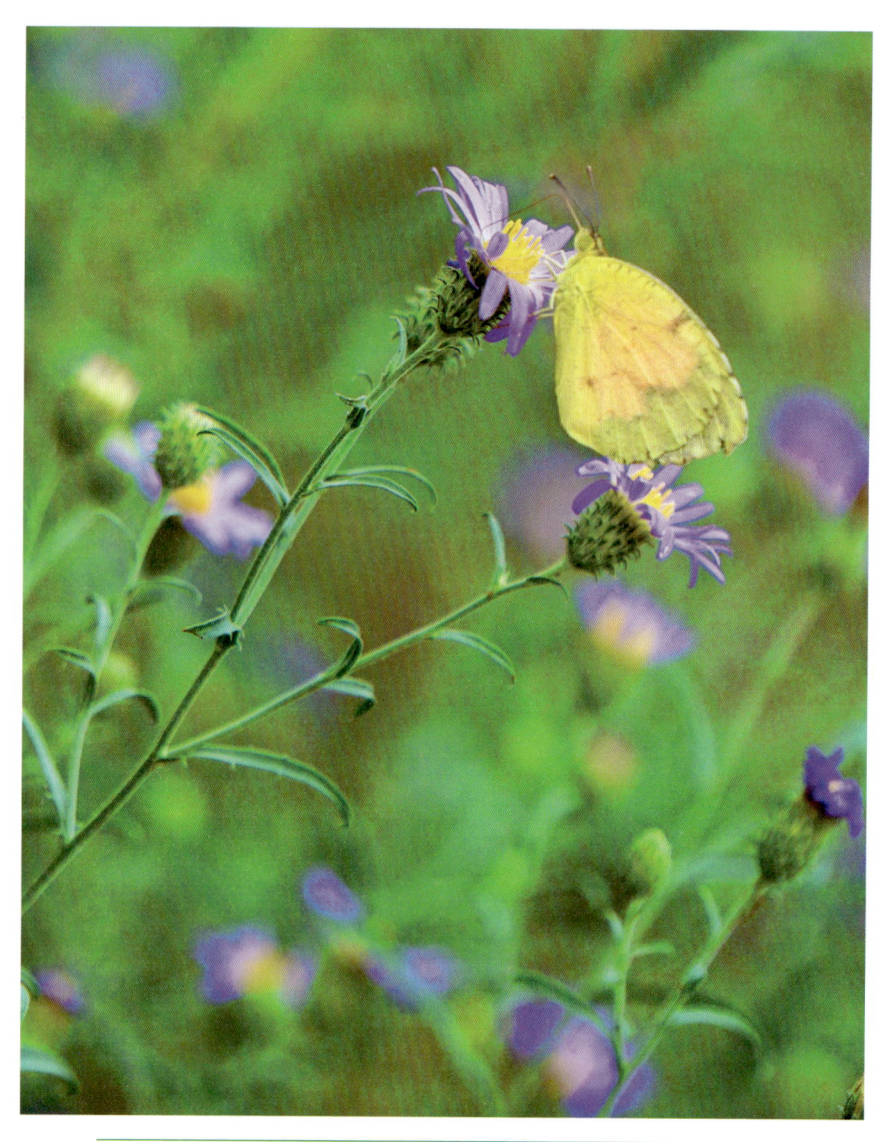

104   The Guiding Voice of Flowers, Trees, and Plants

Aster flowers illuminate their beauty while a moth finds its pollen

ASTER
(Dieteria asteroides)

Primary quality: insight
Energy impact/chakra correspondence: third, sixth, and seventh chakras

Voice of the Flower

Embrace my graceful presence and simple beauty. Let yourself be guided by my energy. Trust your intuition. Listen to your inner voice. Expand your view from within and deepen your insights. Allow yourself to stretch beyond time and space. The radiant yellow glow from within the center of my eye shines at you. Feel its warmth and let light in. Like a shining star, I guide you to turn toward the brightness of your own illumination. As you fill yourself with light, feel an opening in your mind's eye. Let your intuition and higher vision expand as my purple rays radiate outward to begin a new path of natural evolution. Come fully into the presence of this moment guided by your intuition. Trust your insight. Feel connected within all aspects of yourself.

Become aware of any insights or intuitive sensations that help you see or help you heal. Let a new doorway open. Invite the wisdom of your inner gifts in and see how you respond to them.

Allow yourself to tap into this vibrational frequency and trust your inner guidance. Notice the energy you take in and what you give out.

Insight

Aster invites illumination and insight to guide you on your path of personal growth and spiritual evolution. It offers balance and inspiration through vision and wisdom, allowing you to see more deeply from within.

Aster's foundation is strong, though its many branches are flexible, light, and uplifting. The flower's starlike shape represents simplicity, light, and grace. Its rays reach out as if to embark on the path of the flower's joyful spirit.

The purple hue of aster is a unique signature. It draws attention to the third eye of higher consciousness. It reminds us to live in the here and now, to plant and nurture your thoughts from a place of insight. It offers you an opportunity to embrace an expanded awareness of what it truly feels like to trust your insights in all the ways you are living in the world.

There are numerous species of wild asters varying in color, including purple, white, and yellow. The entire plant has been used in Native

American traditions as a smudge to cleanse and uplift consciousness and to furnish smoke in the traditional sweat lodge. The various species of aster have been used as purgatives, to treat eruptive skin diseases, and as aromatic nervines. Aster attracts many pollinators, especially various birds such as sparrows and hummingbirds, and a variety of insects—in particular bees, butterflies, wasps, flies, beetles, and moths.

Aster's flower essence offers a sweet, strong, earthy, green taste. Occasionally the flower essence water turns a soft purple hue like the color of the flower.

✦ *Affirmation* ✦

> I listen to my inner guidance. I awaken to a new vision within myself and trust my insight.

Bells of Ireland 107

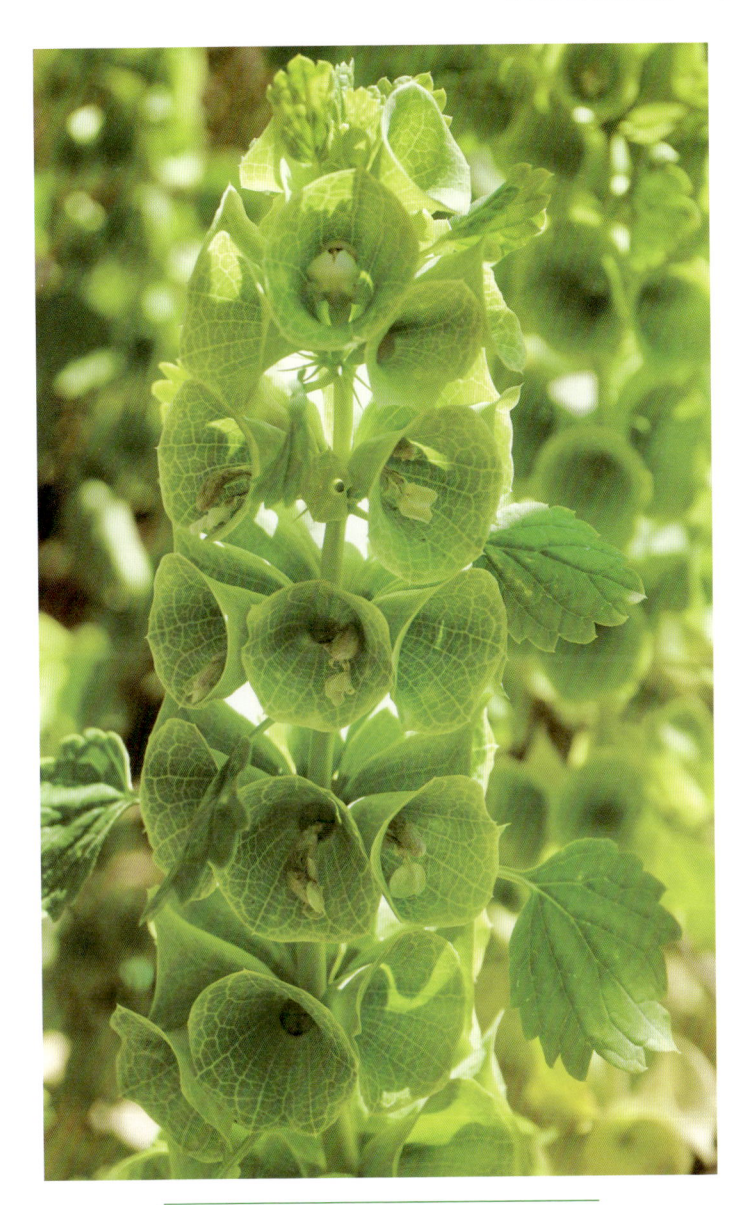

Bells of Ireland flowers' mystical presence

BELLS OF IRELAND
(Moluccella laevis)

Primary quality: healing the inner child
Energy impact/chakra correspondence: fourth and seventh chakras

Voice of the Flower

I stand out among other flowers due to my unusual flourishing green presence. I'm not flashy in terms of color, though I am quite unique.

My root is sturdy and resists pulling. My stem is square with rounded corners. It is light, hollow, and fibrous. My green, bell-shaped leaves grow in opposite pairs in each cluster of flowers. They are veiny and look like spiderwebs. They offer a feeling of protection for the flower that lives inside each bell. My whitish-pink flowers smell slightly sweet and offer a subtle, spicy, minty odor. Like the four-leaf clover from Ireland after which I am named, I carry within me the presence of green magic and mystery.

Welcome to my nature kingdom. I offer you protection in my inner sanctuary. Feel a deep silence and security here, along with the magical presence of my nature spirits. Allow yourself to be nurtured and guided. Communicate and connect with them. Hold the power of their gentle presence in your heart and trust their strength. Feel a deep sense of strength rise within you. Let love pour through your heart. Heal your inner child.

Insight

Bells of Ireland builds and secures a nurturing environment. The flower is seated protectively inside the bell-shaped leaf. If you look closely at the flower, it resembles a spritelike being wearing a hood, sitting inside the shell and facing out toward the opening. It is as if a small, vulnerable child is sitting inside the soft, protective, bell-shaped cup. The child feels nurtured and protected by nature spirits. This signature speaks of closeness and communion with nature.

Bells of Ireland guides you to connect with nature spirits. This enchanting plant offers a feeling of magic and wonder! Take time to sit in a garden or under a tree, or simply to find a safe and quiet place to be in nature. Allow yourself to open to your own natural instincts. Find the strength needed to trust these instincts and to gently act on them. Perhaps this is a time to explore inner-child issues and to cleanse emotional wounds of the heart.

Bells of Ireland is a showy, attractive addition to the garden, although it can be difficult to grow. The leaves have been known to treat digestive issues, reduce inflammation, and support healthy skin. A member of the mint family, the flowers and leaves are edible and can be made into a tea. It is considered a plant of magic and good luck. The leaves of Bells of Ireland smell sweeter and are more flavorful than the flower itself. Their taste is full, aromatic, and pleasant.

Bells of Ireland attracts hummingbirds, bees, and butterflies, offering even more magic to your garden delight!

Bells of Ireland's flower essence tastes pleasant and aromatic, offering a smooth sensation in the mouth.

✦ *Affirmation* ✦

> I feel secure to let love pour into my heart, to help me heal my inner child.

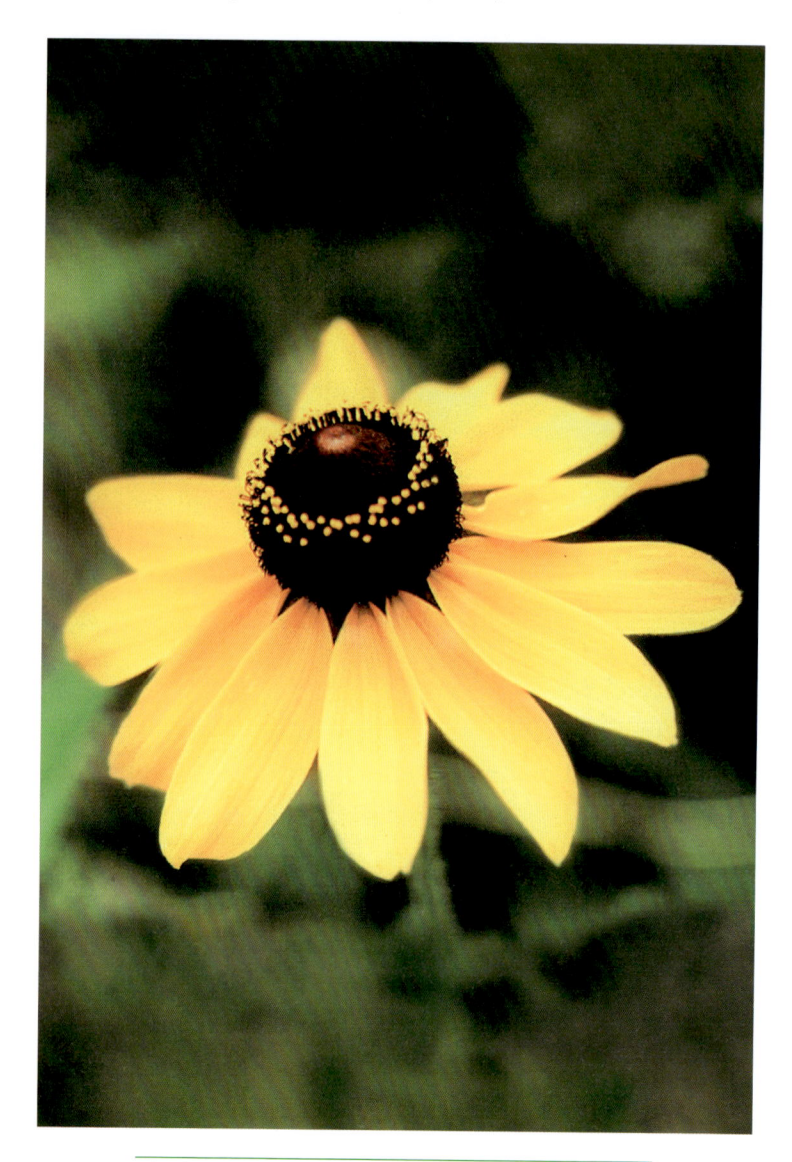

Black-eyed Susan flower stirs your inner radiance

BLACK-EYED SUSAN
(Rudbeckia hirta)

Primary quality: authentic self
Energy impact/chakra correspondence: first, third, and seventh chakras

Voice of the Flower

My flower head grows in a circle of golden-yellow rays. Seeds grow around and up toward my dark chocolate–colored center disk, which is surrounded by up to twenty golden-yellow daisylike petals. Tiny florets encircle the disk in successive bloom and create a yellow halo when the pollen is ripe.

My flower petals have several layers, creating an alternating effect. As the outer layer dies, a younger layer takes its place.

My dark core spreads out into petals of light rays. This symbolizes my ability to help you embrace your inner darkness, your shadow self, and bring it into the light. My golden-yellow crown invites you to embrace your inner radiance.

I invite you to enter the darkness of my inner circle and feel your shadow within my core. Allow it to merge with mine in the void. Experience your awareness of this void without judgment as you stretch outward toward the rays of my golden halo. Feel the warmth and radiance of my halo. Fill your body-mind-soul with that which gives you peace and light. Allow yourself to be permeated with the power of authenticity. I support you to feel free, whole, and at peace with yourself. In this place, give yourself permission to be real.

Insight

Black-eyed Susan reveals your shadow self. Accept and embrace any darkness and fears you may be holding. Release them to your higher source. Trust in the mystery of your darkness. Bring your attention to the positive role that darkness brings to your personal growth. Be real with yourself.

What does your inner voice say to you? What are your thoughts? What may be hidden within you that you are ready to uncover? Explore your thoughts and feelings. Find out what it is you may be hiding from living your true and authentic self. Face whatever that is and connect with it. Relive an experience through your imagination if need be. Take a close look and get in touch with all the levels involved: physical, emotional, mental, and spiritual.

Black-eyed Susan helps you heal by understanding who you are now.

Find purpose and hope in yourself and your life circumstances. As you experience the liberating principle of this plant, inner peace awaits you.

Feel the freedom to be your authentic self.

Black-eyed Susan is a diuretic with the possible side effect of mild cardiac stimulation. It can be used to stimulate the water volume in urine, but not the solids. In the Southwest, the root was historically used to relieve menstrual pains. Native Americans used the root to make a tea to treat colds and chest congestions.

Monarch butterflies—as well as many other butterflies, honeybees, beetles, and flies—are pollinators of the black-eyed Susan family.

The scent of black-eyed Susan is musty, similar to that of a sunflower. The taste of its flower essence is light and sweet, with a gentle sweet aftertaste

✦ *Affirmation* ✦

> I am empowered to believe in myself.
> I feel at peace with who I am.

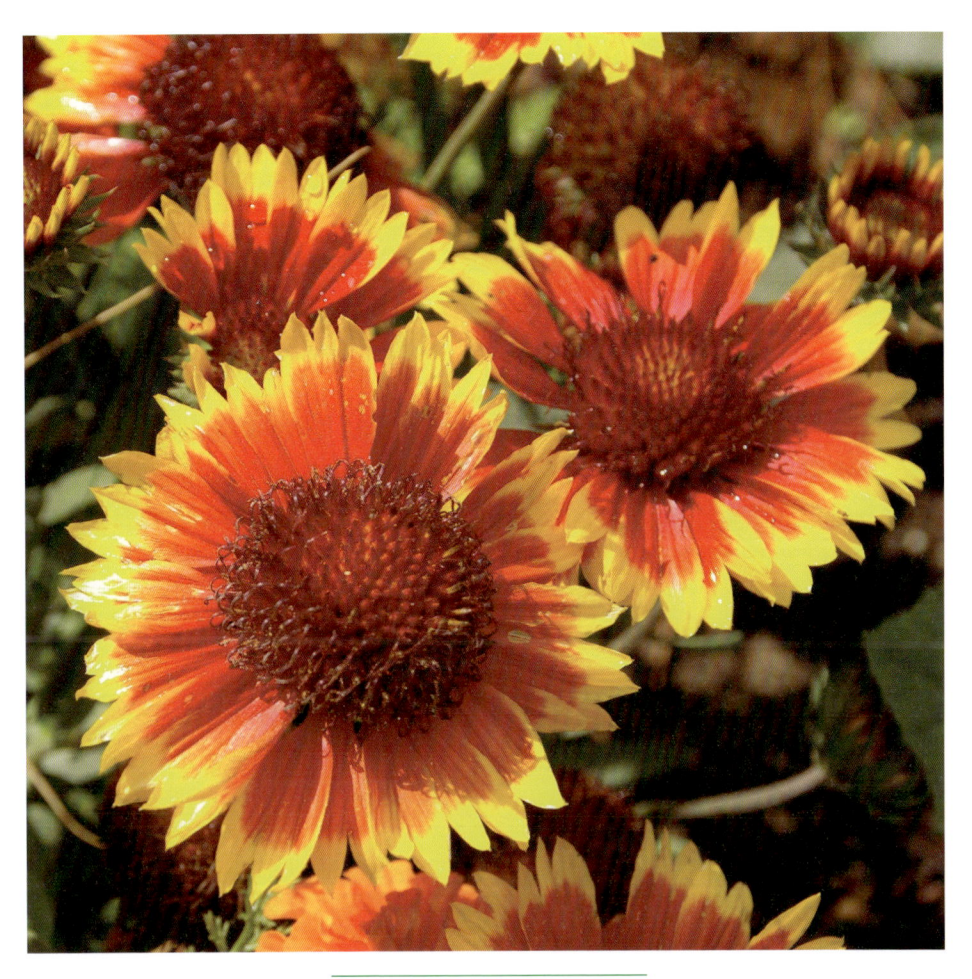

Blanketflower blooms joyfully

BLANKETFLOWER
(Gaillardia pulchella)

Primary quality: enthusiasm
Energy impact/chakra correspondence: first, second, and third chakras

Voice of the Flower

My showy, bright yellow and reddish-orange flowers call to you. I appear as a vibrant and fiery pinwheel. My reddish-orange ray flowers have bright yellow tips. The outside ray flowers are divided into lobes of three. Within each divided petal of the lobe are three symmetrical, wedge-shaped creases. My disk is also reddish-orange, with a golden-yellow dome-shaped center. Red stamens with golden-yellow anthers grow in and around my disk. My center dome is packed with many individual flowers.

I attract those who seek pleasure in living. I invite you to step inside my vibrant colors. Feel my warmth and exuberance. Let yourself experience the sensations and radiance of my vibrant presence. My joyful and creative expression can arouse your vital life force and move even the tiniest cells in your body-mind-spirit.

Let me stir your passion for life. Feel the power of your emotions and the energetic impact they have in your life.

I invite you to experience a newfound freedom of thought, emotions, and actions. Experience the freedom to take new steps in the dance of life to stir your passion, excitement, and enthusiasm.

Insight

Blanketflower reminds you to embrace the radiance within yourself, to kick off your shoes, let your hair down, and feel the freedom to take new steps in your dance of life.

The bright yellow and reddish-orange colors of blanketflower resemble the radiance of the sun. This flower is like a warm fire glowing from deep within your solar plexus, abdomen, and spleen, offering strength and vitality.

Blanketflower offers a fun-loving attitude and the willingness to choose the brighter side. It awakens you to the power of your emotions and the energetic impact they have on your life. Empower your thoughts with purpose and enthusiasm for life. Be inspired to do something fresh and new.

Blanketflower's fiery colors attract beneficial insects as pollinators to your garden, especially bees, hummingbirds, moths, songbirds, and butterflies. The flowers offer a bright and cheery disposition. The Hopi used the *Gaillardia* species as a diuretic. Blanketflower's roots make a tea that treats inflammation of the stomach or intestines, and they can also be ground into a powder and used as a poultice to treat skin disorders.

Blankeflower's flower essence offers a tingling and warm sensation in the belly. The color of its essence water is slightly golden-yellow and it gives off a musty odor.

✦ *Affirmation* ✦

I awaken the fire within me to move forth in life with warmth and exuberance.

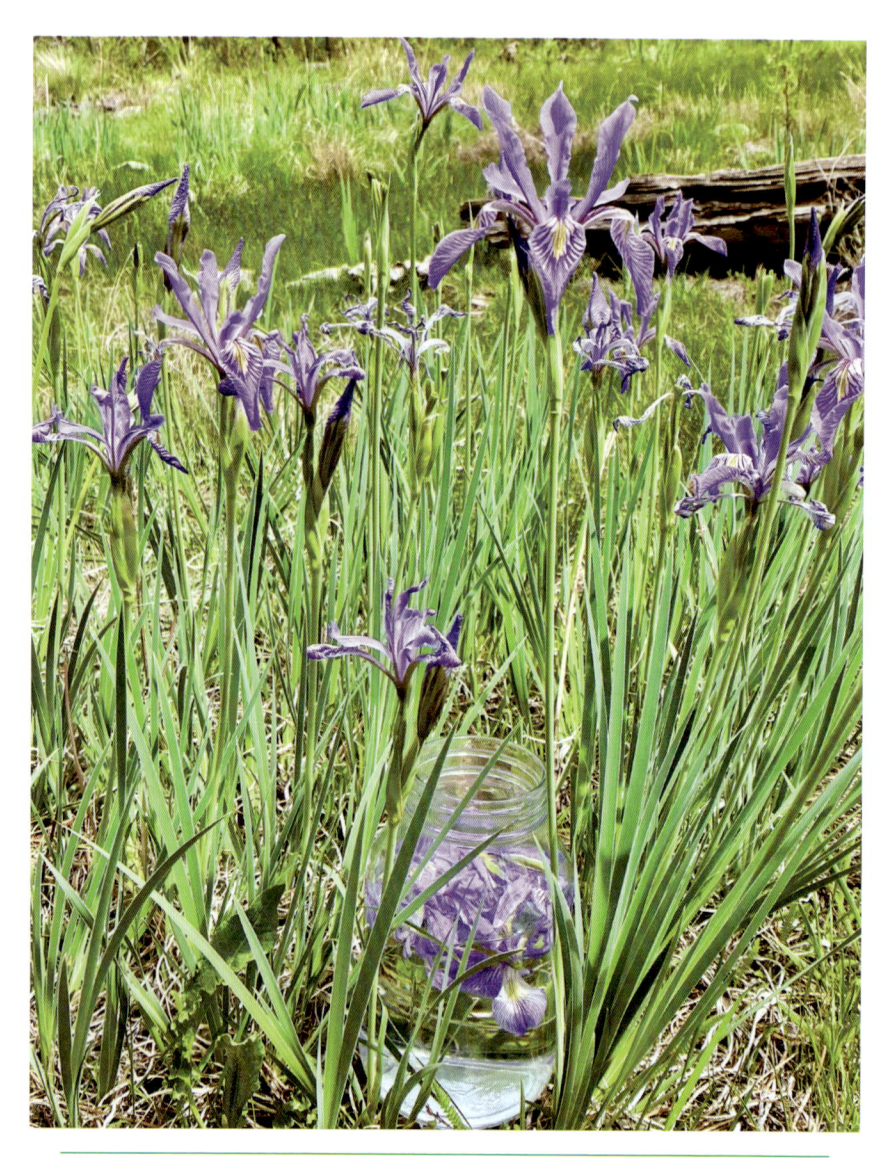

Blue flag iris flower essence in the forest of the White Mountains, Arizona

BLUE FLAG IRIS
(Iris missouriensis)

Primary quality: perseverance
Energy impact/chakra correspondence: third, fifth, sixth, and seventh chakras

Voice of the Flower

My creeping rootstalk grows in clumps along the edges of swamps, wet meadows, marshes, and forested wetlands.

Native to the gloomy bog, I live for several years creeping along the outer edge of the bog to collect enough nutrients to nurture my roots so that I can shoot up my long, tall, slender stem topped by an elegant flower of beauty and simplicity.

My graceful stem is protected by a covering of leaf scales from former growth. Notice my distinctive and subtle, rainbow-colored flowers of pale blue, lavender, and violet. My flowers are six-petaled, with three outer hanging petals and three inner upright petals. The petals are veined, with a deep violet or purple hue tinted with white stripes, and they have a yellow center in each flower petal.

Although I may be challenged by the barriers that present themselves to me, my growth continues at a slow and steady pace. I have learned that skillful pacing of my life's journey helps me build stamina and perseverance when facing hardships or stress. From beneath the bog I am able to rise above any preconceived limitations and self-centered aspects of myself, including the mundane, the material, and the world's inflictions. The divine in me is an infinite resource and prime doer. I am inspired by the beauty of divine grace and divine timing.

My subtle rainbow colors build a bridge that brings harmony. I share with you my uplifting nature and inspire your creativity, simplicity, and imagination. Receive my gifts. You, too, can build your resilience and rise from the bog.

Insight

Blue flag iris prompts you to slow down and pace yourself to build stamina and perseverance. The graceful flower offers the inherent beauty of its nature in its ability to rise from the bog, reach toward the sky, and honor beauty in all its forms.

Blue flag iris, highlighted by the colors of the rainbow, inspires you to make a bridge between what enters you and what leaves you—a bridge that connects your physical, emotional, mental, and spiritual aspects. Blue flag iris inspires you to build your stamina and freely express your creative self.

The three layers of the flower correspond to the three levels of the psyche, commonly known as the higher Self, the conscious self, and the lower self. Iris represents your choice—to be stuck in the bog or lower self of addictive behavior and lack of awareness, or to build your stamina and rise above the mundane to reach a higher way of conscious living and being. Blue flag iris offers further unfoldment of your evolution, which can occur on any or all levels. May you rise from the bog and be inspired to move upward!

Due to its powerful properties, it is generally recommended that blue flag iris be used in combination with other herbs such as burdock root, chamomile, or yellow dock. Fresh, raw roots of blue flag iris are not to be used internally as they could cause nausea and vomiting. The diversity of this plant's healing properties varies. The rhizome has been known to treat conditions such as fluid retention, liver problems, bloating, and swelling, and as an emetic, but should always be heated and steeped before drinking as a tea.

Various insects such as bumblebees, butterflies, and moths are attracted to blue flag irises, however they don't always remove pollen.

The scent of blue flag iris is uniquely sweet, as is the taste of its flower essence. It offers a tingling sensation in the crown chakra and the pituitary, feeling like energy connecting all the way around the head.

✦ *Affirmation* ✦

> I trust that through perseverance I will rise from my bog and be inspired to move forward.

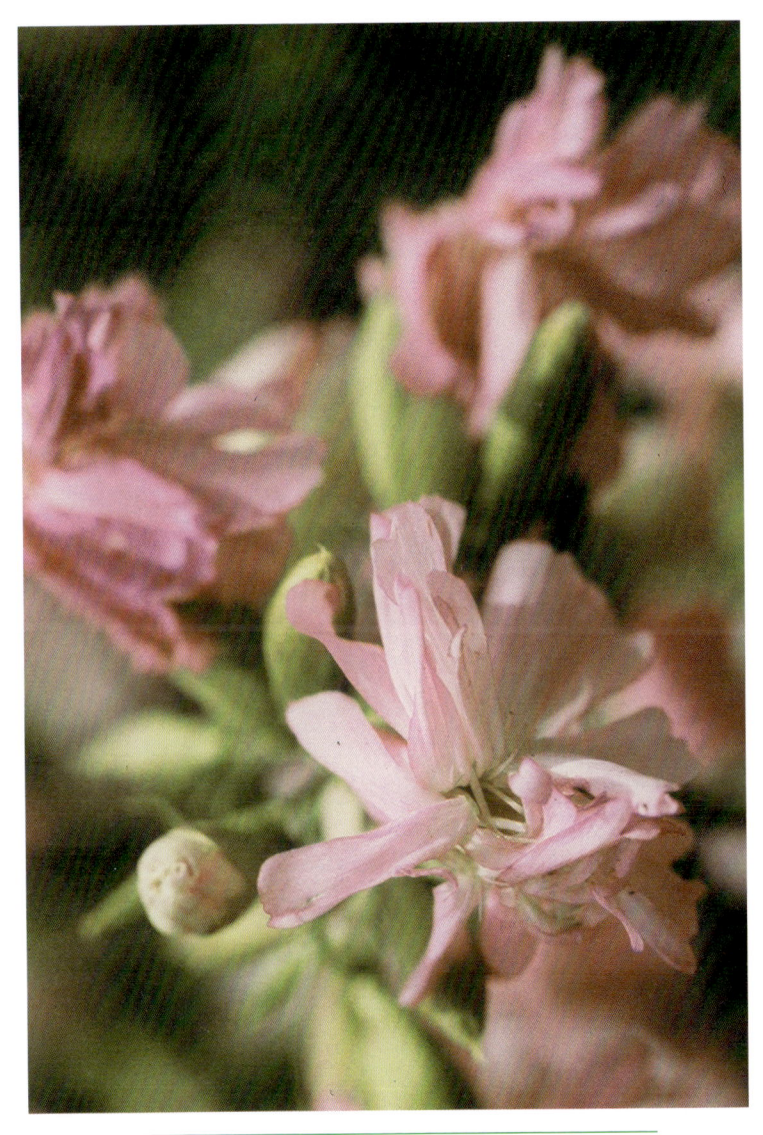

Bouncing bet flowers are aromatically intoxicating

BOUNCING BET
(Saponaria officinalis)

Primary quality: blissful union
Energy impact/chakra correspondence: first, fourth, and seventh chakras

Voice of the Flower

My fibrous rootlets grow on runners and contain a high concentration of lathering saponin. My stout and erect stem grows up to three feet tall. My leaves are oval-lanceolate, pointed, smooth, soft, and pale green. They grow in pairs. Both my stem and leaves contain saponins too.

My showy, creamy lilac and pale pink flowers are sweet, spicy, and aromatically intoxicating. They form dense terminal clusters with five pink and whitish petals with ten stamens. My flowers grow in single and double forms. Each flower petal has two identical, mirror-image parts. If you look closely, the two parts form a heart shape. They give a feeling of balance, union, and harmony. Their soft, creamy pink glow radiates compassion, bliss, and love.

My buds are coated with a creamy white liquid, which are my saponins. As they open, they become very feminine-looking flower heads. Oblong, toothed capsules follow after my flowers have fully bloomed.

I am the power of love within you singing deep into your heart. My compassion and bliss harmonize the divine union of opposites within yourself as well as within your beloved. This divine union is the union of self and Self. As you feel the wholeness of love within, you are more capable of loving unconditionally.

It takes a great love to love yourself and your beloveds without interfering with the natural laws of human nature. Allow the mystery of your union with others in your life to unfold. Accept your imperfections. Change your conditions to create greater harmony and love within yourself first, and then allow this to flow out to your beloveds.

Insight

Bouncing bet offers receptivity, openness, and union of your inner male and inner female. This plant helps you to receive and give love, bringing to your awareness the sacred inner marriage within yourself. Bouncing bet awakens sexual energy. It makes a wonderful flower essence for those who consciously work with their kundalini energy in love-making, allowing it to rise up along the spine to the heart. It opens you to passion, channeling and circulating erogenous energies of ecstasy. It helps you to consciously experience the vibrant energy of all the chakras working together harmoniously.

Bouncing bet allows you to appreciate the mystery of who you are, to find ways that bring harmony into your home and heart. Experience the blissful and loving nature of this precious flower. May the doorway of your heart open wide for love to flow freely within you.

The active ingredients of bouncing bet are saponins found in the leaves and roots of the plant. Boiled leaves and roots produce a sudsy solution that creates a cleansing lather that can be used in the treatment of burns or skin infections.

Medicinally, bouncing bet is an effective expectorant that can be used for treating bronchitis and dry coughs. It is also used as a dynamic laxative and as a mild diuretic. A lotion can be made for soothing sore, irritated skin caused by eczema, acne, or poison ivy rashes. The edible flowers of this plant can be added to salads and have been used to increase the foamy "head" in beer. They can also be dried and used in potpourri.

Bouncing bet's flowers appeal to beneficial pollinators that include hummingbirds, butterflies, hummingbird moths, and bees.

Bouncing bet's scent is spicy and bittersweet, and its flower essence is full, sweet, and spicy.

✦ *Affirmation* ✦

I allow my heart to open and let love flow freely through me.

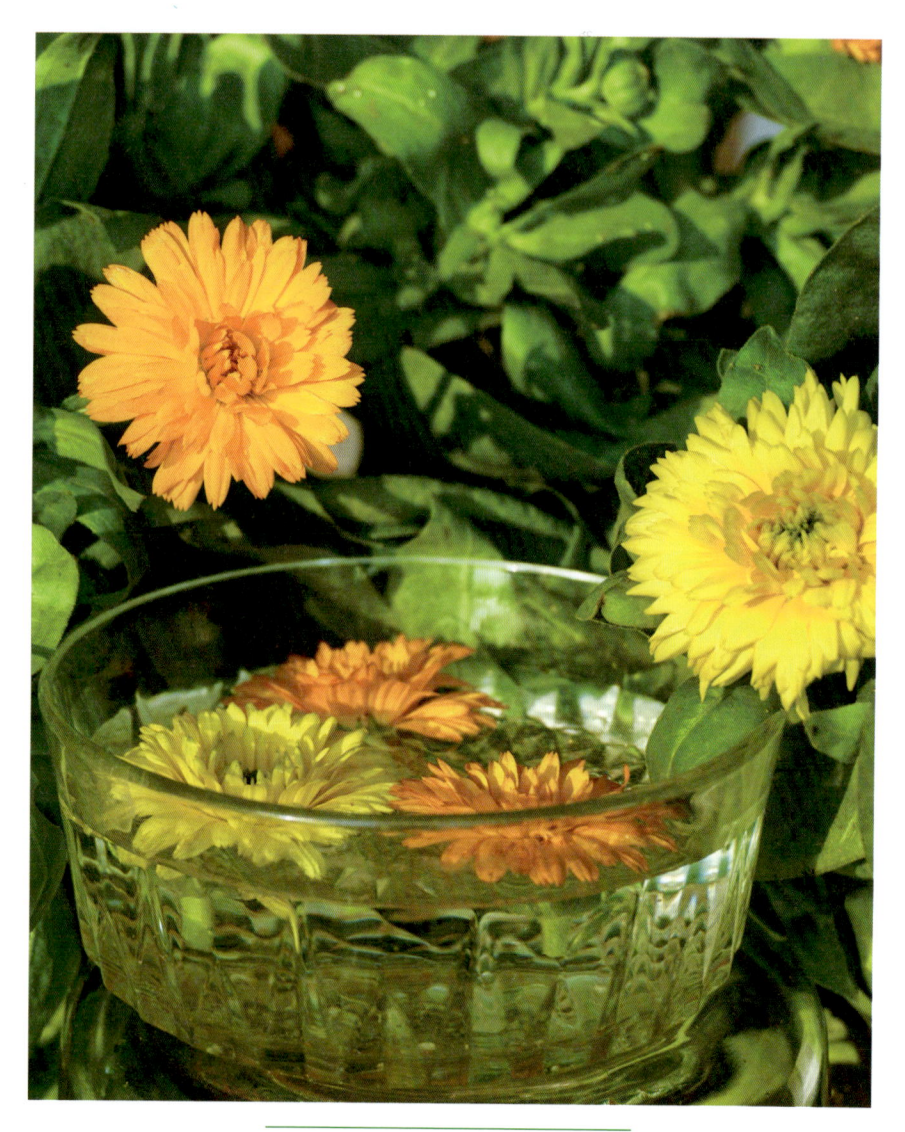

Calendula blossoms' gentle nature

CALENDULA
(Calendula officinalis)

Primary quality: peacefulness
Energy impact/chakra correspondence: second and third chakras

Voice of the Flower

I stand erect with many branching stems that grow from the same root. My green, succulent, angular stems are thick and sturdy, yet flexible. They are covered with fine hairs that are slightly soft and fuzzy. My green lower leaves are paddle-shaped, and my middle to upper leaves are oblong with lemon-lime centered veins. They are hairy, soft, and fuzzy on both sides, and they alternate along the stems.

My golden yellow–orange ray flowers are layered and multipetaled, with single or double flower heads. My ray flowers radiate from a pronounced center of golden-yellow florets. I am known for my long flowering period. As my flower petals die, they become stringlike, appearing as nerve endings to show you that you need to let go of any tensions you may feel. They signify my ability to let go and bring a peaceful presence of calm.

I bring to you a softness that quiets your mind and emotions. I will fill you with the radiance of my gentle presence. My soothing orange and yellow glow warms your inner world and nurtures that place inside that yearns for peace. In this state of calmness, you will become more aware of your thoughts and feelings. Allow an inner warmth and glow to fill your being and radiate outward. Experience my deep healing gifts as you gain inner confidence. Trust in yourself and make choices that bring to you a sense of inner peace and calm.

Insight

Calendula peacefully guides you to ask yourself, What circumstances in life cause me to feel nervous and tense? What can I do to bring more calmness to myself and to my life circumstances?

Calendula calms nervous, anxious feelings, bringing a quiet centering to the abdomen and solar plexus area. It provides an inner warmth and radiance that promotes sensitivity and understanding in the way you relate to yourself and others. It has the energetic power to deeply heal the emotions and the mind.

Calendula's soft, fuzzy hairs on its leaves and stems highlight its soothing, calm nature. The golden glow at the center of the flower invites you to feel warm and fuzzy inside. Visualize calendula's golden-yellow petals reflecting a soft glow within you. Feel peace enter your body-mind-spirit.

Calendula is a versatile herb with a wide array of uses. It is used to treat skin problems such as cuts, inflammation, cracked and blemished skin, minor burns, scalds, skin cancer, frostbite, and athlete's foot. Calendula supports lymphatic circulation and contains carotenoids, strengthening eyesight and the heart as well as treating digestive inflammation, ulcers, cramps, and fevers. Calendula flowers can be eaten in salads and used to flavor soups and stews. Most everything about calendula offers a variety of healing treasures.

Pollinators such as bees and butterflies offering plant reproduction are attracted to calendulas.

The scent of calendula suggests hints of mint, sage, and thyme. Calendula's flower essence is stronger than its scent, yet emits a refreshing and calm feeling that is peaceful to the belly.

✦ *Affirmation* ✦

I allow calm and peace to radiate within me, soothing my body-mind-spirit.

California Poppy 125

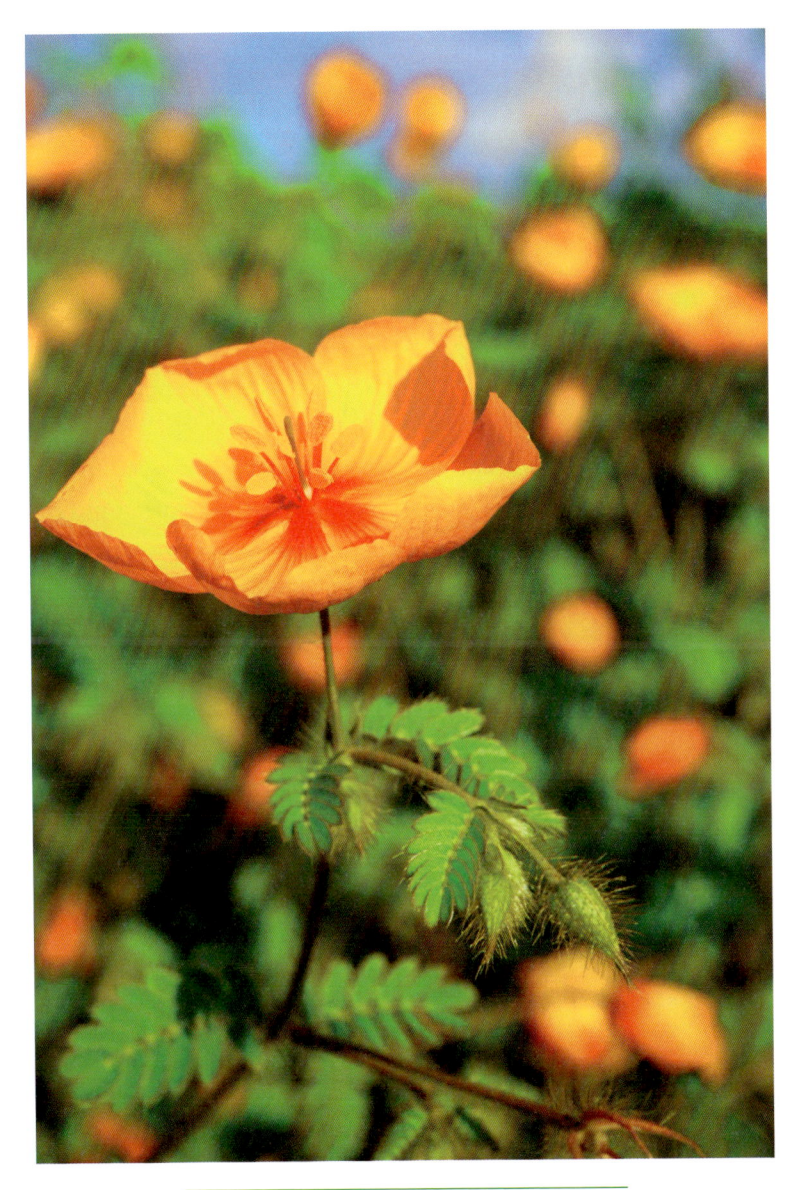

California poppy flower opens to the light

CALIFORNIA POPPY
(Eschscholzia californica)

Primary quality: emotional clearing
Energy impact/chakra correspondence: second chakra

Voice of the Flower

Many stems cluster from my one root. They are smooth, juicy, and moist—sturdy yet bendable. Clumps of well-dissected bluish-green leaves grow at my base. They are light, airy, feathery, and fernlike.

My showy orange flowers have four wide, overlapping petals. A reddish-purple and pink-like ring can be seen at the base of my flower, which appears like a tea saucer. Thin orange stamens come into sight at the center of the flower.

My flowers are highly sensitive and phototropic. They open only in sunlight and stay closed on cloudy days and at night. Without the light of the sun, I form a shielding swirl of protection around me, and yet with the radiance and warmth of the sun, my petals swell and curve outward. They yield to the presence of light, giving and receiving the splendor of magic and grace, offering freedom from the pains you may carry. My petals are thin, delicate, soft, and velvety. They fall off easily and require gentle care.

Let me wrap my petals around you and hold you inside my deep rich orange presence. Feel my protection. The fiery glow of my presence may stir your thoughts and feelings, and awaken your awareness of your emotional field.

Surrender to my shielding embrace. Allow your inner knowing to trust your journey. As I slowly unfold my petals in the morning sunlight, may your thoughts and emotions be lifted. Let the warmth of my gentle radiance embrace you. Surrender to freedom as you clear out old emotions and thoughts. Notice my voluptuous seed pods. Listen to the whispering pop as they burst forth and fall to the ground. Imagine that you are planting new seeds of awareness to bring you to your emotional field within. Embrace the light within you.

Insight

California poppy supports you to take care of yourself emotionally. If you are feeling emotionally shut down, California poppy offers cleansing and purification of stuck emotions or emotional patterns that no longer benefit you.

California poppy taps into your inner knowing of when to be receptive and open and when to protect your vulnerability. It offers you a sense of calm and an opportunity to look at your emotional patterns without judgment. Allow yourself to experience an emotional release in some way.

California poppy is an excellent relaxant and a sleep agent.

Native Americans use California poppy to treat colic. An infusion of California poppy roots and flowers is used as a mild sedative and analgesic to treat overexcitability and sleeplessness. California poppy contains flavone glycosides that are nonnarcotic alkaloids, which support calm in the nervous system. This plant is known to relieve pain, is used to treat gallbladder colic, and as an antispasmodic.

Bumblebees, honeybees, and butterflies carry significant amounts of pollen on their bodies and they are the primary pollinators of California poppies.

California poppy is subtly spicy with a sensual smell. Its taste is strong and refreshing.

✦ *Affirmation* ✦

I breathe deeply and fully to bring peace and calm in the ways I think and feel.

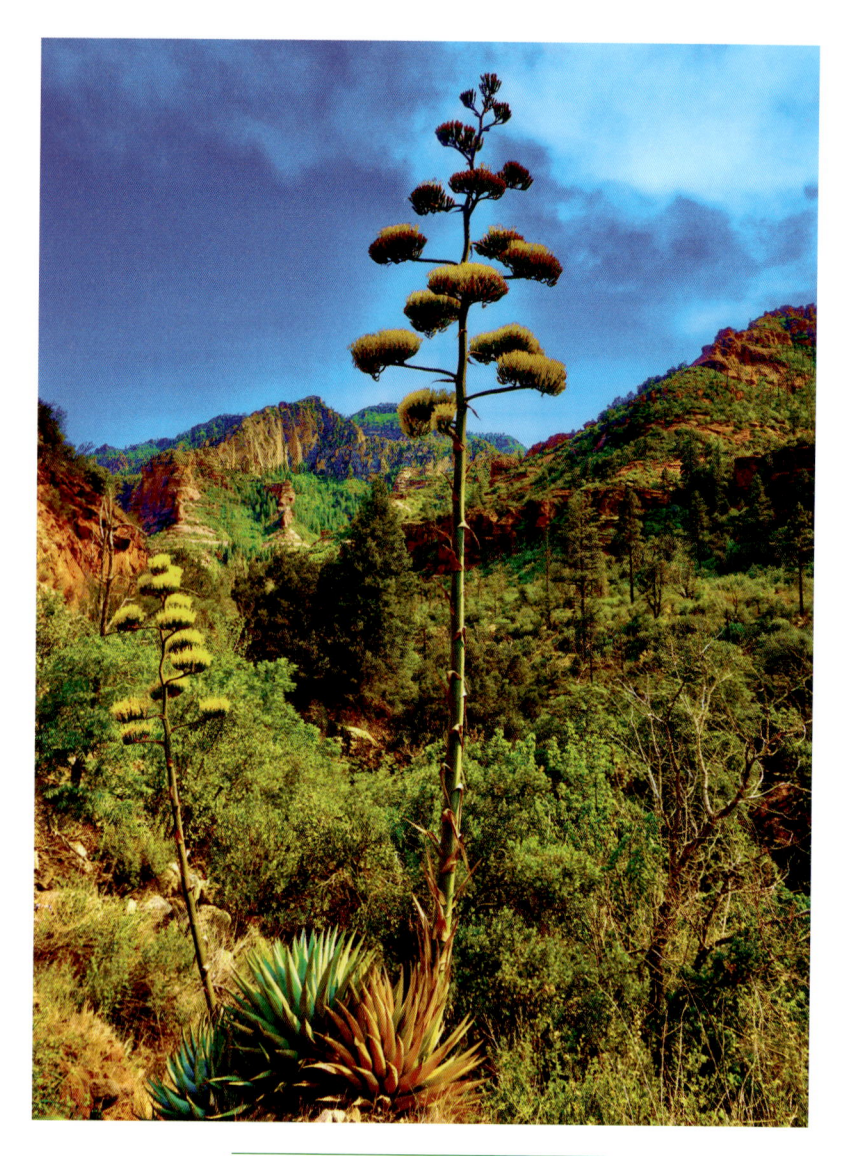

Century plant stands with fortitude

CENTURY PLANT
(Agave parryi)

Primary quality: transformation
Energy impact/chakra correspondence: first, second, and third chakras

Voice of the Flower

Many seasons I have waited—in spring rains, in the hot desert sun, in winter frost and snow. And still I wait. The base of my spiny armor protects me from would-be predators for many years.

I reach deep within my roots in order to live long. I take each moment with care. My life is a journey of surrender and discovery while growing into my strength. Slowly I emerge. In the midst of the silence of flourishing desert harmony, all of nature observes my bold and inescapable transformation, for it is in my rising glory in this final midsummer season that my sacred purpose is served and the highest good prevails. I shudder not, nor do I recoil from this glory that finds its end. I bring to completion a deep connection with all. Surrendering with ease, I prepare my seeds for new birth, for another lifetime.

Insight

Century plant suggests that a breakthrough is on its way! Its massive clusters of reddish-orangish-yellowish flowers reach toward the sun. They offer a feeling of strength, fortitude, and exaltation, and symbolize guidance from the light of the sun. Empower your personal transformation as you stretch the horizons of your mind.

It takes from eight to twenty-five years for this plant to produce its only flowering stalk. Eventually, in its season of glory, a thick, erotic, reddish-purple shaft emerges from the heart of the agave as it gradually forms its branches and flowers, stretching into a majestic being as it embodies its full character.

This signature of century plant is its ability to help you to grow into and feel a new sense of freedom. It gives you the strength needed to break through your barriers. Century plant teaches courage, patience, strength, and survival as a natural process.

Stay focused on your life goals and the ways you feed your strength and how you express yourself. Honor yourself. There may be something you need to let go of so you can move on. Embrace a new cycle of birth and celebration. Decide what it is in your life that calls out to be transformed.

The century plant stalk and agave stalks in general are known for their high alcohol content. They are collected, fermented, and roasted in a fire pit to make alcoholic beverages, some of which are distilled, such as mezcal, pulque, and tequila. As Gary Paul Nabnan and David Suro Pinera say in their book *Agave Spirits*, "The second meaning of the word *mezcal* metaphorically implies transformation of a wild, sometimes caustic plant into a dreams domain, not just a delectable beverage."[1]

The inner mucilage in the leaves and root of this plant contain soapy substances used in manufacturing steroids. The leaves generate strong fibers that are traditionally used to weave baskets and sandals. The tips of the leaves are sharp and thorny, and they have been known to be used for needles and pins.

You can't help but notice the artful mandala-shaped rosette leaf base of the agave family. Its enticing energetic impact brings you right into the center of yourself and the center of all things.

Century plant's expressed leaf sap boiled in a tea is used to treat indigestion, stomach fermentation, and chronic constipation. Burns, cuts, and skin abrasions can also be healed with the fresh sap.

Bees, hummingbirds, and bats feed off century plant blossoms for nectar and pollen.

Century plant flower essence tastes strong and powerful, sweeter than the musky odor it produces. A feeling of strength and tingling may be felt in the belly.

✦ Affirmation ✦

I embrace my life as a journey of surrender and discovery as I grow deeper into my own strength.

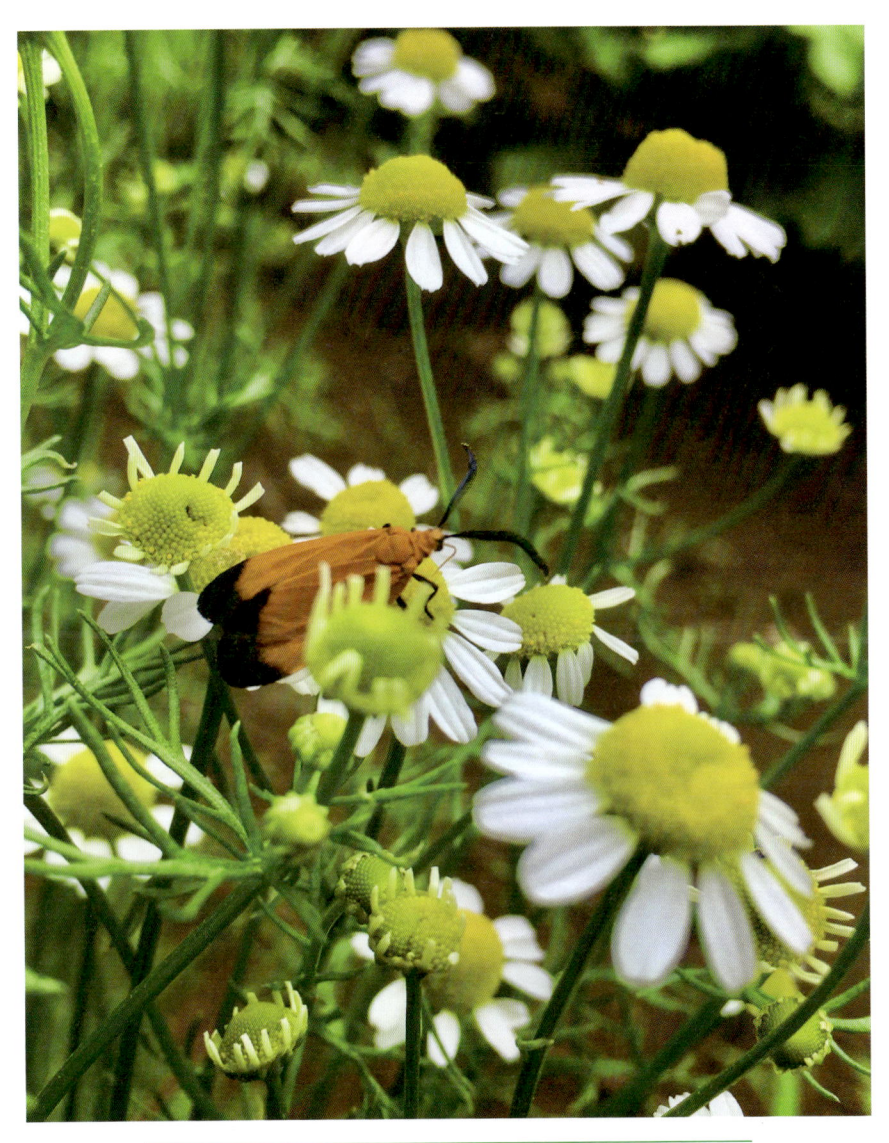

Chamomile flowers emanate their soft and loving nature

CHAMOMILE (GERMAN)
(Matricaria chamomilla)

Primary quality: emotional harmony
Energy impact/chakra correspondence): third and seventh chakras

Voice of the Flower

Come be with my sunny nature and lightheartedness. My white ray flowers open and extend upward toward the light of the sun as my yellow center shines within. I am here to help you feel brightness and joy, and to share your happiness with others. I give you comfort and remind you to slow down and relax.

My creeping rootstalks spread and create a carpet-like surface. My smooth, round, and slender stems bend and ease even in the slightest breeze. You will notice that my bright green leaves have a lacey, fernlike appearance with no stalk. They are light and airy, and may alternate or grow in parallel on my stems. My touch is soft and delicate. Experience the lightheartedness of my nature as I exude a gentle presence of calm and harmony.

Become aware of the pleasant things in life that bring you joy and peace. Take time to love and appreciate yourself. Find ways to relieve tension and stress. My tranquil disposition offers you a serene way of living, giving you emotional balance and stability.

Insight

Chamomile calls you to spend time with yourself to relax and center. Notice how you feel. You are being given an opportunity to become more aware of the ways you build tension and stress in your life.

Chamomile uplifts and releases tension. It promotes peace and balance within. If you have difficulty sleeping or are feeling restless, drink chamomile tea or take a chamomile flower essence. In fact, Tasha Tudor (1915–2008), an American writer of children's books, captured the spirit of this plant when she famously said, "Nowadays, people are so jezzled up. If they took some chamomile tea and spent more time rocking on the porch in the evening listening to the liquid song of the hermit thrush, they might enjoy life more."

This plant's single, daisylike, symmetrical flowers have marked conical, fuzzy, hollow, yellow centers and grow on long stems. The flowers have a bitter yet pleasant taste. Tiny seeds of chamomile flowers produce pollen for the bees. This little flower holds many forms of medicine and is a very useful plant to get to know.

Chamomile contains a blue volatile oil that is derived from the flowers. Over the centuries it has been known for its sweet apple scent and its soothing qualities. Baths and poultices of chamomile can be used to treat headache as well as kidney, liver, and bladder dysfunctions. Today, chamomile is a favorite among herbs. In addition to its traditional folk uses, it is known as the "baby remedy" for its use in treating colic and as a sedative for whining, crying, impatient, irritated babies, and children with earaches, teething pains, and difficulty sleeping. Chamomile in general is for the irritated and restless person and offers many uses.

Chamomile's fragrant foliage as well as its flowers attract a variety of bees, butterflies, and other insects.

Chamomile flower essence is fruity and earthy, calming to taste and experience. Its flowers' scent carries a hint of honey-lemon and apple, and its essence tastes similar to its fragrance. It offers a soothing sensation to the body.

✦ *Affirmation* ✦

I take time to slow down and feel calmness within, bringing emotional balance into my awareness.

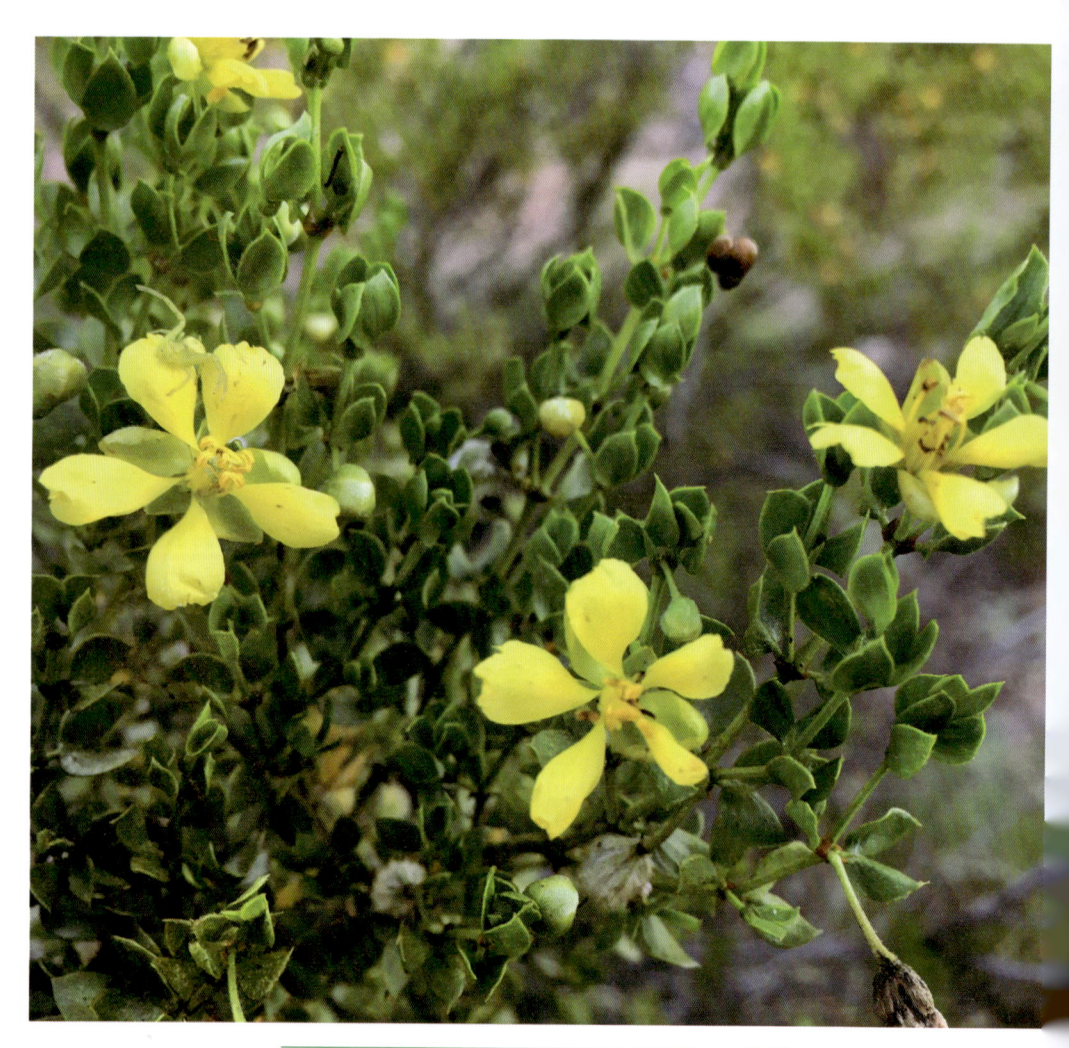

Chaparral flowers give an aroma of purification

CHAPARRAL
(Larrea tridentata)

Primary quality: cleansing and survival
Energy impact/chakra correspondence: first and third chakras

Voice of the Flower

Here I am—take in my distinct cleansing presence. I invite you to walk through my stands and feel refreshed by my healing energy. Experience my power as it surrounds you with a feeling of security and survival.

Take a deep breath and let my spicy aroma fill every cell in your body. I offer a cleansing from deep within, helping you to experience a profound connection to Earth energy. Awaken the energy within yourself and understand the ways that you survive. I support you to strengthen your awareness and the ways you want to cleanse from deep within.

Drink my flower essence water. Breathe in the aroma of my fresh and uplifting, golden-yellow, five-petalled scented flowers. Allow my healing presence to offer you a deep sense of purification and rejuvenation. I welcome you to step through new doorways within yourself. Let go of something old. Receive the clarity that brings in the power of your cleansing and survival.

Insight

Chaparral invites you into an unseen world of aromas and healing energy. Experience the etheric nature of chaparral to facilitate your soul's journey.

Across the Southwest, native chaparral stands grow as many-branched and leafy large shrubs with greenish-yellow foliage. The small, resinous leaves curl and appear similar in color to its photosynthesizing branches. The small, yellow, five-petalled flowers and pinnately divided leaves are a signature of the Caltrop family. This plant is also known as creosote because of its distinctive scent, which is similar to true creosote derived from coal or pine oil.

Chaparral is known to be one of the oldest plants on earth, with some individual plants living up to ten thousand years! It contains a sticky and distinctly resinous smell. It is especially effective for storing fats and oils to offer a longer shelf life in various ways due to its antioxidant ability to prevent rancidity.

Chaparral is used as an antiseptic and antimicrobial for skin conditions, cuts, and wounds. It slows down the progression of bacterial growth, making it a good remedy for long-term dressings.[2] It is also used as an antioxidant to treat liver and blood disorders.[3] Chaparral treats many conditions, among them, the treatment of brittle nails and hair, dry skin, joint pain, cracked feet, allergies, eyesight, and autoimmune diseases. Chaparral is known to treat arteriosclerosis and hardening of the arteries, and it has a reputation for both inhibiting and stimulating the growth of cancer cells.[4]

Chaparral offers many healing and cleansing properties, and can be made into tinctures, salves, ointments, essential oils, and even a tea if you can handle its strong and pungent taste. No wonder chaparral has been used in Native American ceremonies and sweat lodges for smudging and purification.

We have made numerous visits to the chaparral stands here in the Verde Valley of Arizona with our students. We have circled, prayed, meditated, and journeyed with chaparral throughout the years, and everyone has consistently noted how powerful this plant is and how it offers a feeling of security and survival.

Bees are the primary pollinator responsible for pollinating chaparral plants.

Chaparral's flower essence offers a deep cleansing, especially when made after a fresh rain, and the taste of the water and the presence of the plant is felt throughout the body.

✦ *Affirmation* ✦

I breathe in energy of cleansing and renewal from deep within.

Cliff Rose 137

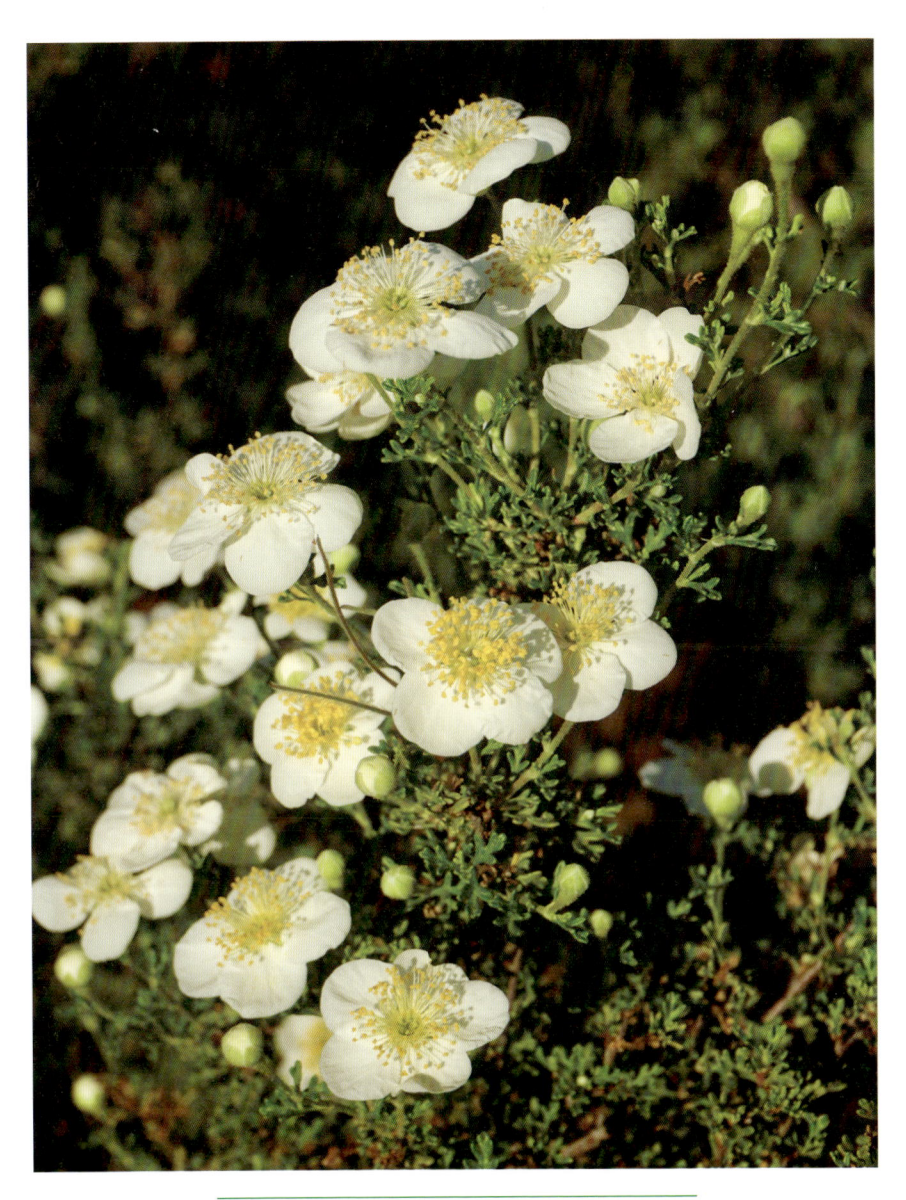

Cliff rose blossoms offer a soothing fragrance

CLIFF ROSE
(Cowania mexicana)

Primary quality: self-acceptance
Energy impact/chakra correspondence: third and seventh chakras

Voice of the Flower

Step inside my creamy-white, five-petaled, open flowers, and you will see a flurry of yellow stamens arising from my center. Feel my gentle embrace. My alluring roselike and orange blossom fragrance is soft and sweet. Its presence will soothe your mind and body. You may take in my scent even before you notice me.

I bring to your inner realms a way of recognizing who you are so I can help you value all that you are. My foundation is strong. My roots can grow between rocks and on dry earth. Each of my flowers securely join at the tips of my freely branched and tiny-leafed, dark evergreen shrub. My palmate-shaped leathery leaves appear like succulent little hands opening to the sky.

I have the power to help you reflect on your own inner strength and self-worth. My healing presence is strong, yet humble. I attract those who notice me, who honor their inner gifts and nurture their self-worth and self-acceptance from a place independent of others. Sip my nectar and feel the power of my love.

Insight

Cliff rose offers a gentle, uplifting boost. When in full bloom, the entire shrub or tree is covered with creamy-white flowers. It is quite picturesque.

The sweetly fragrant orange blossom and roselike scent of the abundant flowers is a pleasant attraction to the eyes and the senses. The flowers first bloom a pale yellow and evolve into a soft creamy-white color. Each flower is about one inch wide and has five petals, with a cluster of short, golden stamens inside.

While collecting pollen from the stamens, insects casually brush against the pistils and transfer pollen from flower to flower. A single-seeded fruit called an *achene* emerges from the fertilized pistil. Each achene has a long, fuzzy, stringlike, feathery tail called a *plume*. Up to ten plumed achenes can grow from one flower head. As the wind catches them, their seeds are scattered. This signature reflects the plant's soft and gentle nature and reminds us to flow with the wind and plant our seeds for new growth.

Cliff rose's soothing flowers lure you into a place within yourself that is soft and loving. Here you are given an opportunity to connect with how you accept who you are from a place of love and acceptance.

Create an intent that encourages you to build your self-acceptance, self-confidence, and your ability to love yourself. What is your relationship to yourself? What do you do to feel that you are accepting and loving yourself? Cliff rose awakens you to empower and love yourself. Be guided by your "higher good" and create positive self-awareness.

The traditional peoples of the Southwest have used cliff rose in a variety of applications. The tea is an emetic used by traditional singers during sweats and in various ceremonies. Cliff rose leaves and stems can be ground along with juniper branches to make a yellowish-golden dye. A tea can be made to treat sores, wounds, backache, and to address the first signs of a chest cold. The Hopi used the wood to make arrows. Basket makers of various tribes made clothing, sandals, mats, and rope from the shredded bark. Elk, deer, and even cattle chew the leaves of cliff rose for sustenance.

Sweat bees, honeybees, and masked bees are pollinators of cliff roses in the Arizona desert.

Cliff rose flower essence tastes subtly fruity and roselike, similar to its smell. The essence feels soothing and relaxing in the throat.

✦ *Affirmation* ✦

My true image of myself is unblemished by the judgment of others.

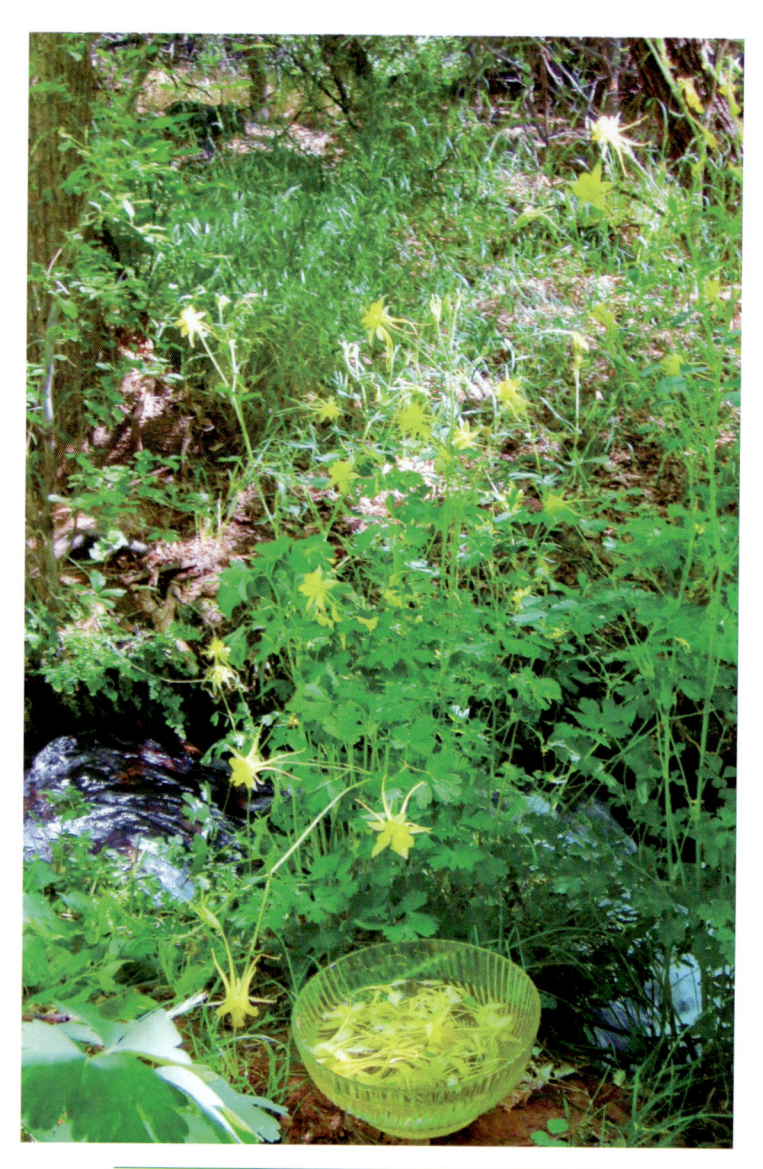

Yellow columbine flowers twinkle with merriment

COLUMBINE (YELLOW)
(Aquilegia vulgaris)

Primary quality: inner beauty
Energy impact/chakra correspondence: third and seventh chakras

Columbine (Yellow)

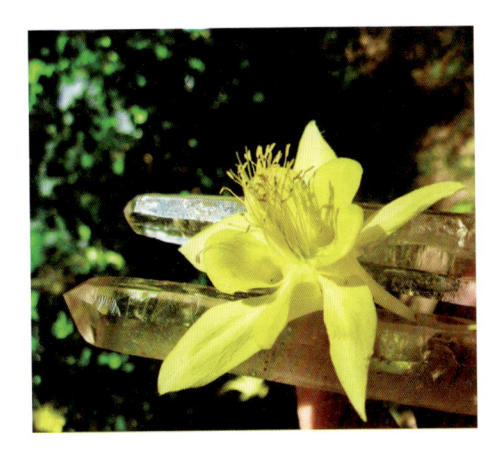

Yellow columbine flower vibrates its essence

Voice of the Flower

My graceful elegance resonates with the golden treasure of my divine beauty. My light-filled vessel twinkles with cheer, goodness, and beauty for all. I will help you discover, nurture, and unveil your own inner beauty.

Like a hummingbird, imagine that you have landed on my sweet, juicy nectar deep inside my long, extending spurs. Breathe in my sweet fragrance. Swim in my nectar. Allow yourself to laugh and play. Capture your own essence of pure enjoyment and beauty. Feel it and embrace it. Give yourself permission to keep it, to treasure it, and to share it. Feel and see my light shining down on you. Take in all my treasures and goodness. Feel them within you.

Accept and love your own true expression of beauty. Honor all that you are. Let your inner beauty be felt and shine out for all to experience.

Receive all the goodness that life has to offer you. Give it back in the expression of your authentic nature.

Insight

Columbine is calling you to discover and claim your inner beauty. Columbine's flowers emanate a strong, honey-sweet scent from each bloom's five yellow, soft, fuzzy, petals. The cuplike golden petals appear open and receptive, emanating light and the goodness of life. A clump of golden stamens emerge from the center.

Its long, funnel-like, tubular spurs hold a sweet nectar, a treasure held deep inside the bloom. The entire expression of the flower captures the magic and beauty of life—like a fairy who comes and sprinkles cheerful fairy dust in your face and helps you connect with your own beauty from deep within.

Columbine reminds you to appreciate, nurture, and love yourself and all the goodness life offers you. It offers healing energy right where it is needed. This plant reflects the beauty of life in general and the beauty within each of us. It wakes up your senses so you can feel and express your inner beauty.

Traditionally, columbine has been known for its use as a love potion; sweethearts would mash the seeds and rub them on their bodies. Columbine root, with medical direction, has been used to treat external skin diseases. Fresh roots can be mashed and rubbed on swollen, aching joints. The boiled leaves and roots have been used to treat scurvy, plague, fever, dizziness, diarrhea, and bladder problems. The leaves, eaten raw, have been used to treat swollen glands or adenoid problems, and were commonly used in potions to treat sore mouths and throats.

The sweet nectar of columbines especially appeals to hummingbirds and bees, as well as nocturnal hawk moths.

Columbine flower essence is fragrant, powerful, and full. Its odor is full-bodied and fragrantly sweet. It can heighten the senses!

✦ *Affirmation* ✦

I capture the beauty of life and I open to my inner beauty.

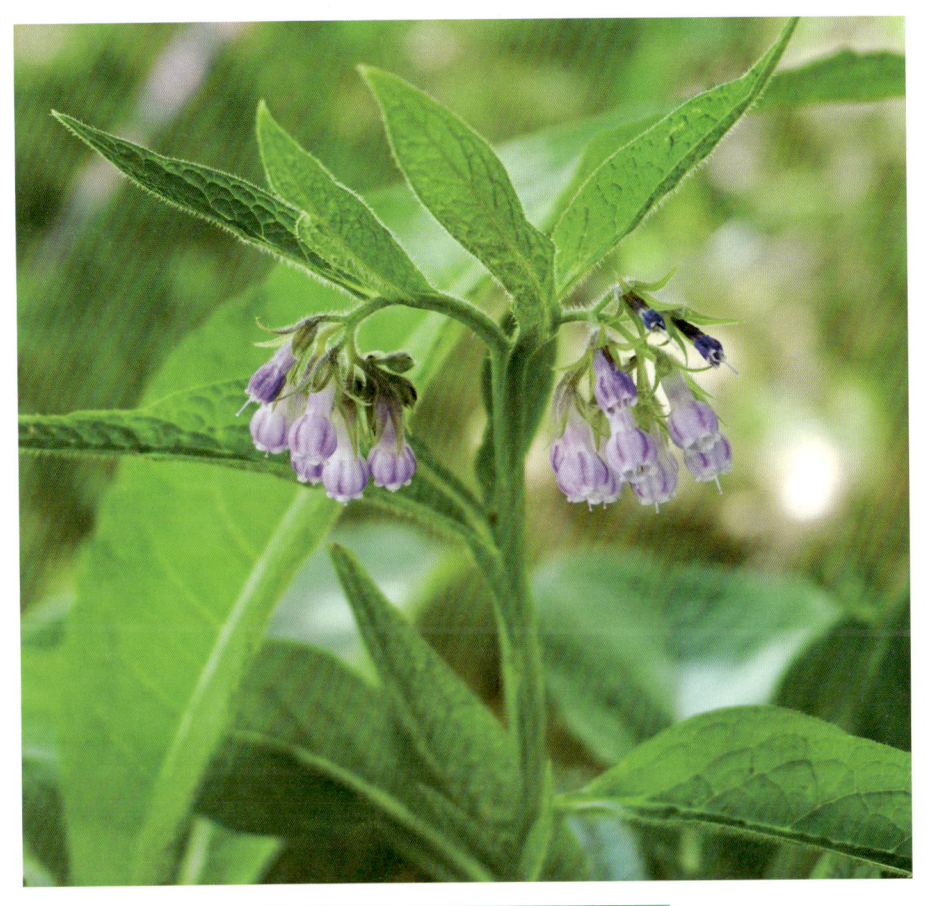

Comfrey blossoms for personal retreat

COMFREY
(Symphytum officinale)

Primary quality: support
Energy impact/chakra correspondence: third, fourth, fifth, sixth, and seventh chakras

Voice of the Flower

I am a member of the Symphytum genus, a group of about thirty-five species of flowering perennials. My thick, hearty, penetrating taproot grows up to one foot long or longer. It carries moisture and valuable nutrients to the upper soil levels. My stem is winged and three-sided. It is liquid and fibrous inside, rough and hairy on the outside. My stem branches near the top and can grow several feet or more.

My dark green, hairy leaves are thick-ribbed and alternate on the stem until they reach my flowers. My leaves are oval-shaped on a nearly sessile stalk, with the underside rough and prickly, and the top side soft and fuzzy. Near the base of my flower cluster appears two smaller leaves that grow in opposites. They are shaped like wings.

My flower colors range from creamy yellow, pinkish-lavender, to mauve, and they may be striped. They are bell-shaped with stems that grow in terminal or one-sided clusters on a short, drooping raceme. They taste and smell slightly sweet and earthy green.

Visualize the inside of my drooping, tubular flower. Take a peek and look inside from below. Look at the colors inside my flower's wall as they shine from the outside light. Notice how my flower is individual yet participates as a whole, connected in a circle with other blooms for support. Feel my humbleness and strength. Get in touch with the support you will need to benefit from the whole of your situation.

I am a strong, wise, and sensitive helper who is here to support you unconditionally, yet I need to take time out for personal retreat. It is necessary that I protect myself to balance the energy that I give out. It may be difficult to get to know me, but once you find the doorway open, you will discover my capacity for endless support. It is through my sustenance that I am so very drawn to offer my loving assistance to you.

I offer you the gift of support and understanding to see the greater good of your situation. By doing so, freely give of yourself. Offer your support when needed. Support is a gift that comes from the heart, free of conditions, free of entanglements.

Insight

Comfrey guides you to ask yourself if you are feeling the need to receive support in some way or if there is someone or something that needs your support.

Comfrey's tubular, clustered flowers droop toward the ground. They are protected by the plant's leaves and make a statement of protection and surrender. The flower's drooping position shows how each flower is supported by its cluster, yet each individual flower also offers its own support.

The main life support of comfrey is carried by its long taproot, which offers support and feeds all the chambers of the entire plant. Clusters of blossoms are fed and supported by the many branches that in turn are supported by the taproot.

Imagine that you and your loved ones are growing together on a cluster of flowers. You each carry your own individual power and strength, yet you also need support from the other blossoms on your cluster. Over time, you take turns supporting one another and supporting yourself as you move through life. Let love guide you in harmony and balance in those times of need when you are called on for support, or when you are calling out for support. As the saying goes, "It takes a village to raise a child." See the cluster as your village.

Comfrey has been known for centuries as an invaluable remedy and is claimed to be a miracle worker as a wound-healer and bone-knitter. Poultices, oils, and teas can be made from comfrey's roots and leaves. The leaves contain useful substances and more protein than any other herb or plant. Use with caution.

The stunning drooping petals of comfrey flowers attract a variety of bees, butterflies, and hummingbirds—and especially bumblebees—as pollinators.

Comfrey flower essence is slightly sweet, similar to clover, fruity, and earthy. Its scent is similar. It offers a warming sensation throughout the body.

✦ *Affirmation* ✦

I lovingly support who I am.

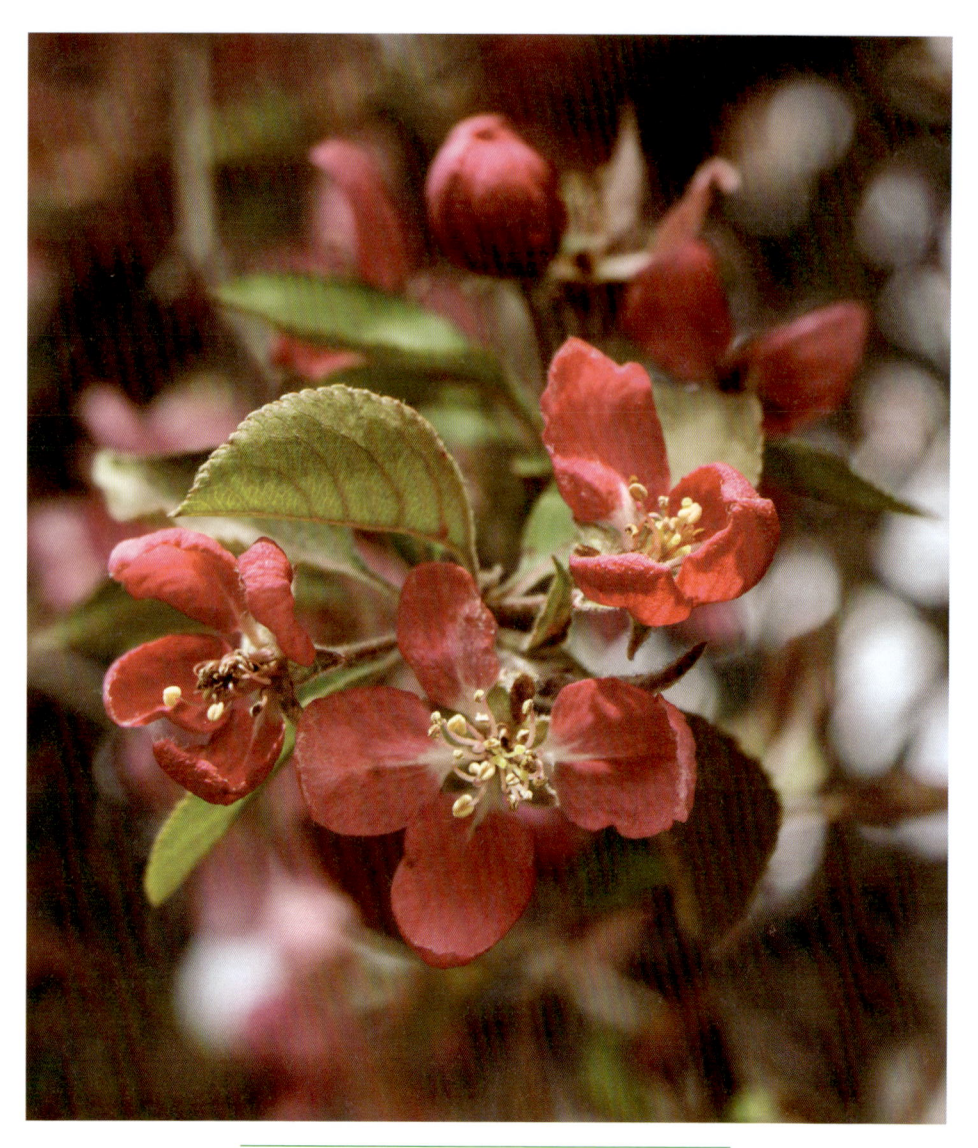

Crabapple flowers show their clustering jewels

CRABAPPLE
(Malus spp.)

Primary quality: open heart
Energy impact/chakra correspondence: first and fourth chakras

Voice of the Flower

It's no wonder that I've been called the jewel of the landscape. I produce the most beautiful, elegant, attractive, and showy fuchsia and deep pink blossoms. My aromatic blossoms are filled with a fruity fragrance in the spring that will make your heart sing!

My flower buds first appear small and tight. In this state of growth it may remind you of what it feels like to experience a closed heart. When my flowers open, they appear in their cluster as a perfect floral arrangement, with five symmetrical petals and a burst of stamens with golden-yellow anthers that produce pollen. They have a half-interior ovary where the lower half is embedded in the stem and the upper half is exposed.

My flowers grow in a cluster, bursting forth from my seeds, the source of energy that stimulates my growth. Much in the same way, your heart is the seed from which you evolve your being. Your heart is the first organ formed in the development of the embryo, followed by blood and the circulatory system, which allow nutrients and waste to be transported in the budding embryo. Your heart, as a living organism, continues this process throughout your life. It takes all the right nourishment to support your heart, helping you grow from a place of loving awareness.

Step deeper into the portal of your heart. Trust the constantly changing rhythms that occur within you and in your daily life. Listen to how your heart communicates with all parts of your being. Imagine your heart as a powerful pump, circulating the life force in every moment, all day long. With each heartbeat, bathe in the presence of your love. Let your heart open wider and deeper. Feel the love within you. Extend your love out to the universe.

Be in the presence of all that I am. Feel your heart open and awaken your soul.

Insight

Crabapple's buds appear tight and closed. Inside they are percolating with energy. You can't help but feel the presence of life that is ready to burst forth.

The opening of the flowers in their clusters yields an energetic presence and awareness of the heart field. The flowers offer a joyful, uplifting, and connected feeling from deep within the heart. Can you remember a time when you could feel your heart opening? Perhaps a special experience brought you into the sensation of your heart bursting forth.

Crabapple's flowers offer the power of divine mind and childlike innocence, beauty, and the mystery of the soul. Bask in this power place in your heart. Allow the rhythm of your heart, mind, and emotions to flow as one. Activate this flow from a place of love rather than a place of control or fear. If in your mind you are letting go, you can freely expose your heart and soul by trusting the heart shield from within to similarly open.

Crabapple fruits are similar to an apple, though they are much smaller and have a sour taste. The colorful fruits appear in the fall and often endure through the winter. They are rarely eaten raw as they contain malic acid, which causes the sour taste. Crabapple fruit reminds you that life's circumstances can leave you with a sour taste in your mouth, which can lead to a sour feeling in your heart. However, the new blossoms that come forth in the spring show you that even a sour crabapple comes from beauty. Its presence can remind you that no matter how sour your life is, if you come back to your heart, you can feel love and support, and overcome that nasty sour taste.

As you feel replenished, welcome wisdom into your heart. Embrace the natural rhythms of your heart as they consistently change throughout the day. Feel your heart beating. Send love to your heart, and from your heart to every cell in your body. Allow the electromagnetic currents in your heart to radiate creative force and power.

It's a natural condition of the heart to always be in love. It is only our mind and life experiences that smother it. When you identify with love, it instantly opens your heart more. Your heart recognizes the feeling of love that's already there.

If you see love in everyone, that doesn't mean that you approve of what they're doing or feeling or the ways they're treating you. Rather, acknowledge that every human being comes from a place of love in their heart, and it's only their words and actions that cover this up. Realize that everyone has love in their heart. If you do, that is what you will see.

Crabapple reinforces the ability to trust and surrender to your heart. Through your heart, trust the wisdom of how you feel and let it guide you.

Crabapple fruits are high in antioxidants and can support your body to get rid of harmful free radicals. Similar to other apples, they have many healthy nutrients. Avoid eating the seeds and core, though.

Crabapple flowers offer spring forage and pollen for many kinds of bees and flies especially.

Crabapple's honeylike flower essence tastes and has a scent similar to its blossoms. Its sweet, fragrant presence lingers on the palate.

✦ *Affirmation* ✦

I love and support the rhythm of my heart.
I open to the flow of my heart's wisdom.

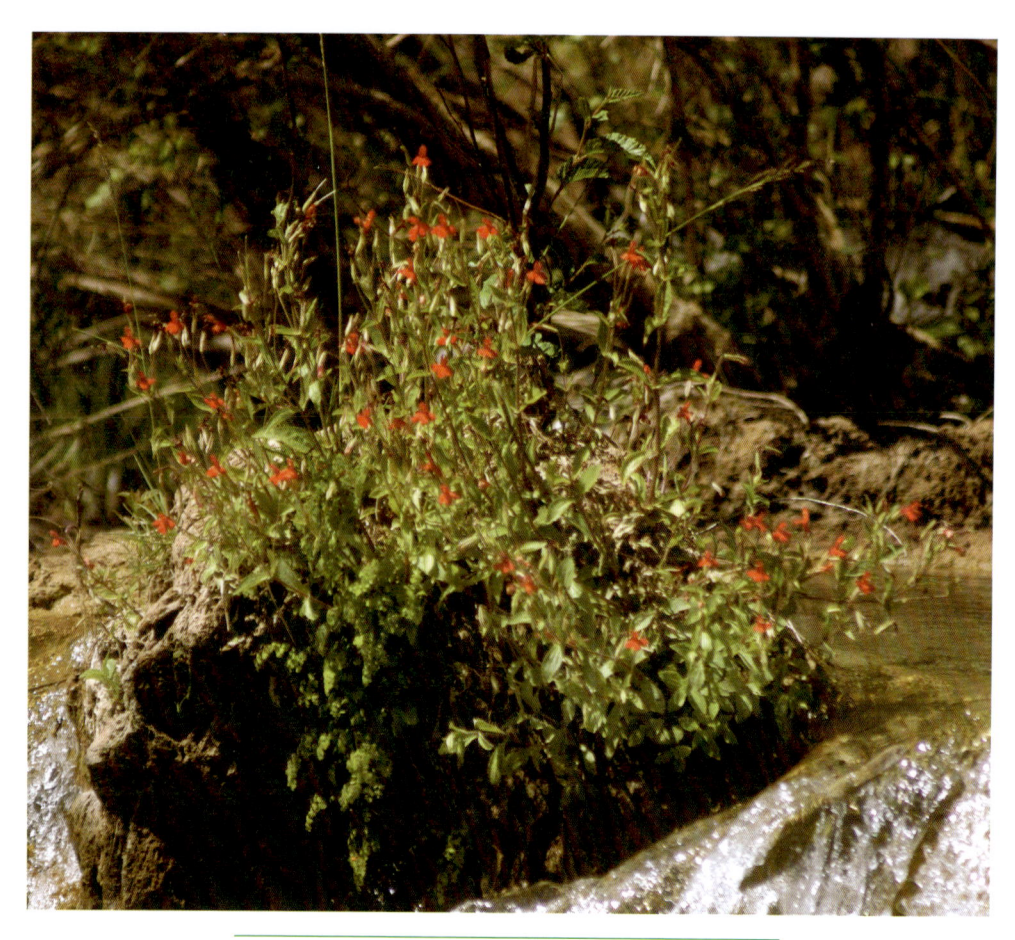

Crimson monkeyflower plants teach us how to flow

CRIMSON MONKEYFLOWER
(Mimulus cardinalis)

Primary quality: emotional power
Energy impact/chakra correspondence: first, second, and fifth chakras

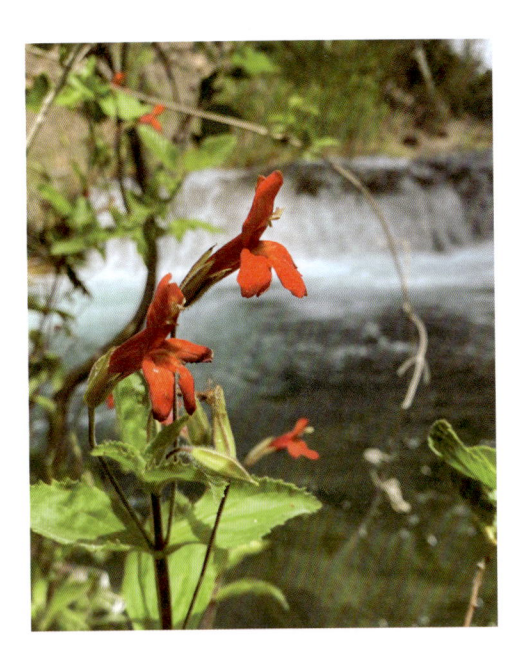

Crimson monkeyflower blossoms invite you to join them

Voice of the Flower

I thrive in or near flowing water, which cleanses and frees me to move with the flow of life. I am here to guide you with your emotional shifts.

Notice my bright red presence as I sway with the natural currents of water. My flowers offer a spicy smell, yet taste sweet. My irregular, two-lipped sticky flower has five petals or lobes. My petals join in a long tube or funnel. My upper lip's two broad lobes point upward, and my lower lip's three notched petals point downward. Two sets of fuzzy yellow stamens line my throat. As a member of the snapdragon family, I resemble a mouth with an open throat, suggesting communication and expression.

My sticky leaves grow in opposites. They are a vibrant shade of green and contain a resin that is sticky and viscous—a reminder to let go of sticky relationships or situations you may find yourself in.

You will realize in me there exists a doorway beyond your personal limitations. Recognize that portal to your emotional power that is opened through your awareness and connection with your higher Self. As you drink the nectar of my free expression, wash away any burdens that you carry that have weighed you down. I am the doorway through which you can speak your truth, heal old wounds, and invite the new in.

> *Come inside my red funnel and taste my nectar deep inside. An opening awaits you. I call out to you to gather your strength. Claim your emotional power and personal fulfillment.*

Insight

Crimson monkeyflower calls you to step into your emotional power. It loves to grow in or near flowing water. As water represents emotions, moods, and feelings, monkeyflower's favorite location demonstrates the movement and cleansing of emotions. The sticky, hairy leaves and stems of the plant signify any sticky relationships or situations that you may want to extricate yourself from.

The crimson and reddish-orange colors of the flower represent the root and spleen chakras, which are linked to emotions and the water element in your body.

Crimson monkeyflower energetically takes you back to your roots or past to heal any emotional pain and helps you tap into your own sweet nectar. Here you have the ability to gain or regain your emotional power by working with your core emotions. Let yourself experience the creative power of this plant.

Crimson monkeyflower roots have been used as an astringent. The leaves taste somewhat buttery and are included in the diet of Native Americans, who crush the raw leaves and stems to use as a poultice to treat rope burns and wounds. The fresh greens can be eaten raw in salads. The entire plant is edible. What a profound plant to discover in watery landscapes!

Crimson monkeyflowers' bright red color attracts pollinators and their sweet nectar provides a wonderful source of food for hummingbirds and bees as their primary pollinators.

Crimson monkeyflower carries a somewhat bittersweet fragrance. Its flower essence is fruity and light.

✦ *Affirmation* ✦

I swim freely in how I feel, continuously moving and flowing.

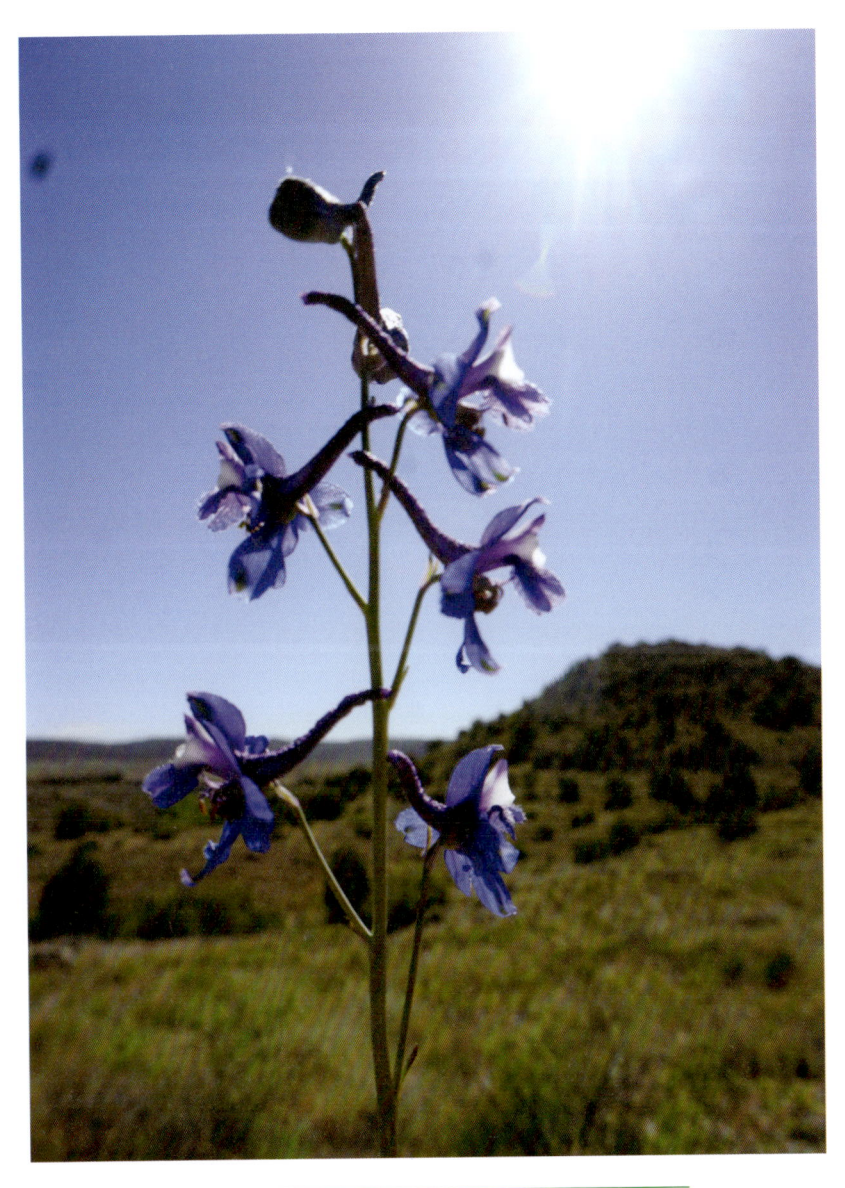

Desert larkspur flowers breathe in the soft breeze

DESERT LARKSPUR
(Delphinium scaposum)

Primary quality: self-expression
Energy impact/chakra correspondence: fifth and sixth chakras

Voice of the Flower

Breathe in silently through your nose with your mouth closed, placing your tongue on your upper palate for a few moments. As you inhale, slowly breathe deep into your belly, allowing it to swell. Then extend your breath by breathing out through your mouth for a few moments longer, allowing your belly to pull in. Follow the flow of air into and out of your body with the rise and fall of your belly.

Visualize my elegant spike and colorful, five-petaled, royal blue blossom and purple spur. Inside the spur is a hint of white. My flower gracefully moves with the wind and offers you a sense of freedom, song, and breath. Feel air pass through you like a soft breeze caressing your throat. Send your breath down through your heart and into your belly. Let my breath carry you deep inside my blue chamber.

As you connect deeper with yourself, listen to the voice in your heart. Let your senses be soothed by the natural rhythm you have created, aware of all the parts within you. Let the power of your voice emanate with the power of love in your heart. Hear my voice and song. My message is of change and movement. Be as one with me. Breathe deep into the mystery of life. Use the power of your imagination and the clarity of your thoughts to fashion a new direction. Feel the energy of your body and be present with it.

When your body is relaxed, it helps you to connect deeper with yourself so you can hear the voice in your heart. Notice how the rhythm of your breath echoes your body, feelings, thoughts, and vibrations.

Feel your connection with sound and frequencies. Let your senses be soothed by the natural rhythm you have created, aware of all the parts within you. Let the power of your voice emanate with the power of love in your heart. As you awaken your senses, become more aware of your inner calmness.

Envision riding the currents of your own rhythm and voice. Express your authenticity from a place of love and wisdom. Take freedom in your flight, and move with gracefulness as you ease into your life's journey.

Insight

Desert larkspur gives the gift of attuning to your inner rhythm. Be at ease in the way you express your voice and your authenticity. Be willing to let go of the past and embrace the currents of energy you are now aware of.

Desert larkspur enriches the power of your voice and stirs your imagination to express yourself in ways that bring clarity to your direction. Allow yourself to step deeper into your awareness to bring about a transformation. As you cultivate your self-expression, listen to your inner voice and follow what you feel in your heart. Your life is an adventure without limitations. Embrace it fully and gracefully.

The Hopi grind the flowers with corn to produce blue cornmeal and use this blend in sacred ceremonies.

Hummingbirds, bees, and butterflies are attracted to desert larkspur, although bumblebees are the plant's primary pollinators.

Desert larkspur flower essence smells and tastes full and sweet, and offers a cooling and soothing sensation in the throat.

✦ Affirmation ✦

> I express myself with grace and ease for the highest good of self and others.

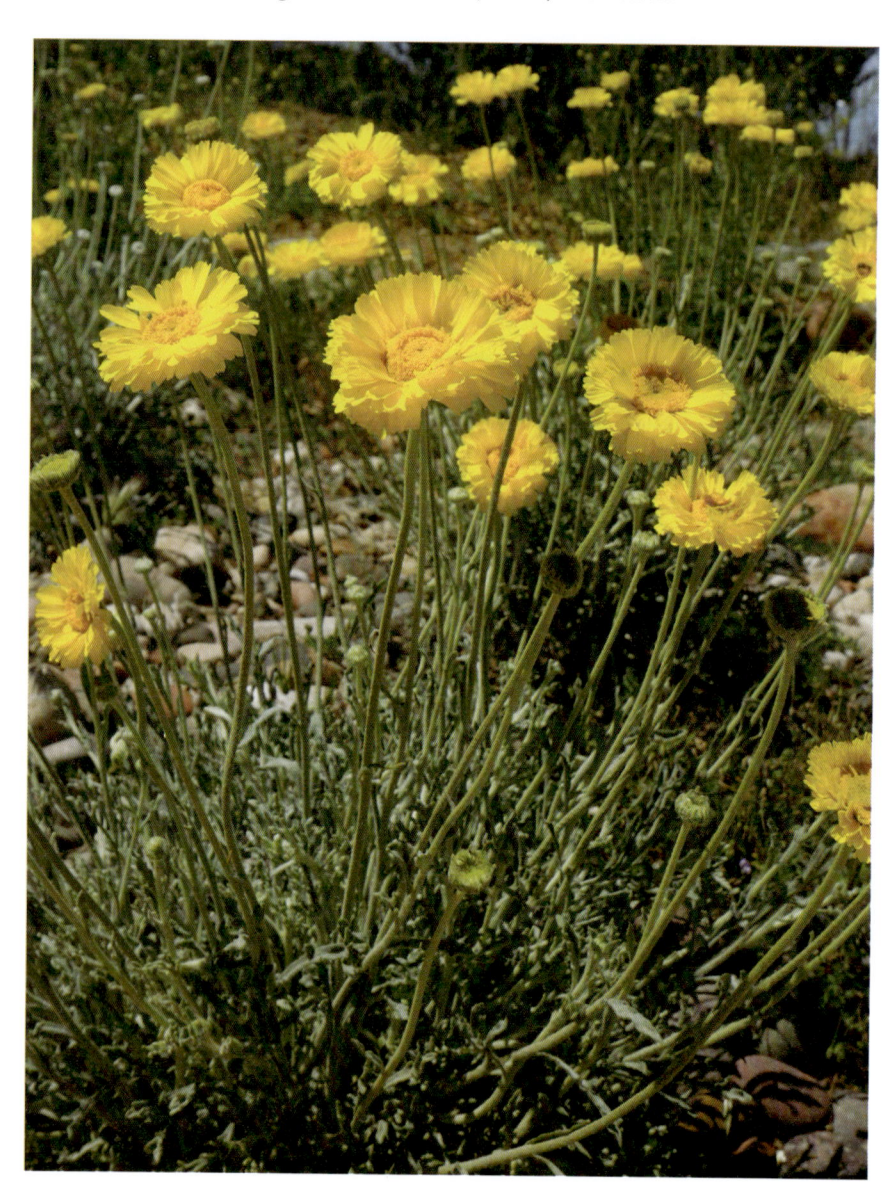

156 The Guiding Voice of Flowers, Trees, and Plants

Desert marigold flowers exude their warming presence

DESERT MARIGOLD
(Baileya multiradiata)

Primary quality: experience with ease
Energy impact/chakra correspondence: third chakra

Desert Marigold

Voice of the Flower

My golden-yellow flower heads are daisylike, with a deep, rich, golden-yellow center. My outer rays often bleach out and turn papery in the sun. I bloom sporadically over a long period of time and am one of the showiest common bloomers of the sunflower family.

My graceful presence dances on the desert floor. My long, woolly stems and brilliant flower brighten the desert's dry, sandy washes. My velvety soft, well-divided leaves are mostly clustered at the base of my fuzzy, pastel green stem. My long stems grow in clumps, and each stem bears a single flower.

Let my bright color fill your mind and body with my warming presence. From my center I reflect back to you the wisdom that comes from deep within your soul. Trust this wisdom, and let your thoughts, emotions, and actions flow in your life circumstances. Honor your flexibility to move with any challenges or choices facing you in your daily life.

May your heart and mind be filled with my yellow halo. Experience your life with ease. Feel the ability to be receptive and bend in even the slightest breeze.

Insight

Desert marigold urges you to be flexible. The intensity of desert marigold's bright, golden-yellow hue heightens your awareness and reminds you to silence your mind. Become aware of your body and your present environment. From this place of heightened perception, allow yourself to be accepting, flexible, and willing to flow with life's circumstances.

Desert marigold is here to teach you to balance your analytical mind with your intuition. Within this balance resides a fountain of wisdom. Let this wisdom guide you to nurture yourself, and to find softness and ease as you experience life.

Desert marigold can be found growing on rocky slopes, sandy mesas, washes, roadsides, and upper desert grasslands in the U.S. Southwest and northwest Mexico. It is a wonderful pollinator in desert habitats, offering wildlife cover and erosion control, especially in disturbed areas. The small white hairs that cover the plant retain moisture and support its sturdy nature and long growing season.

Due to its compounds containing anti-inflammatory and antiseptic properties, desert marigold leaves have been used among traditional peoples of the Southwest to treat conditions such as skin irritations, wounds, and digestion. Desert marigold is also known for its spiritual and healing influences in Native American traditions.

A variety of bees and butterflies are attracted to desert marigolds as their leading pollinators.

Desert marigold's subtly sweet flower essence offers ease and solace throughout the body. Its scent is similar.

✦ *Affirmation* ✦

> I experience my life with ease. I am receptive and can bend in even the slightest breeze.

Desert Willow 159

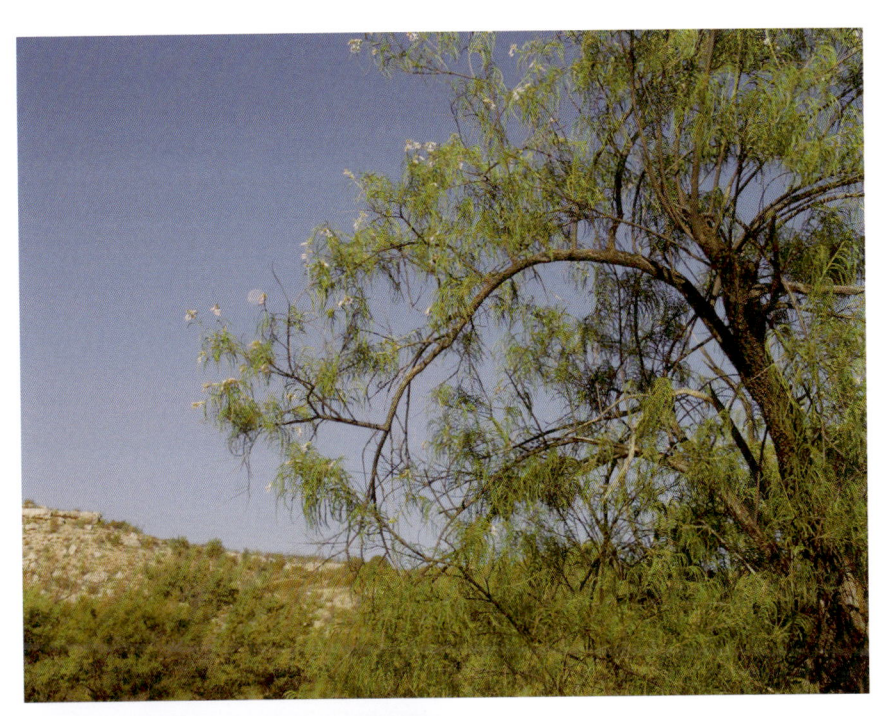

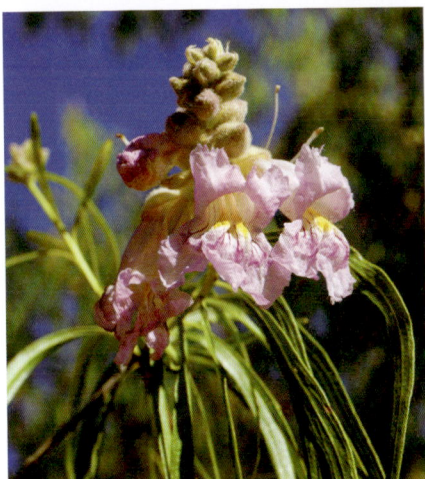

Flowering desert willow tree dances in the wind

Desert willow flowers show their grace and elegance

DESERT WILLOW
(Chilopsis linearis)

Primary quality: nurturing love
Energy impact/chakra correspondence: first, third, fourth, fifth, and seventh chakras

Voice of the Flower

My loving and sensual flow calls you to step closer to me and explore who I am and the feeling I awaken in you. My pinkish-violet flowers and soft colors, along with my flowing branches, express my sensuality and nurturing nature. My artistic beauty, grace, and elegance catch your eye.

As you explore the depths of my pinkish-violet, trumpetlike flower, imagine being in its center. Take in my sweet and spicy fragrance. As you are embraced by my sensual aroma, experience the gentle sweetness and strength inside my petals. Let my scent surround you as you connect deeper. Look around and see my deep magenta colors brush against my soft pink and lavender petals. Listen to my deepest sounds and the power of my vibration.

Embrace all that you can—the beauty of my soft elegance, the movement of my sensual flow, the strength of my abundance, and the wonder of my creative life force. Feel my passion. Allow your heart and voice to open to my compassion and nurturing love.

Insight

Desert willow asks you to walk the path of compassion. Search deep within to discover new ways to nurture and love yourself.

Desert willow's flowing branches, leaves, and flowers come forth in abundance. Its soft shades of pink and lavender bring a feminine grace that nurtures the soul.

Experience the beauty of desert willow. Let your heart open to its kindheartedness and love. In the center of your heart space, imagine an opening, a doorway for you to step into and beyond. Give yourself permission to love and nurture yourself no matter what. Feel what it is like to love yourself unconditionally.

As you explore deeper within, feel the stirring in your heart and your soft and gentle nature. Become secure in how you can nurture and love yourself, and your love of life will be joyfully renewed.

The leaves, bark, and flowers of desert willow, when made into a tea or tincture, can be used as an antifungal and anticandida to treat infections of the intestinal tract. Native American peoples used the wood and branches to make bows and dream catchers and to make framing structure in sweat lodges. The beauty and grace of the flower of desert willow is very eye-catching, and the plant can be cultivated as an ornamental.

Desert willow trees are a wonderful addition to the pollinator garden, attracting hummingbirds and bees to their sweet nectar.

The scent of desert willow is sweet, full, and sensual. Its flower essence is strong and earthy, and its taste somewhat bitter. The authors find this essence to especially heighten the senses and bring attention to the heart energy field.

✦ *Affirmation* ✦

I unconditionally love myself and nurture my entire being.

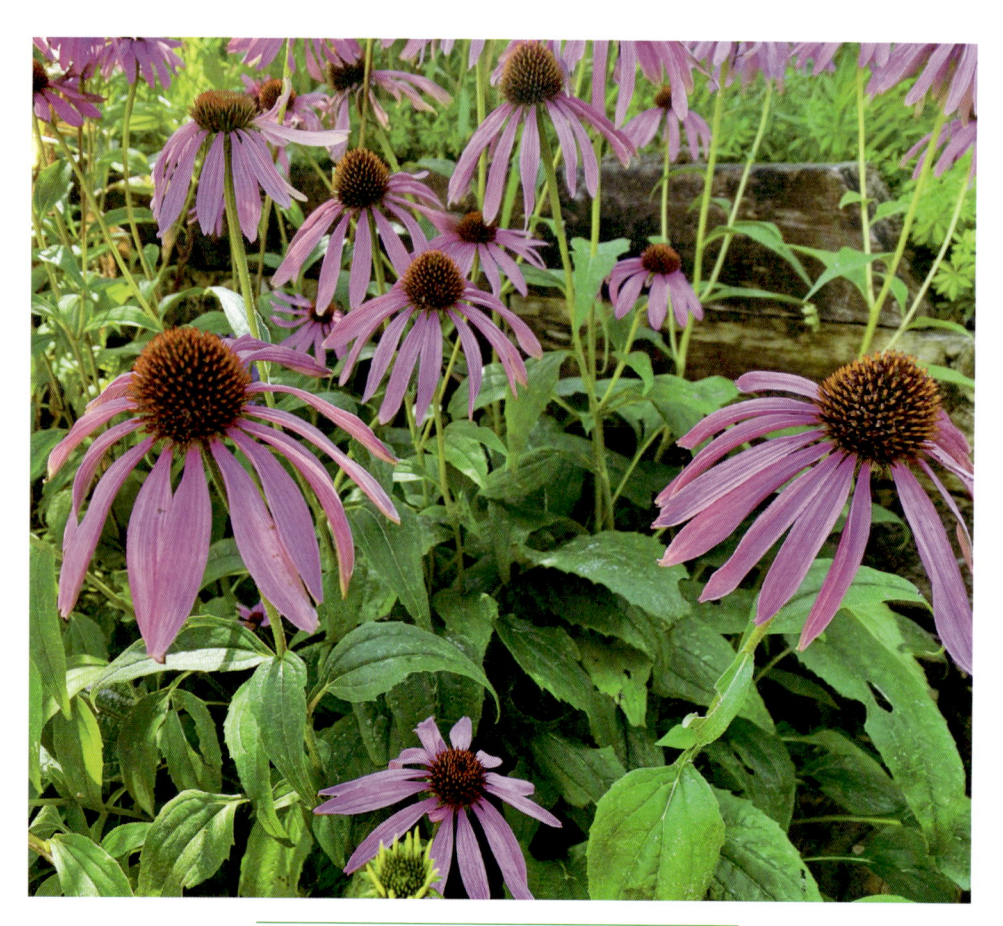

Echinacea flowers revitalize your whole being

ECHINACEA
(Echinacea angustifolia)

Primary quality: vitality
Energy impact/chakra correspondence: first, second, and sixth chakras

Echinacea

Voice of the Flower

My deep taproot takes several years to mature, similar to your own development of learned behaviors, habits, emotions, and personality traits. Over time you become more conscious of who you are and what you want to let go of. Explore and uncover your own taproot as you restore and revitalize your true essence.

The center of my flower head, an orangish red, symbolizes my vital life force. The core of this center protrudes outward, and its fiery colors represent the sun. My inspiring lavender to purple ray flowers extend outward in a circle. Imagine my purple rays all around you. Each of my petals symbolize the stages of life of my journey. Bring your awareness to your own life journey and what you are experiencing now. Be inspired by me to recognize your higher Self.

I invite you to connect with your higher Self to discover whatever it is that holds you back. Explore what keeps you from renewing your energy and strength. I am here to help you eliminate whatever it is that you need to let go of, to restore you to wellness and wholeness. The wind carries my seeds and yours to foster a new place of growth, a refreshing place of becoming and being. Take this opportunity to renew and rejuvenate yourself. Celebrate your vitality!

Insight

Echinacea encourages you to revitalize your health and energy. Restore your body-mind-spirit to its natural vibrancy. What your body really wants from you is to slow down and take care of it, to find ways that energize and renew your whole being. Restore your connection with yourself. Listen to your inner voice and discover what it is that your whole being is calling out for.

Echinacea reflects what it is that uplifts your energy. With this awareness, create natural, healthy ways to enjoy life. Offer self-care to your body, mind, and emotions. Experience your life in a new way that brings you strength and rejuvenation. Stir the richness and vitality that you have brought into your life.

Feel refreshed by echinacea's full, strong, aromatic taste and smell, which energizes and rejuvenates.

Echinacea was the medicine of choice of the traditional peoples of the Plains. They used it to treat the bites of snakes and rabid dogs and to treat fever, stings, septic sores, and poisoning. The root was chewed or made into a powder to treat toothache, mouth and gum sores, and swollen glands. A juice of echinacea can be made to treat burns.

Echinacea offers a multitude of medicinal uses. It is considered as one of the best blood cleansers, is a natural antibiotic, helps boost the body's immune system, fights infections, and is used in various forms to treat the common cold and flu.

Do you want to create and conserve a monarch waystation? Echinacea flowers offer a magnetizing effect to monarch butterflies, as well as many other kinds of butterflies and bees. Plant echinacea to protect monarch habitats and embellish your garden buffet!

Echinacea's flower essence odor is aromatic and pleasantly strong. Its taste is full and strong, mildly tart, yet pleasant, offering an energizing and refreshing effect throughout the body.

✦ *Affirmation* ✦

I experience life's richness and vitality.

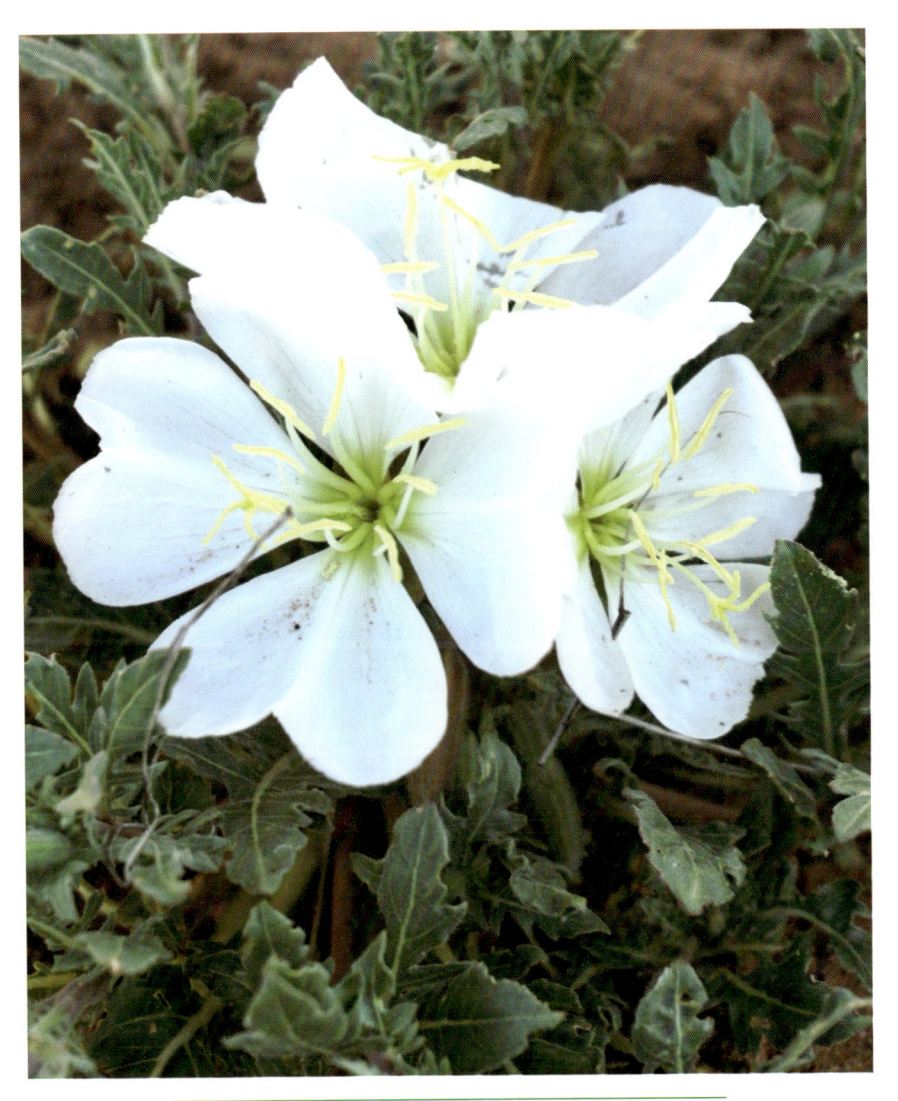

Evening primrose blossoms forth its feminine nature

EVENING PRIMROSE
(Oenothera caespitosa)

Primary quality: self-worth
Energy impact/chakra correspondence:
fourth and seventh chakras

Voice of the Flower

My sweet-scented flowers open in the evening and close when the morning sun bursts forth. My showy overlapping petals appear delicate and emerge from a slender floral tube that rises from a tuft of narrow leaves. I hold deep inside of me a pool of sweet nectar. When all else is sleeping and all around me is calm, I am stirred by the moon's light. As I awaken in the night light, my petals blossom in their fullness and radiate out. The soft light of the moon brings comfort to me.

The shadows created by the moonlight across the desert floor mirror back to me my own sense of inner worth. It is here, in the silence of the night, that I sink my roots deep into the earth. I trust my inner strength and the purity within me to find value and meaning in my relationship with myself and all of life. Feeling safe within myself amid the moonlight and its shadows, I trust my self-worth and awaken to my power.

I call on you to awaken to your sweet nectar within.

Insight

Evening primrose calls on you to heal any unresolved issues centered around your self-worth.

Evening primrose's flower appears delicate, yet it is stronger than it seems, since it is able to take root and grow in dry, rocky ground. In those rocky times in life when you feel unworthy, evening primrose reminds you to delve deeper into the essence of who you truly are. Imagine the nectar you hold deep inside. Be in your strength. Step into your roots.

Evening primrose's showy, sweet-scented flower has four white overlapping petals that appear very delicate. The thin flower petals have slight veins. The center of the flower is yellowish with eight long white stamens and yellow anthers. Each flower lives for only one night. The following day it turns pink as it wilts.

Only long-tongued hawk moths, the pollinator of evening primrose, can reach the nectar. Hawk moths have stout bodies with long, narrow forewings and shorter hindwings. They have the longest tongue of any other moth or butterfly—a large hawk moth tongue can extend up to fourteen inches, long enough to get at the nectar tucked deep inside the blooms. This is a reminder that we too carry a sweet nectar within us. Evening primrose reflects that purity and goodness, like the innocence that we were born with.

Life experiences can tarnish your sweet nectar and drag down your sense of self-worth, how you see yourself. Awareness of your intrinsic purity and goodness can get buried by life situations. But you have a right to acknowledge your self-worth and goodness.

Some days you may have to dig deeper to find the nectar within. You struggle to find your sweet nectar. It may only take one special event, one thought, one person, or one situation to help you see your sweet nectar, which is always within you. When it gets buried, evening primrose reminds you to dig deeper until you find it once again.

It's your lack of self-worth that keeps your nectar buried. Sometimes you can scratch the surface of it and get a snippet of nectar. It whets your thirst for that nectar and gets you to start looking for another flower, each time going deeper.

The hawk moth shows us the perseverance we need to keep trying to find our nectar. The nectar is its only source of nourishment. The flower lasts only one night. What will trigger your response to dig deeper into yourself, to reach deep inside to find your nectar? Nectar comes in different strengths, just as does your awareness.

Trust your senses. Whatever has been hidden is about to be revealed. If it is buried, then dig some more. If it doesn't come up, then dig deeper. The beautiful part about it is that you may only have a moment to find it, but if that moment passes you by you will always have another chance when a new flower blossoms.

As a night-blooming flower, evening primrose illuminates in the darkness of the night. People with low self-worth tend to live in their own shadows. Trust that in the darkness you will find the light of your self-worth. Shine your light out into the world.

Evening primrose offers you an opportunity to reconnect with what it is that you truly value and honor most in yourself. Listen to the voice of this subtle flower from deep within. Drink its sweet nectar. Awaken to your inner strength and worth.

The primrose family offers diverse interactions for healing. Hildegard of Bingen recommended gathering a bouquet of fresh primroses and placing them on the heart to sleep and calm the nerves. The root can be pounded into a pulp to reduce swelling and used as a poultice.

The scent of evening primrose flower essence is subtle and sweet. Its taste is also subtle, similar to fresh spring water. Its essence offers a quiet and soft energetic impact on the body.

✦ *Affirmation* ✦

> The stillness of the moonlight feeds my soul with comfort and strength.

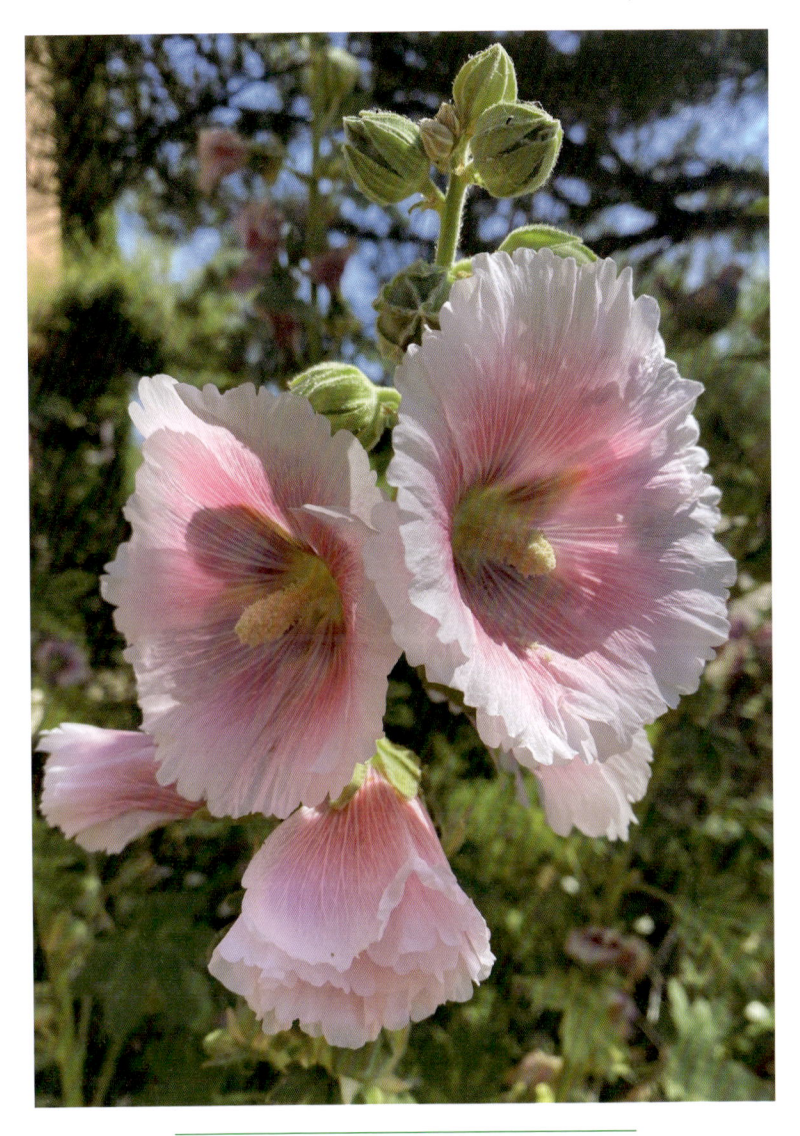

Hollyhock flowers reveal their hidden spirits

HOLLYHOCK
(Alcea rosea)

Primary quality: circle of life
Energy impact/chakra correspondence: first, fourth, and seventh chakras

Voice of the Flower

Notice the sway of my sturdy yet yielding flower spikes as I move with the breeze and wave at you. Hear my call. I beckon to you to step into my radiant energy field. I speak to you from the center of my blossoms. Listen to my magical story . . .

One bright sunny morning while visiting Grandma, Emma awoke with excitement. This was the day they planned to spend in Grandma's flower garden with the hollyhocks. Grandma loved hollyhocks and grew hollyhocks of many colors.

After breakfast, Emma and Grandma entered the garden. Emma was filled with wonder as she walked along Grandma's floral garden path. Some hollyhocks had magnificent spikes with alternating blossoms and buds. Their halos glowed in the sunlight. Other spikes had an abundance of seed pods with withered flowers growing along the stem.

Emma's excitement continued to build. Grandma told Emma that the Latin name for hollyhock, Alcea, comes from the Greek altho, which means "healing." Grandma said to Emma, "Let's be really quiet. Gaze into a flower, put an ear next to a hollyhock blossom, and close your eyes. Feel the presence of the hollyhock. The hollyhocks have a special message to share with us." Emma bent in toward the flower to hear what it had to say:

"In the center of my silky, five-petaled flower, notice my five-pointed star that reaches outward to each of my tender, flexible petals. Feel my magic! A soft wind has sprinkled me with pollen, which is my fairy dust. Imagine that you are given five wishes to help you realize your dreams. Imagine a fairy riding on a hummingbird or a bee, attracted to the pollen that drips onto my petals, sweetening my nectar and spreading a richness within you and all around you. See my beautiful fairies in my blossoms, showing off their precious, spirited skirts.

"I am honored to share my flourishing blossoms to help you feel the happiness and freedom that I show. May my playful appearance bring out the spirited nature in you! Let your voice and song amplify with me!

"Growing near others in my family, I stand proud and tall. Feel supported and hopeful as you reach out to fulfill the unlimited possibilities of your dreams!"

Emma opened her eyes and felt the warmth of Grandma's hand placing hollyhock's brown, wheel-shaped seeds in her palm. Feeling the power of the seeds in her hand, Emma understood the circle of life and the importance of planting seeds that lead to evolutionary growth.

Insight

The poet and painter Lloyd Mifflin is believed to have written in 1916: "They rise behind the fountain rocks, these spinsters robed in dainty frocks, so stately, prim, and tall; their hue the very rainbow mock, these quaint old-fashioned hollyhocks against my garden wall."

The symbolism of hollyhocks goes back to ancient times. Hollyhocks characterize the cycle of life, and as such, they have been and still are used in rituals for death, rebirth, and fertility.

The fairy realm has long been associated with hollyhocks. Fairies were thought to use the blooms as skirts. The seed pods were known as "fairy cheese" because they look like a cheese wheel.

Hollyhock flower petals feel gentle and delicate, yet they are firm, and the plant stands tall. When you touch a flower blossom you can feel its ability to yield and bend. This signature of the flower tells us to stretch beyond our limitations. Its playful dance, as seen in the swaying of its tall stalks, shows us the value of enjoying and being grateful for our own life cycles.

Several stalks can grow from hollyhocks roots or rhizomes. Although the root feels tough on the outside, it is actually viscous on the inside. The finely bristled stems or spikes reach upward of five to eight feet high, with palmate, lobed leaves alternating along the sturdy stems.

When the leaves and stems begin to lose their life force, the hollyhock produces a disk-shaped seed pod that contains many seeds, so that the plant reseeds itself in great abundance and with vital energy for the next generation.

If you are drawn to hollyhock, let your heart open wide to new possibilities. Notice where you are in your life's cycle. Feel into what may stir you to let go of something old. Allow your life to unfold naturally. Bring a new cycle into your life that you can be grateful for. Bring an abundance of happiness, friendship, and love into your life!

Hollyhock roots, stems, leaves, and flowers all contain a mucilaginous substance that offers a silky texture that can be used for skin creams and to treat sunburn. Hollyhocks have a variety of medicinal uses. The leaves and roots can be made into a tea to treat intestinal, kidney, and urinary tract infections, as well as sore throat, ulcers, vaginal soreness, and more.

Hollyhocks naturally reseed themselves. The force of their seeds offers evolutionary growth. If we don't plant seeds, we have no future. This plant represents the cycle of life.

Although hollyhocks offer very little or no smell, hollyhocks' rich nectar draws many a pollinator, such as hummingbirds, bees, and butterflies.

The flower essence has a subtle taste and offers a silky sense of softness and comfort.

✦ Affirmation ✦

> I stand tall with gratitude as I bend with ease and dance with the wind.

Honeysuckle 173

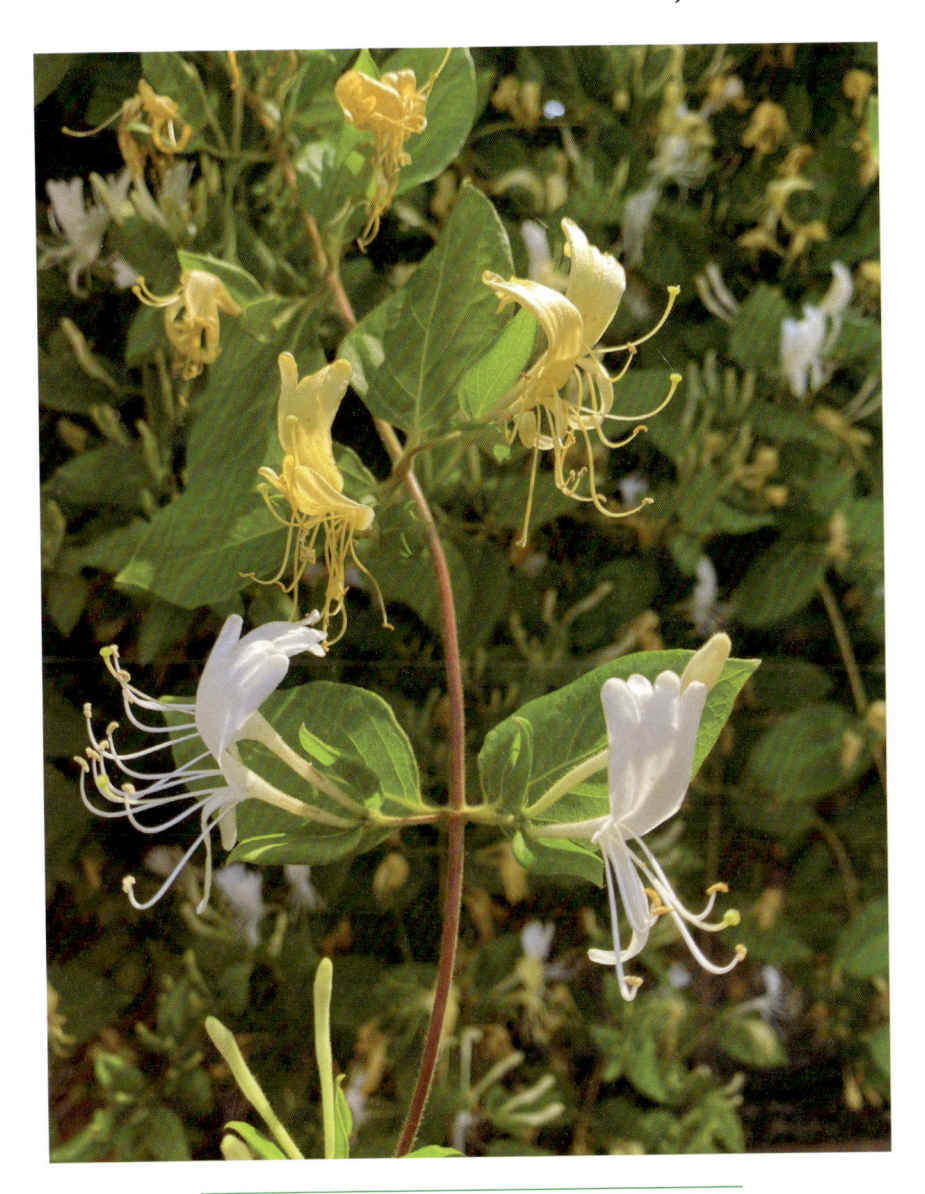

Honeysuckle flowers fill your senses with sweetness

HONEYSUCKLE
(Lonicera japonica)

Primary quality: balance
Energy impact/chakra correspondence: third and seventh chakras

Voice of the Flower

Open your hands as if to receive the warmth of the sun's brilliant rays, as the soles of your feet sink into the cool, moist earth. Let the flow of energy move from your hands all the way to your feet. Now let the energy flow back from your feet and be received by your hands. Experience this connection between your hands and feet that I offer you. Let it fill your senses. Feel the balance that it brings to you. Notice that my leaves grow in pairs, providing balance for my flowers to emerge. The joining of my leaves indicates the bringing together of opposites.

My flowers carry a rich, powerful, sweet fragrance. They are creamy white and tubular, breaking forth into pairs and dividing into five lobes that split into two diverging lips. My upper lip consists of four uniting lobes, and they look like little feet or hands with four toes or fingers. The lower, single lobe or lip arches backward. Five long, white, spindly stamens with yellow anthers and one pale green, pin-headed pistil emerge from my center.

My sweet, powerful aroma and the taste of my flower's nectar offer the sensation of grace and balance. I invite you to feel the presence of being in the moment now. Let the sweet flow of life harmonize naturally within you. Feel union within yourself. Enjoy and nurture the balance that you hold inside of you.

Insight

Honeysuckle offers you a sense of peace and balance within. Trust and accept the seeming contradictions within yourself. Honeysuckle brings these opposites together to provide balance, integration, and harmony.

Imagine tasting honeysuckle's sweet and powerful nectar. Allow it to bring you to a place of wonderment that you experienced as a child. Let its refreshing taste uplift you and bring harmony within. Fill your senses with its enticing aroma.

Experience the harmony that brings wholeness to you. Stir your passion for new possibilities. Bring sweetness and happiness into your life. Feel your inner balance.

Honeysuckle is known to be a cooling herb that clears heat, along with other medicinal applications. The flowers are used in perfumes, essential oils, and potpourris.

Many nectar-feeding pollinators love the sweet food source that honeysuckles provide. These include especially hummingbirds and varieties of bees and butterflies.

Honeysuckle flower essence tastes like it smells—fragrantly sweet and nectarous. Its taste is pleasantly uplifting and refreshing!

✦ *Affirmation* ✦

I live in balance and harmony and arouse the sweetness of life.

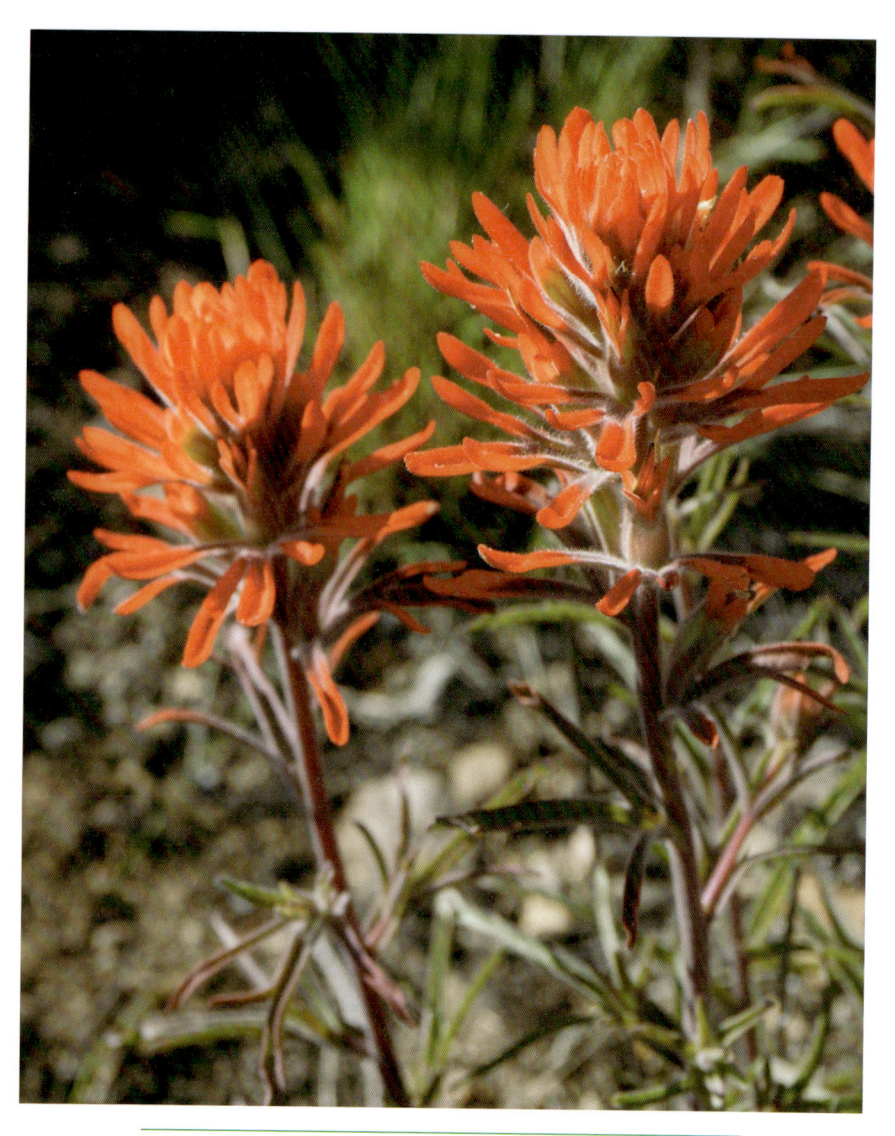

Indian paintbrush's fiery red blossoms artistically appear

INDIAN PAINTBRUSH
(Castilleja chromosa)

Primary quality: boundless creativity
Energy impact/chakra correspondence: first, second, fourth, and sixth chakras

Voice of the Flower

Notice my bright, reddish-orange presence. My appearance is highly artistic. I offer you a sense of warmth and creativity. My soft, fuzzy leaves and flowers reach outward as if to receive and give vital energy.

Imagine peeling back my vibrant red clusters to explore my inner essence. Hidden deep inside, envision my tiny, pale green, rather modest flower blossoms. Visualize these little treasures inside of me. Feel the presence of your own inner core. Take in the scent of my sweet nectar.

Envision what it would feel like to absorb water and nutrients from the roots of a nearby tree, or to host plants that help you to thrive and blossom until you have enough strength to survive on your own. Become familiar with my inner essence and the inner essence within yourself. Listen to my healing gifts.

I invite you to enter the silence of your mind, where no voice is heard and no sound is made. In this deep stillness, feel my presence. Allow your roots, at the deepest core of your being, to draw on my resources. Awaken the power within yourself to lovingly nurture your roots to grow deeper. Encourage your roots to spread out in new directions. Come to realize that no matter where you came from or who you are, you have the ability to create within yourself a new foundation.

Experience the silence in me, and in this place feel the fullness of survival in your world. Discover a newfound freedom. My silence inspires your vision, your passion for life, and your creativity.

Feel a stirring of boundless inspiration. New insights and life visions may arrive at your doorstep. Discover the beauty of living a more interdependent life with others. Stay connected to your roots and the strength of your foundation. Anchor your inner treasures.

Insight

Indian paintbrush reminds you to ground yourself and take time out from your daily life to be still and relax in silence. In silence, feel your inner cohesion. From this place of a silent mind and body, healing happens.

Indian paintbrush burrows its own root system into the roots of nearby host plants. Once Indian paintbrush can hold its own, it no longer needs to struggle for survival. This plant's dependence on other plants demonstrates the virtue of interdependence and the ability to survive and flourish with the help of other plants until it gathers enough strength to survive on its own.

We often need support from others to assist us with our survival needs—getting a job, finding an affordable home, health and nutritional guidance. Once those basic needs are met, we feel relief that we can live life more freely and creatively. Likewise, the sharing of a host plant's vital nutrients with Indian paintbrush, with seemingly no loss or harm to the host, is an example of interdependence and shows the importance of being a humble receiver and a compassionate giver.

Indian paintbrush's true flowers are pale green, hidden inside its reddish-orange bracts. It's these colorful bracts that dot desert landscapes and mountain meadows. They give a sense of creativity, warmth, and vitality. Tucked inside the beautiful reddish bracts lie hidden the true essence and nectar of the flower; its gift is to share with you the power of your own inner treasures. It wants you to thrive on your own sweet nectar and to be creative in all the ways that you live in the world.

With each moment you are creating your life. New insights and life visions may arrive at your doorstep at any moment.

The long, white corolla tube in Indian paintbrush contains a sweet nectar at its base and can be pulled out and eaten. The Diné (Navajo) make a tan dye from the blossoms and a greenish-yellow dye from the stems and leaves, which is used to dye wool in traditional rug-making. The root is used to treat spider bites. Caution: Due to its high selenium content, it should be used internally only in small doses.

The bright red flowers of Indian paintbrush attract pollinators such as bees, butterflies, and hummingbirds.

The scent of Indian paintbrush is slightly bitter, and its flower essence tastes strong and bitter. It offers a feeling of being present and grounded, sending a tingling sensation to the root chakra.

✦ *Affirmation* ✦

I feel relaxed and rooted in who I am,
knowing that my needs are met easily and creatively.

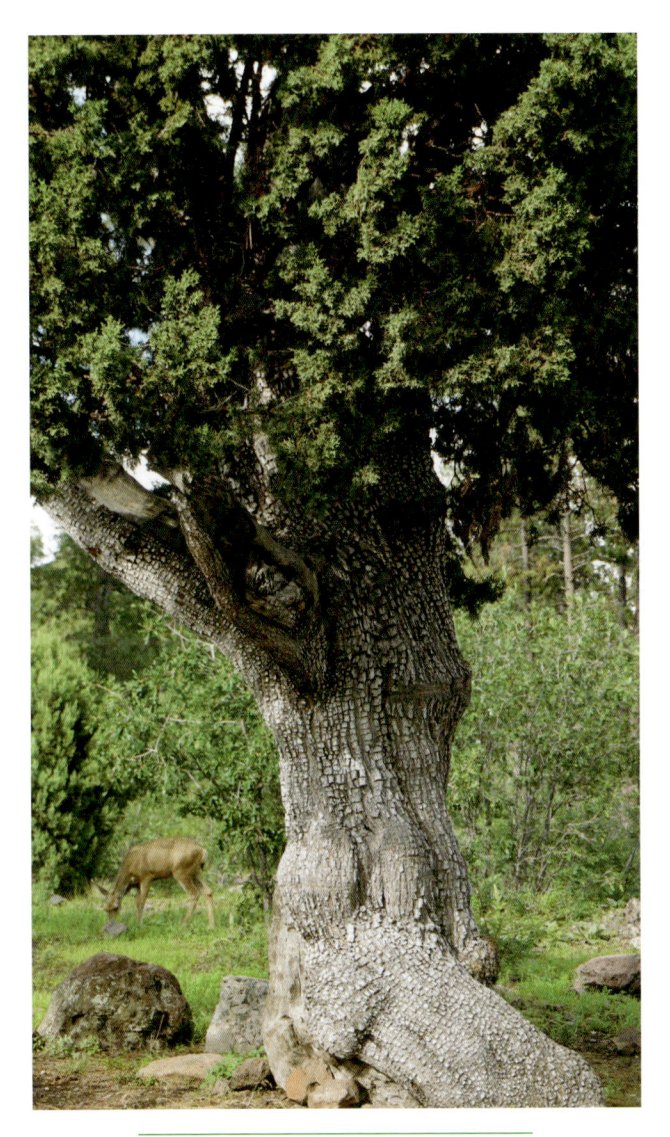

Juniper tree restores your inner being

JUNIPER
(Juniperus deppeana)

Primary quality: deep cleansing and renewal
Energy impact/chakra correspondence: all chakras—first, second, third, fourth, fifth, sixth, and seventh

Voice of the Flower (Needles)

Imagine that you are sitting on the earth, facing my massive, woody trunk. Feel my life force and power, and experience the circle of protection all around you and me.

Let your eyes follow the furrowed patterns in my bark. Place a hand on my bark and a hand on the earth. Feel my rugged texture on your fingers and notice how my bumpy, checkered pattern is largest at the base of my trunk. As you look at the patterns in my bark, notice how they appear smaller as they travel up my branches. I encourage you to explore higher, up high to the greater expanse of my freedom.

I inspire you to face your own internal patterns. Become more aware of your relationship to any unwanted patterns that no longer serve your purpose. As your unwanted patterns release, appreciate the new freedom that awaits you.

Beneath the surface of where you are sitting, imagine my roots burrowing inside the darkness of the earth, finding nutrients for survival. As you connect with my grounding energy, visualize the darkness and mystery of growing and evolving out of the earth. Envision my expansive root system below you as you breathe in from the earth and into my roots. Feel your strength and mine as you become deeply rooted. Become more aware of the many living organisms, elements, and electromagnetic fields below you and surrounding you.

Listen to the sounds made below the earth—electrical signals, sound waves, and communication emerging through my roots and moving upward to my crown. As your breath rises from my roots and upward into my branches, stems, needles, and berries, bring in the woody aroma of my refreshing blue-green needles.

Experience the revitalizing and cool taste of my scent and essence as the slightest breeze moves through your body, mind, and spirit to instigate deep cleansing and renewal.

Insight

Juniper helps you feel your strength and ability to endure. This sturdy tree can survive in drought and thrives in the heat of the day, and in thunderstorms, lightening, rain, and snow. It is able to form a huge network of nutrients that supports and sustains its life force. Allow yourself to feel juniper's protection. Shield yourself with a field of energy all around you and within you. Listen to your breath. Notice how you feel. Let the power of the earth come through to you.

Notice any unwanted pattern that has served its purpose and is no longer needed. Give it a voice. Confront the undesired pattern—acknowledge and embrace it. Show it love and compassion. Then let it go and thank it for the lessons and insights it has shown you.

Become aware of your roots, your foundation. See yourself growing larger and taller, expanding outward, creating a large circle of strength and protection all around you. As a juniper, notice what you see at your highest point. Be aware of your arms as branches of the tree, your fingers as the needles and berries, your sacrum and spine as the trunk, your feet and tailbone as the roots. Take in all that you can.

Juniper offers deep protection, cleansing, and purification. Its presence brings a feeling of being held in Grandmother's loving arms. Its scent fills your body, mind, and spirit with deep cleansing and renewal. Stir the depths of your internal awareness to create healing and rejuvenation. Bathe in the freedom of your new experience.

Dried juniper berries can be crushed and used to flavor foods and are the primary flavor in gin. Juniper berries can be made into bracelets and necklaces to be used for protection, healing, and purification. They can also be thrown on hot rocks in sweat lodges. Juniper essential oil tones the skin and makes for a refreshing, rejuvenating scent to fill your home.

Juniper trees are known to clear negative energy, to lift the spirits of those who are depressed, and to take in a refreshing new outlook. Juniper wood is pleasant and aromatic. It deflects moths, which makes it good for use as a blanket chest. The wood also is commonly burned in Southwestern homes to provide heat during winter months.

Juniper trees are wind-pollinated and people can be very allergic to their pollen.

Juniper needles have a distinct piney scent reminiscent of a Christmas tree. Its essence tastes like it smells and is refreshing and invigorating.

✦ *Affirmation* ✦

> I am aware of my need to take time out, to be present, and to live a life that restores and renews me.

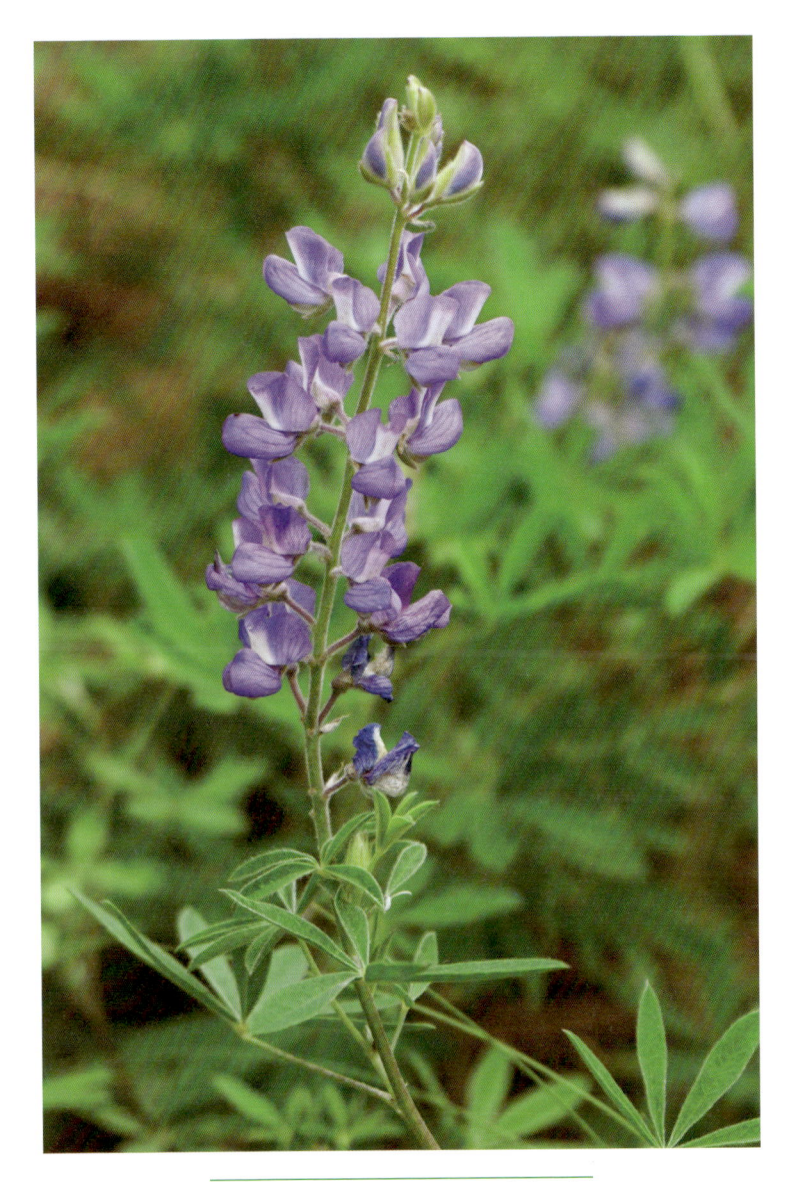

Lupine flowers reach toward the sky

LUPINE
(Lupinus spp.)

Primary quality: higher purpose
Energy impact/chakra correspondence: sixth and seventh chakras

Voice of the Flower

My colorful, showy flowers are pealike in appearance and grow in terminal clusters toward the top of my hairy stem. My flower consists of two petals. The broader upper petal is slightly hairy on its back and seems to fold backward. The smaller petal folds are closed. If you open up the inside of my folds you will see five or six tiny stamens with golden-orange anthers. When ripe, a small, green, fuzzy seed pod appears. You can see the impression of little peas or beans inside my pod. One white spot appears on each fold of the upper petal. The lower petal is solid lavender in color. My flowers carry a sweet and pleasant fragrance.

My broad, bluish-lavender flower petals offer just a trace of being open yet are well-protected. My light-filled flower carries a deep sense of inner vision. My open palm–shaped leaflets face the sun throughout the day to receive water that nurtures me. Visualize your open hands receiving the sweetness of life and guiding you on your journey.

I am here to assist you on your path of higher purpose. Observe the way you receive and use your abilities to make choices. Discover your true path as you walk your life's journey. You will come to understand that the power within you is based on your ability to know yourself.

Receive my guidance and let me illuminate you along your path. Feel the power of my presence entering and energizing your being. In the stillness of this moment, allow a step to take place between what was and what will become. In this place, let light fill your silence and carry your vision. This will allow you to experience your higher purpose. It will take you beyond time and space.

Insight

Lupine leads you on a path of healing or a path to find a higher purpose or deeper meaning to life. A plant journey with lupine carries a deep sense of inner vision, of following one's path of spiritual evolution. Being in the presence of lupine opens you to be filled with light energy. It awakens your intuition and visionary capabilities at a deep level.

The essence of lupine grants you the ability to step beyond yourself. It helps you to achieve your vision and to bring it into physical reality. By doing so, you enrich yourself and others and your life choices.

Acknowledge the silence or space of being that lupine offers you. Allow yourself to be in that space without looking ahead or behind.

A feature of lupine is its open palm–shaped leaflets that face the sun throughout the day. When our hands are open and not clenched, we can feel the power of light entering and energizing us. Open hands depict giving as well as receiving, as well as being in balance.

Feel a natural flow of energy taking place within you. Feel the energy of your body in the present moment. This awareness will guide you on your path toward a higher purpose.

With help from certain bacteria, lupine's root nodules put the nitrogen that they obtain from the air back into the soil. The seeds of some lupine species are used in lotions to treat skin problems.

Effective pollinators for lupine are a variety of bees, hummingbirds, and butterflies. Lupine seed pods can drop up to a dozen seeds.

The fragrance of lupine is soft and sweet. Its flower essence is also sweet, mellow, and smooth.

✦ *Affirmation* ✦

I am open to trusting my journey.
I surrender to my higher purpose.

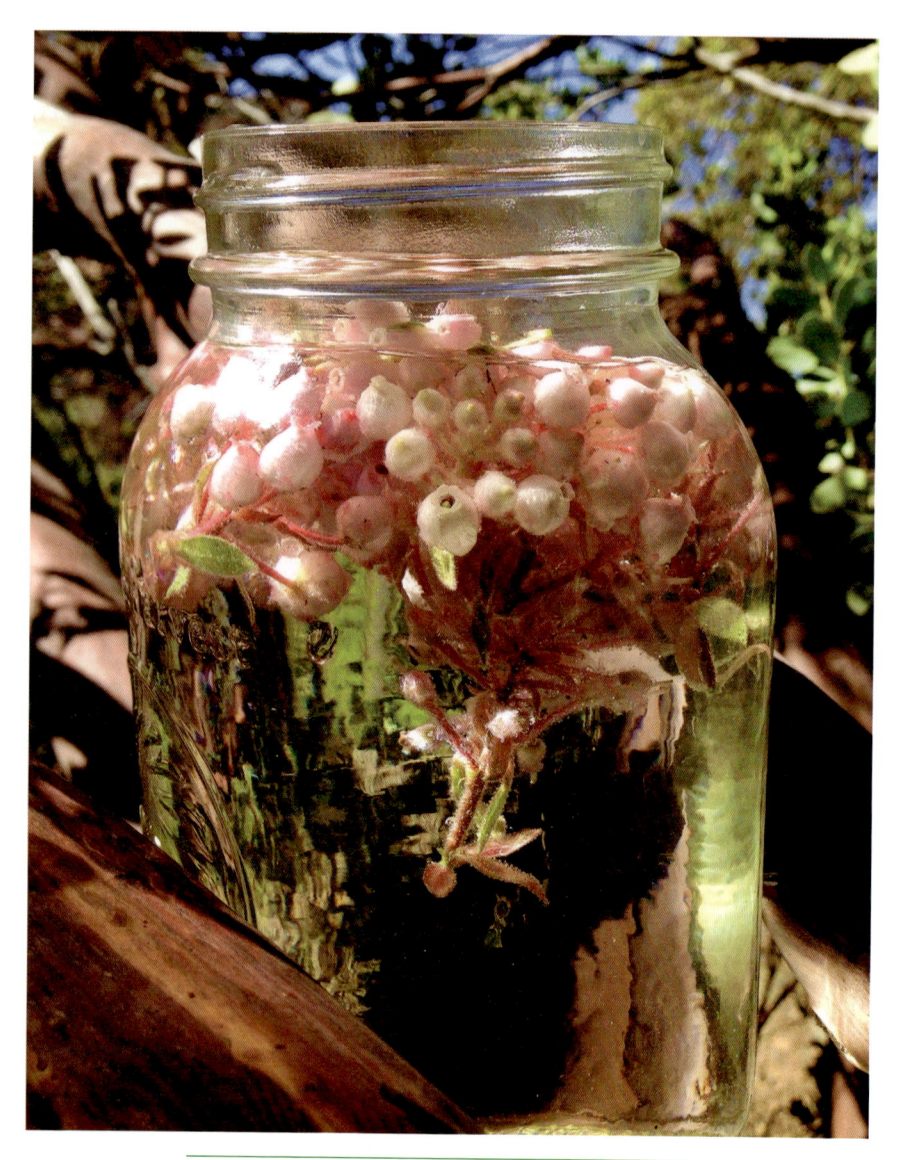

186   The Guiding Voice of Flowers, Trees, and Plants

Manzanita flower essence energizes with the tree

MANZANITA
(Arctostaphylos pungens)

Primary quality: heart-filled vessel
Energy impact/chakra correspondence: first and fourth chakras

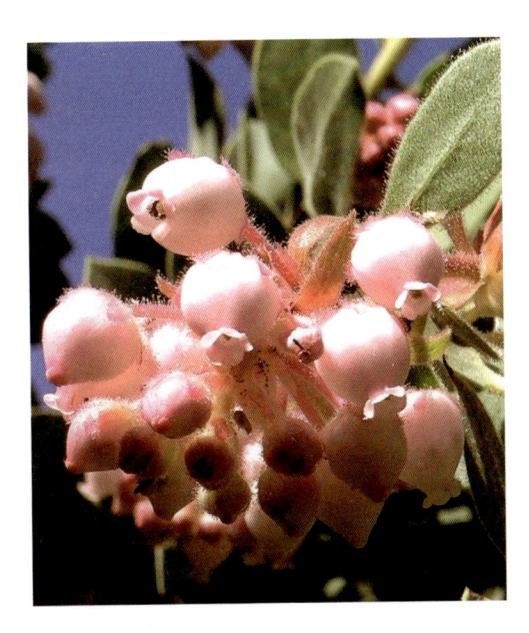

Manzanita flowers burst forth with energy

Voice of the Flower

Imagine you are walking on a wilderness trail. You notice a vibrant shimmering in the sun before you. As you come closer, your wonderment builds, and you feel that something is beckoning you to the rich, reddish-orange bark of my graceful presence before you. My smooth bark calls out for you to touch it. You are instantly drawn to my enchanting beauty and my message. I can survive in drought and appear green and healthy even on the hottest days of summer.

My leaves alternate along my branches. They are thick, evergreen, and smooth. My branches look like arteries extending from my trunk, which you can envision as a heart, pumping blood out to my many branches. I am a reflection of the inner workings of the human body.

My pinkish-white flowers emerge like vessels filled with droplets of nectar. They hang elegantly from my slender stems. They are borne in terminal clusters that are sticky and hairy. Each of my flowers forms a tear-shaped tubular bud with a yellow tip. Five flower petals form a circle at the tip of each flower, and five at the bottom. A flurry of tiny white stamens arise from my center. My sticky resin and fruity-sweet fragrance attracts bees and hummingbirds.

I was named manzanita, Spanish for "little apple." My berries are small, fleshy apples with a thin skin and a large central seed—and they taste like apples, too.

I am here to help you to listen to your heart. My pink petals smell like apples and honey. See the bees and the hummingbirds feasting on my sweet nectar. Listen to their contented sounds as they suck up nourishment.

Whatever behaviors, thoughts, or emotional turmoil you carry, connect to the true heart of the matter. Allow yourself to breathe and listen to what your heart is saying. Stop and take time for yourself and only yourself.

My love and radiance pour through to you. Trust what you feel in your heart. Connect with your natural flow. Live life from a place of self-love. Feel the sweetness of life's flow pulsing through your heart and your whole body. Give yourself permission to relax and experience joyful freedom. Blossom into a gentle release. Enter your heart-filled vessel.

Insight

Manzanita encourages you to form a deeper relationship with yourself, with your heart and the blood that circulates throughout your body.

The life force field of manzanita is characterized by the tree's smooth yet twisted branches and reddish bark. The flow and movement of manzanita offers a feeling of blood flowing through your arteries, enlivening you.

Manzanita's small, pinkish-white, vessel-shaped flowers represent the bursting forth of life-flowing energy. Being with manzanita offers a heart awakening and feeling of vitality. Manzanita reminds you to listen to your heart, to bring peace into your heart. We are all born out of love. It's always in us. Manzanita is about being aware of this and letting your love energy pulsate within you and then radiating it out.

Manzanita promotes a loving relationship with your heart, bringing you joy and compassion.

Manzanita's smooth, rich, reddish-brown branches are a feature of the high desert. Teas and leaves of manzanita are known to help with nausea, upset stomach, and diarrhea. Native Americans soak the leaves and use them as a poultice to reduce inflammation and discomfort related to poison oak.

Manzanita is known to treat mild urinary-tract infections and bladder gravel, and can be used in sitz baths following rectal or uterine surgery, after childbirth, and for vaginitis. Mix the berries with apple juice to make a jelly with a semisweet, tart flavor. Manzanita leaves can be smoked, and its dense root crowns and thick wood can be used for carving and woodworking.[5]

Dried manzanita leaves can be smoked; they "offer a strong body and flavor, astringent, [to] mix in small amounts with other herbs . . . this was one of the plants used as a base for smoke mixes by almost all the First Nations."[6]

Floral visitors that are attracted to manzanitas include hummingbirds, butterflies, wasps, moths, flies, and bees.

According to the Watershed Project: "In a fascinating show of symbiosis and adaptation, bumble bees employ a sonic technique called 'buzz pollination' where, while hanging upside down on a manzanita flower, they vibrate their flight muscles to a pitch of middle C, causing the pollen grains to be released from the anthers and onto the bee's fuzzy abdomen. As the bumble bee moves from flower to flower, it fertilizes the stigmas with the pollen clinging to its belly—brilliant!"[7]

Manzanita's flower essence tastes like the apple-honey fragrance its flowers give out. It provides a lingering note of harmony throughout the body

✦ *Affirmation* ✦

I trust my heart's flow in my life's journey.

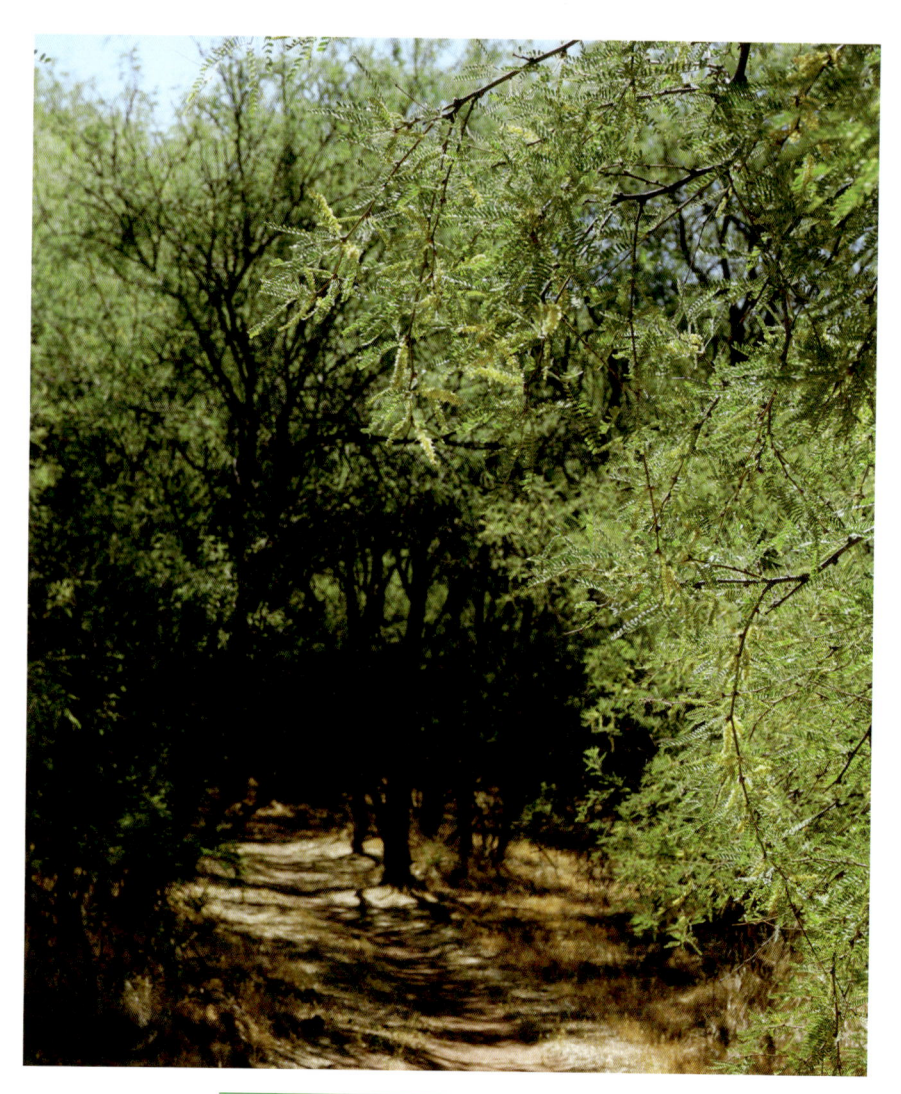

Mesquite forest invites you into its mystery

MESQUITE
(*Prosopis* spp.)

Primary quality: trusting the invisible
Energy impact/chakra correspondence: first and fourth chakras

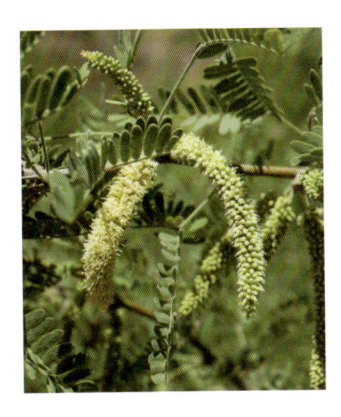

Mesquite catkins adorn the tree with a sweet scent of musk

Voice of the Flower (Catkin)

I invite you on a journey into the underworld of my mesquite forest. Face the darkness of the unknown, any fears or shadows that you may be holding deep inside. Remain awake as you enter my invisible energy field. I extend an offer to you to travel into those untold places within yourself that you may or may not know.

Feel magic stirring throughout your body; it is the power of my magic. Enter the mystical path through my enchanting mesquite forest. Under my canopy, ground yourself, silence your mind, and become still within. Imagine my gnarled and persistent roots growing deep below you. Trust that the mystery of the darkness holds what you cannot see.

Visualize placing your hands on my shaggy, rough bark.

Feel the ridges of my bark between your fingers. Allow my woody, musky aroma to stir your senses. Embrace the excitement that this energy brings.

Now look up into my branches. Though my bark may appear old and my stature twisted, trust the innate nature of who I am.

My dense leaves are fernlike in appearance. My thorns represent the thorns that you encounter in life. What will it take for you to get past those thorns and trust the mystery of the unseen?

As my catkins blossom from my branches, you, too, can trust the unseen energy that is brought forth from my trunk and roots below.

I give you an opportunity to look into your own undercurrents. Step into the invisibility of your underworld and connect with whatever it is that you have buried there over time, the deepest and darkest places of your life's journey. Find the truths that have been buried. Trust the darkness. Support is available on your journey, even in the darkest of times. Give the shadow a voice and bring it into the light. Listen to what your inner voice is saying to you. Receive its message and the opportunity for growth that it brings. It will instill wisdom and shed light on how far you've really come on your life's journey. Feel the power of this transformation and keep it within you. Know that "the truth shall set you free."

In doing this for yourself, you build your trust in the mystery of what is unseen, knowing that it is coming from the richness of your deepest undercurrents.

Insight

Mesquite offers you a deep and enriching presence that you may feel but cannot necessarily see. Mesquite brings in mystery and intrigue that calls on you to trust what cannot be seen but lives deep within.

Mesquite is a small, leguminous, vascular tree, native to the U.S. Southwest and Mexico. It is extremely hardy and drought-tolerant. It draws water from the water table through its long taproot. Mesquite trees leverage similarities and differences in their own microbial makeup. They share their nutrients through a mycorrhizal network with other trees of their own species. Mesquites are quite resilient to changes in the environment due to their symbiotic relationship with fungi and other microbes. Our mesquite forests and their invisible microbes hold an ancient wisdom and keep our ecosystems in balance.

Mesquites can adapt and grow in various kinds of soil. They provide shade and wildlife habitat in areas where other trees cannot grow. Mesquites are much more than what they appear to be—they offer food, fuel, medicine, and much more.

Mesquite's tiny budding catkins are lime green and waxy. They are symmetrical in shape and size, length, and width. Five tiny-petaled, pale green or yellowish flowers emerge in clusters. They draw many pollinating insects.

If you take a bite from a tiny bud of a catkin you may be surprised by its refreshingly fruity taste. This is an example of the power of mesquite's unseen presence—it is something more than what appears on the surface. As mesquite catkins sprout from the tree's branches, this is a reminder that you, too, can trust the blossoms of your inner wisdom. Experience the unseen energy that is fed through mesquite's trunk and roots below as if it is your own.

Mesquite's roots and root hairs branch into the earth to take in water and nutrients. Its underground stems move moisture and nutrients to and from its catkin flowers and leaves.

Mesquite roots support the trunk and the entire growth of the tree. Your own root system supports the trunk of your being and your growth. Your inner wisdom may be hidden from you, buried in your darkest places. It's the pain of what you're still holding onto that masks your wisdom. It's not the wisdom that brings you fear, it's the pain that you shove down. Once you bring it up and are aware of it, you bring it into the light of consciousness and in so doing, you release it.

To trust the invisible in the darkness is to know it from deep within. Trust in the inner wisdom that this tree offers. Apply it to the areas in your life that will help you to trust that what is unseen will ultimately help you grow.

Mesquites are the most common trees in the Desert Southwest. Leaves, catkins, twigs, gum, and bark can all be used in medicine-making. Mesquite seed pods, also known as the fruit of the mesquites, can be ground into a tasty meal or flour; they can also be used whole in decoctions and syrups. Mesquite catkins offer a musky fragrance and fruity taste. A powdered tea made from mesquite seed pods can be used as an astringent, an eye wash to treat pink eye, to treat gastrointestinal inflammation and intestinal distress.[8]

The preparation and extensive uses of mesquite are quite detailed. You may want to explore more of this invaluable plant on your own.

Mesquites' primary pollinators are bees. In the American Southwest, there are over 160 species of bees in relation to mesquites.

Its catkin flower essence tastes refreshing, like what you experience following a fresh rain.

✦ *Affirmation* ✦

I trust the mystery of the unseen.

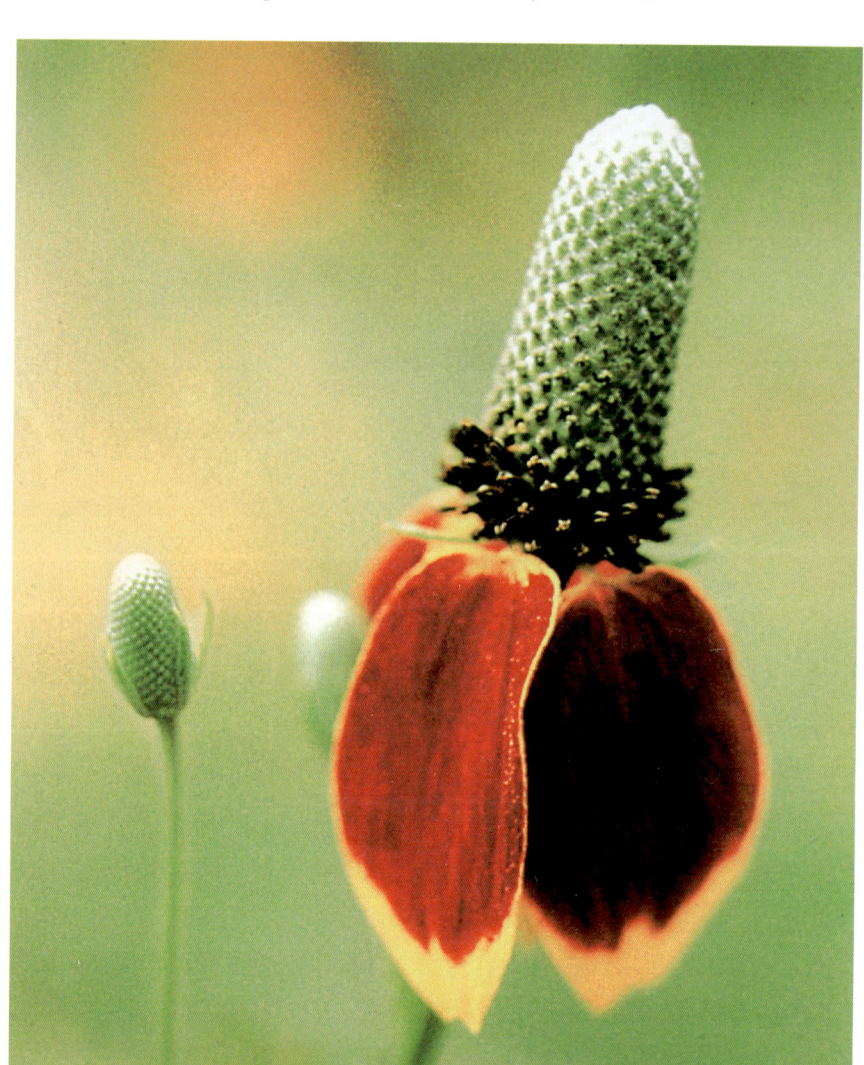

Mexican hat flower surrenders to the earth as it rises toward the sun

MEXICAN HAT
(Ratibida columnaris)

Primary quality: freeing pain
Energy impact/chakra correspondence: first, second, and third chakras

Voice of the Flower

Come sit under my flowering crown. Allow yourself to rest and listen. Feel the nature of my protection and look at my sombrero-shaped flower. Notice how my yellow and reddish-orange petals reach down toward the earth, yet my seeded conehead springs up toward the sky.

I am here to help you experience the freedom of becoming aware of any kind of pain you are carrying. Visualize placing your hands on the earth. Allow the earth to absorb your pain. Feel her strength and support. Become aware of any pain you may be feeling. Embrace the discomfort of your pain. Talk to it. Give your pain a voice. Thank the pain for what it has taught you about yourself. Allow the pain to help you to let go of it. The power it has held over you is now released and transformed.

The simplicity of my individualism shows that each of my petals is a separate unit, yet connected to the whole.

You may feel certain emotions or pain that you choose not to share with others. As I grow in a community of others like me, I acknowledge that each individual plant has its own identity and power to heal. Stand true to your own power as you experience the freedom of releasing your pain.

Insight

Mexican hat guides you to acknowledge and release any burdens or pain you carry. This plant's drooping petals reach down toward the earth. They signify the plant's ability to surrender and its need to be connected to the earth. Mexican hat gives you the opportunity to face your pain. Release the emotional hold it has on you. Surrender to the pain for what it is and what it represents in you. This will help you to connect deeper to your true Self.

Listen to your inner voice as you reach out and connect with the support that the Earth gives you. Embrace your healing process from deep within. There comes a time when you become aware that prolonging the connection to your pain only makes it grow deeper.

Like Mexican hat's seeded conehead reaching toward the sky, you, too, can awaken to the freedom of moving forward as you ground yourself in the earth. Let go of the hold that pain has had on you. Step forward in a new direction that supports your journey.

Mexican hat offers you the feeling of being whole and free in who you are.

Native Americans make a pleasant-tasting tea of Mexican hat by brewing its leaves and flower heads.

Bees, butterflies, and beetles are considered the main pollinators of Mexican hat flowers.

The scent of Mexican hat flower essence water is slightly fruity, although its taste is bitter and pungent. It asks your gut to free yourself of your burdens.

✦ *Affirmation* ✦

I let go of the thoughts that hold me back.
I am empowered and free.

Morning Glory 197

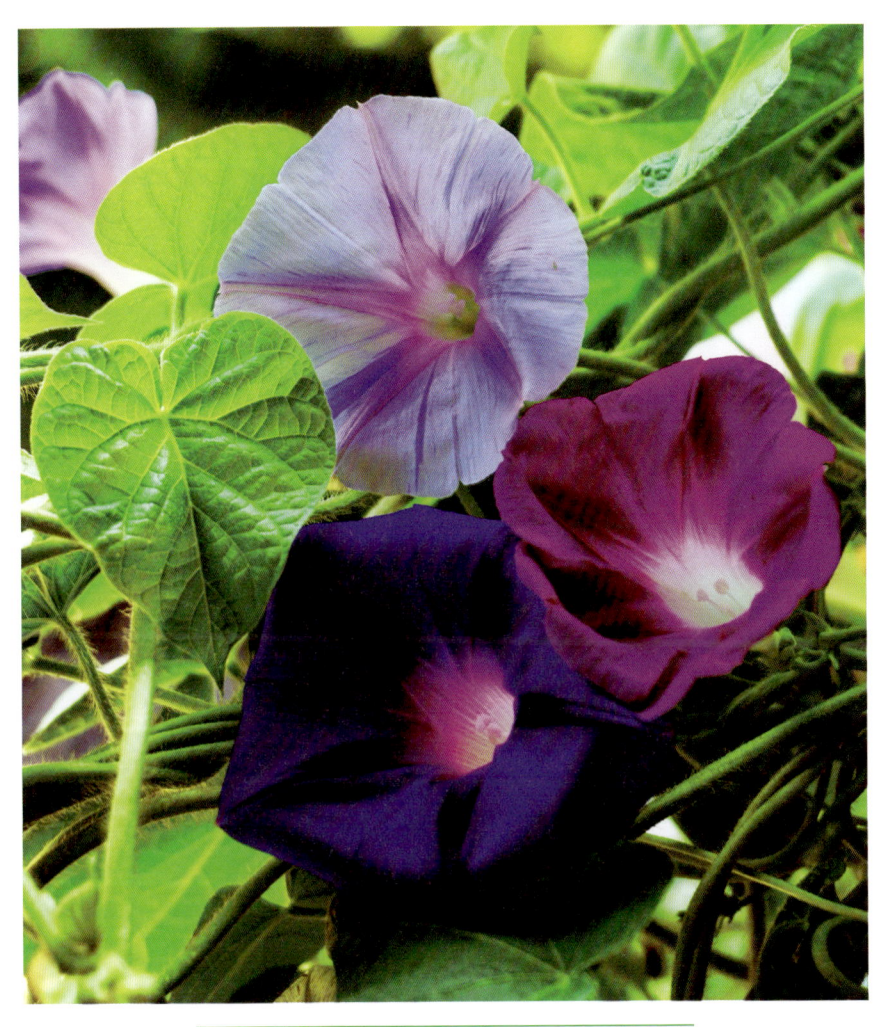

Morning glory flowers shine forth with new life

MORNING GLORY
(Ipomoea purpurea)

Primary quality: new beliefs
Energy impact/chakra correspondence: fourth, sixth, and seventh chakras

Voice of the Flower

My name, glory, speaks of the splendor of my luminous colors. A glowing light emerges from the center of my flower. I offer illumination, inspiration, and higher vision.

My splendor shines forth in celebrating the dawn of a new day. As the sun begins its journey in the east, I, too, open up my violet-purple petals. I embrace the beginning of a new day. I offer you the awareness to begin anew.

Experience the feeling of being liberated in this moment, completely free of worries and doubts. Let this moment guide you to begin a new way of exploring your beliefs. I offer you an opportunity to make a fresh start and begin a new way of living.

Receive the wisdom of my glorious nature. I invite you to give yourself permission to break away from old patterns. Embrace your light. Let my essence help you move toward self-liberation.

Insight

Notice the soft and gentle glow in the center of morning glory's flower. Feel the presence of this glow within you, and let it enter your being. Bring your awareness to the deep magenta star that reaches toward the edges of the flower and the violet-purple color of the petals.

A morning glory flower begins anew every day, unfolding a fresh blossom with the rising sun. Once it has experienced its full bloom in the morning it closes up, and despite their brief existence morning glories leave behind new seeds for new growth.

Morning glory says that every seed you gather in your life carries new life. You are encouraged to plant your seeds one by one as you grow your bouquet of wisdom that leads to freedom.

Morning glory helps you to be in touch with your natural rhythms. It stimulates your ability to make a fresh start as you begin a new day or explore a new thought.

Perhaps the beautiful glowing colors of morning glory will beckon to you to get up in the morning to watch a sunrise.

There are over six hundred species of morning glory. Because of the wide variety of species and the different effects produced by the use of the seeds as opposed to the roots, it's difficult to document this plant's use as an herbal remedy. The species of morning glory shown here is a common cultivated garden plant that doesn't produce hallucinogenic effects, unlike the seeds of the wild plants, which have been used by shamans to support people on their spiritual journeys.

Morning glory flowers provide various vitamins and minerals and are known to reduce stress, improve sleep, treat digestion, and support the immune system. The roots have a purgative effect due to their fatty acids. We do not suggest ingesting morning glory seeds, as they can produce ill side effects. This is not a plant to abuse.

Bees and butterflies are effective pollinators of morning glory. There are bees called *morning glory bees* that are associated with morning glory flowers.

Morning glory flower essence offers a subtle scent, although the essence water itself is stronger and slightly sweet. The authors have experienced an intensification of visually seeing brightness and colors of light when taking moring glory flower essence.

✦ *Affirmation* ✦

I celebrate this day with a new thought,
a new feeling, and a new activity.

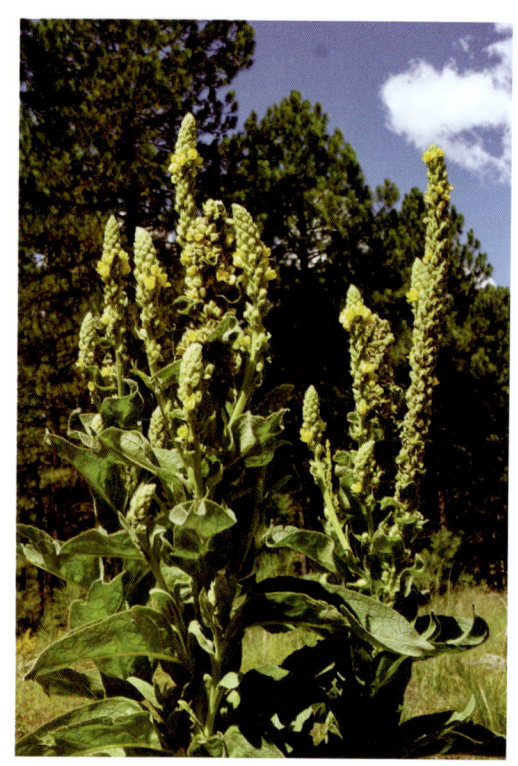

Mullein plants soothe, calm, and nurture

Mullein flowers help you to listen to your inner self

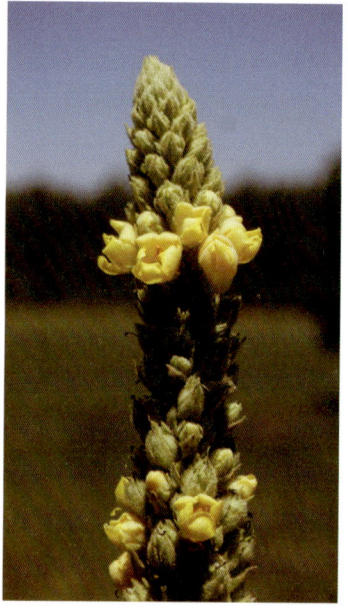

MULLEIN
(Verbascum thapsus)

Primary quality: intimacy
Energy impact/chakra correspondence: second and third chakras

Voice of the Flower

I have a powerful ability to take in and absorb that which feeds my life, my spirit, and my growth. I will show you the benefit of taking in and absorbing all that is you.

My stalk is stout, thick, and tall, and my base especially strong. My leaves grow in a basal rosette. They are velvety and densely hairy. The entirety of me is soft and fuzzy. My stalk rises from the center of my rosette-shaped leaves and reaches toward the sky. My strength of character along with my softness offers protection all around me.

As my five-petaled, lemon-cupped flowers and seeds are securely shielded in my soft and woolly flesh, I offer you security and protection. In this place, trust your own personal intimacy. Listen to your inner voice and inner truths. Empower your ability to go deeper inside yourself. Trust your own inner resources. Feel safe within yourself. Listen to your inner voice. Experience my intimate nature, my gentle strength, and my soft touch.

Insight

Mullein leads you on the path of wholeness that seeks intimacy and security within yourself as well as in your relationships.

Mullein's densely packed, lemon-yellow flowers and buds circle around and upward toward the top of its spike, giving off a yellowish light. This is a signature of the plant's ability to promote focus, purpose, and lightness. It guides us to the awareness of our own inner light and encourages us to share our light with others.

The woolly, earlike signature of mullein reminds you to listen to your inner self and to likewise listen to others in the ways that you communicate. This plant teaches you to listen to your inner voice, to live and act according to your truth and your values.

The enormous absorbency of mullein leaves is a powerful signature of the plant. They act as a relaxant and promote absorption. On another level, this signature is related to your process of assimilating emotional and mental states that no longer serve you. Through the process of assimilation, you are able to take in and incorporate what you are able to absorb at the highest level possible.

Mullein is especially helpful for anyone who wants to strengthen yet soften their masculine nature. Mullein promotes strength with gentleness, encouraging you to build a tender closeness with your innermost self and invite intimacy into your life.

Mullein is a powerful, multifaceted plant, known as a natural wonder herb that dates back to ancient times. The leaves and flowers, prepared in teas, syrups, extracts, tinctures, infusions, and gargles, are used as an antispasmodic, mild diuretic, mild sedative, demulcent, emollient, expectorant, and tonic.

Mullein offers a plethora of medicinal uses. Herbalists use it to treat coughs, colds, bronchitis, asthma and catarrh, nervous disorders, hemorrhages in the lungs, shortness of breath, diaper rash, tonsillitis, migraine, earache, glandular swelling, pulmonary diseases, venereal disease, swollen joints, emphysema, nerve pain, burns, sprains, incontinence, edema, dysentery, and more.

The flowers can be used in a facial cream to soothe the skin or as an infusion to brighten hair. The seed oil soothes chapped skin, and the plant can also be used as a dye.

Smoking the leaves offers relaxation and serves as an expectorant. Our friend Mairi Ross characterizes mullein as "one of the friendliest smoke plants" and "traditionally one of the most frequently smoked plants."[9] It is known to be used in the Navajo Deer Way ceremony.

The soft-scented floral attributes of mullein flowers attract bumblebees as a vital pollinator among a few other kinds of bees and flies.

The scent of mullein is more prevalent in its flower essence water, where it carries a profound honeylike scent. Its taste is similar and stronger. Mullein's flower essence is soothing, cool, and gentle. It offers a relaxing feeling in the abdomen and solar plexus.

✦ *Affirmation* ✦

I give myself time each day to listen to myself.
I value my self-worth and the intimacy I feel within myself.

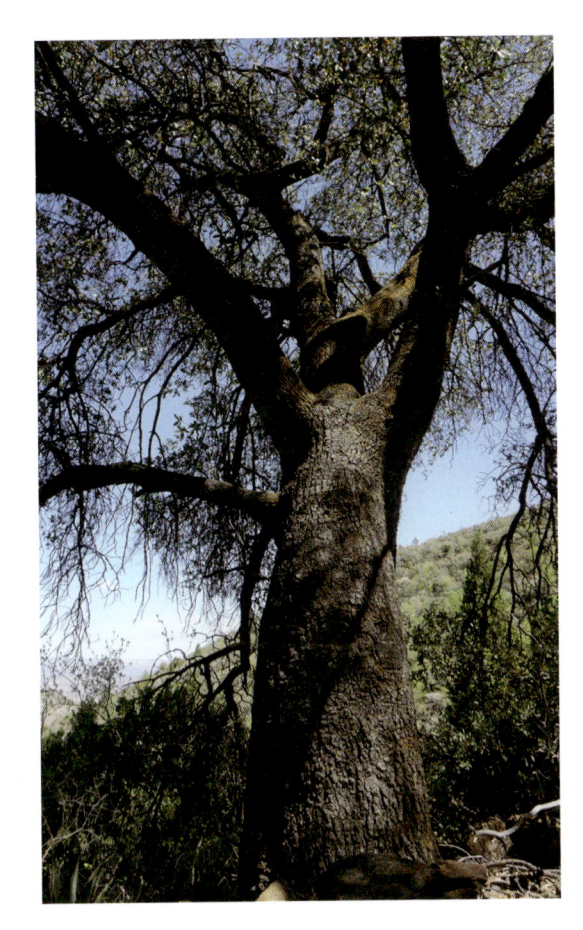

Oak tree's formidable presence (Grandfather Oak described in chapter 7)

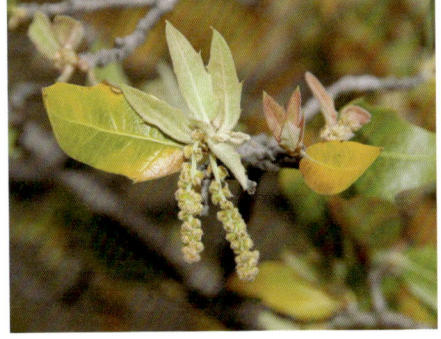

Oak catkins release their pollen to the winds

OAK
(Quercus gambelii)

Primary quality: grounding strength
Energy impact/chakra correspondence: first, second, and third chakras

Voice of the Flower (Catkin)

I am here before you in all my strength and beauty. Find a place below my branches that calls to you. Stand with me, wrap your arms around my trunk, and rest your cheek against my bark. Breathe in my woody scent.

As my roots grow deep into the underworld, pulsating, surviving, and thriving in the earth's rich soil, so too do my branches reach outward and upward, extending to the heavens.

Close your eyes and listen to the winds swirling through my catkins and branches. My catkins are strong and fuzzy. They find their hold on the stem, showing us how to grab on to our strength to empower who we are.

Often you will find small oak galls—abnormal outgrowths of plant tissue—on my branches and leaves. They enclose the larvae of nonstinging wasps. These galls are a signature of what it takes to have the "gall"—the nerve—to stand up for yourself, to speak your truth, and to move through a transformational chrysalis state. Follow your own inner guidance as you transform and move through life, leaving only a slight imprint of the past behind.

I want to share my enduring strength with you on your journey. Recognize your own strength and beauty within.

Insight

Oak offers the ability to anchor, protect, and be conscious of your own inner strength. Oak tree roots spread from root sprouts and grow from an underground, deep-feeding system. Rhizomes interconnect clones that intervene with the root system. It is fascinating that oak has the strength and ability to thrive under both morphological adaptations (physical changes that occur over generations based on environmental conditions such as water deficiency), and physiological adaptations (how the oak's internal response for survival reacts to external stimuli, especially to drought and moisture cycles, to gain and maintain homeostasis). Oak's deep root system supports the tree to sustain soil stability and reduce erosion.

Oak has the ability to thrive and survive climate changes and varying soil and moisture conditions. Oak paces itself slowly in its own steady growth cycle by tapping into its deep root system. This demonstrates the nature of oak's strength and its ability to gain, sustain, and maintain homeostasis.

Oak forms a strong foundation. Its strength comes from the inside, forming a structure of "strong bones," which teaches us the importance of what it means to anchor and hold our energy from a place of strength and endurance. Oak's enormous trunk and massive branches show the tree's strength and fortitude. Imagine that you can hear the hum of oak's power through the heart of its trunk.

The bark of the oak tree provides a sturdy shield, reminding us to guard the boundaries of our inner strength. By trusting our shield, we are reminded that we too can be strong and enduring, and find ways to adapt to our environment and life situations while nourishing ourselves.

Male flowers appear as drooping and fuzzy catkins or tassels. Their purpose is to release pollen that is carried by the wind to the female flowers.

Smaller female flowers grow in clusters with a ring of small leaves or bracts at the base. They produce a short spike with a cup-shaped growth that evolves into an acorn. When there is a lot of moisture, both male and female flowers gain their strength. They produce in abundance.

As the fruit and seeds of the tree, acorns offer yet another creative endeavor that displays strength and fortitude. This developmental stage of true originality sparks inspiration and encourages new ideas. It helps you to be aware of the forward motion that is derived from your own inner strength and steady pacing.

Oak nourishes strength from deep inside yourself, helping you find security in all the ways that you survive and endure in the world. It supports a feeling of being grounded and strong in who you are. Use your strength and energy to lend endurance to your life's journey.

Galls that grow on the gambel oak are highly astringent and can be used in the treatment of chronic diarrhea, hemorrhage, and dysentery. Oak acorns, sufficiently soaked or boiled to remove their tannins, can be eaten for sexual potency, and the root is an analgesic and cathartic, as well as a vulnerary.

Oak catkins carry a powerful musky, earthy, bittersweet scent. The catkin essence water tastes similar and is even stronger, offering a sense of grounding strength.

✦ *Affirmation* ✦

I feel anchored in and true to my own inner strength.

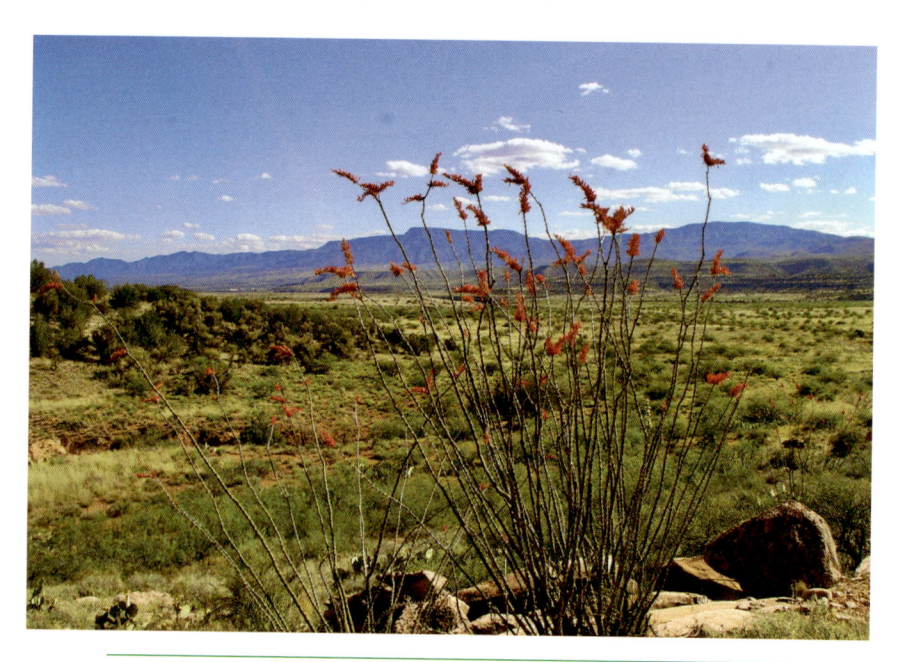

Ocotillo plants are luxuriant and exhilarate the desert landscape

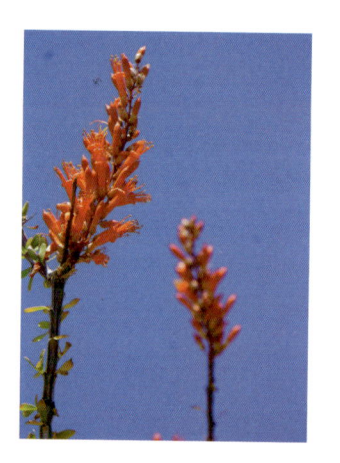

Ocotillo flowers' sweet nectar attracts hummingbirds and bees

OCOTILLO
(Fouquieria splendens)

Primary quality: creative life force
Energy impact/chakra correspondence: first, second, and third chakras

Voice of the Flower

I am a showy, flowering, spiny shrub of the rocky desert.

Near the bottom of my base my stem divides into many slender, erect, spiny branches. Small, rounded, drought-tolerant deciduous leaves grow from my branches and fall in the winter. They leave behind leaf stalks that develop into stout spines. My bright scarlet flowers branch out in terminal clusters.

I invite you to step into the vitality and creativity of my vibrant nature. Let your curiosity be stirred by my passionate red flowers and long spiny arms. My aura of protection bathes you with confidence, exuberance, and security.

Visualize a hummingbird entering my tubular crimson flowers and drinking my sweet nectar. Likewise, I invite you to explore the nectar deep within you that sustains and nurtures all that you are.

I am here to show you how to survive in the heat of the desert. Learn how to survive in your own conditions, both physically and emotionally.

I empower you to experience your emotions from a place of retrospection, to respond from a place of love. I offer you inner strength to accept yourself unconditionally. Like the hummingbird sipping my nectar, you, too, can gather resources to soothe and rejuvenate yourself.

Awaken your life force within. Open new doors for living a creative and light-filled life.

Insight

Ocotillo teaches you to become more aware of the life force driving your emotions.

Notice how ocotillo's spiny arms sway loosely in the wind, much like the wave motion that emotions ride in your energy system. Release your emotions and unconscious patterns to the wind. Feel the freedom of giving those patterns away. Ocotillo encourages you to ignite the creative life force within.

The word *ocotillo* means "little pine" in Spanish and is derived from Nahuatl, an Aztec language that describes this plant's torchlike cluster of crimson tubular flowers growing at the stem's tips. Let ocotillo's illumination guide you on whatever it is that you would like direction with.

Feel the sustenance and survival of ocotillo. Its presence shows you its strength to survive and the creative life force that you too possess. Ocotillo's bright red flowers arouse emotion and passion from a place of strength and endurance.

Ocotillo offers a variety of botanical treasures. Its branches are traditionally used to provide a living fence of protection around homes and gardens in desert environments. Imagine that you are able to protect yourself by creating your own living fence of protection as you choose creative ways to express yourself emotionally.

Ocotillo flowers and leaves are used as a lymphatic decongestant and to treat spasmodic coughs. The bark and leaves treat swelling and sore muscles and are used for abrasions, wounds, and bruising. Ocotillo blossoms, placed in a bowl of water overnight, make for a delicious tea.

The clusters of ocotillo's bright red flowers draw hummingbirds and bees to pollinate in the Desert Southwest. It is a captivating experience to walk among the ocotillos and hear the sounds of fluttering and buzzing all around.

Ocotillo flower essence water is slightly sweet and fully fragrant, similar to its scent. It offers a sensation of peace and calm in the sacral energy field.

✦ *Affirmation* ✦

I recognize the rhythm of my emotions.
I have abundant resources to follow my creative path.

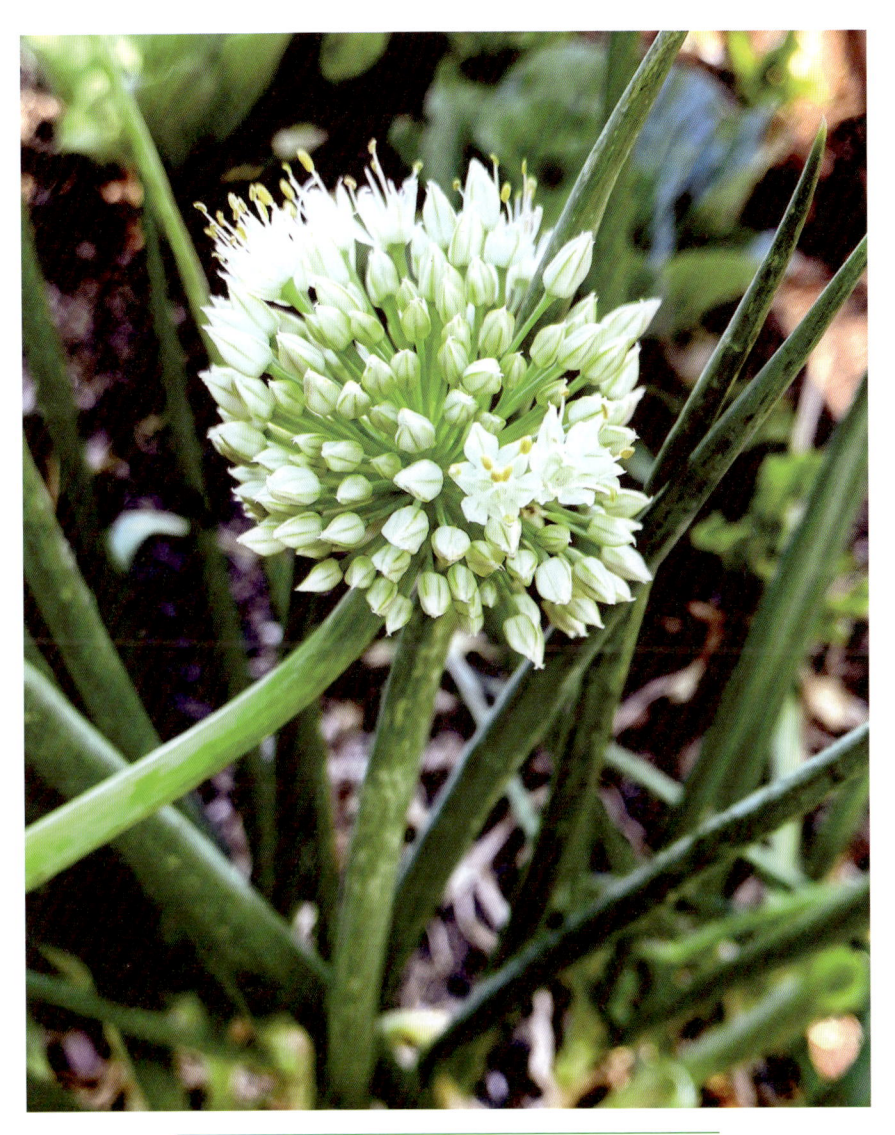

Onion flowers help you peel away your inner layers

ONION
(Allium cepa)

Primary quality: healing from grief
Energy impact/chakra correspondence:
fourth and seventh chakras

Voice of the Flower

I am one of the oldest cultivated plants in the world. I welcome you to explore what lies beneath the surface of your being. Grief can be all-encompassing. You hold it deep within. You may not even realize that it's grief that's taken over. Grief comes in many forms. It may include the loss of another person, a lifestyle, or something that you hold dear that has been taken or given away.

I am made up of many layers that form my whole. I am here to help you discover the layers within yourself beyond the illusion of fear and separation. Bring to your awareness the corners where you hold grief. It is in these places where grief may be hidden or stuck. Acknowledge and explore any grief that you may be holding. Listen to your emotions and your body-mind for the places that call out to you in discomfort or confusion. Give any discomfort a voice. Allow yourself to go into those areas so that you can connect with what it is you're feeling. Let your discomfort speak to you. Go deep into the core of your grief and pain. By doing so, you are peeling away your grief or discomfort in a deeper way. Now you can understand it and make peace with it. By being aware of your grief and processing it, you are peeling off the layers within you that will lead to inner peace.

As each layer dissolves, become more and more aware of your true nature. I offer you an opportunity to give your grief a voice—to know where it came from, to understand it, and to grow from it.

Insight

Onion gives you an opportunity to become aware of any grief you may carry so that it can be released. It helps you get to the heart of the matter of whatever it is that you are grieving about or holding onto in some way.

A signature of onion is its distinctive odor and vapor that causes the eyes and nose to "cry." Onion helps you peel away a layer of discomfort or sadness that grief may bring to you once it has been uncovered. You may then discover a new depth of understanding about yourself. Give grief a voice and connect with its root cause. Allow healing to take place.

As you feel a deeper connection with yourself, allow your heart and mind to open further. Embrace a deeper understanding of your relationship to your whole self. By letting go of grief, you can be where you naturally belong.

Onion is one of the world's oldest cultivated plants. Medicinally, onion contains antibacterial and antifungal components that in a paste or juice form can be used to prevent infection in wounds and burns. A volatile oil in the onion stimulates the tear ducts and mucous membranes of the upper respiratory tract. Onion skins make a pretty dye of yellow, oranges, and browns.

Honeybees are the pollinators for commercial production of onions. Onions aren't able to self-pollinate because the plant's male anthers produce pollen before the female stigma has the ability to be receptive.

Onion flower essence water tastes and smells just like an onion! It offers a feeling and an insight of getting to the core of the matter.

✦ *Affirmation* ✦

> I peel away my inner layers of discomfort and discover a newfound sense of peace and freedom.

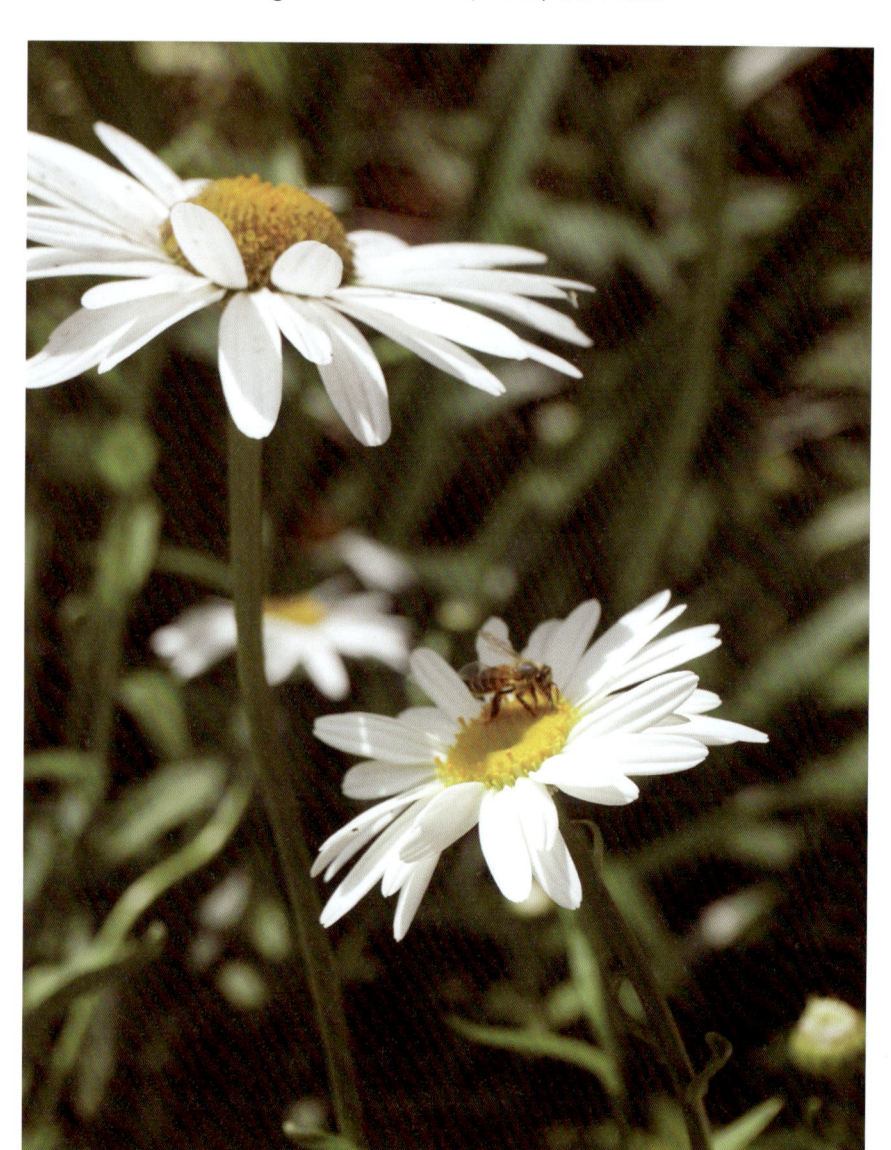

Ox-eye daisy flower's insightful nature attracts a honeybee

OX-EYE DAISY
(Chrysanthemum leucanthemum)

Primary quality: inner awareness
Energy impact/chakra correspondence: third and seventh chakras

Voice of the Flower

Each of my stems has only one large, solitary flower. My simplicity and individualism signify the safe and comfortable feeling of being alone without being lonely. Despite my simplicity, I offer characteristic patterns that magnetically attract you to my yellow center, which is a golden head with a white halo, giving a feeling of deep peace and relaxation. It is here where I offer a balance between intuition and the intellect.

Listen to my insightful nature and stir your creative intuition and inner knowing. I offer you awareness of the center of your being, your higher Self. From your center, let peace come in. My trancelike nature offers you a sense of expansion and fullness. From this place it brings you a depth of awareness about yourself and what it means to trust your inner knowing. Discover balance between what you feel intuitively and what you know intellectually, for each carries the other. Honor the wisdom that comes from within your mind's eye. Allow wisdom to support and nurture what it is that you feel inside.

As you get to know me better, experience my bright and joyful nature. Let yourself feel happiness deep inside. My flower essence water gives a feeling of energetic youthfulness, optimism, and inner awareness.

Insight

Ox-eye daisy beckons you to listen to what you feel and know within. In times when you feel uncertain or lonely, ox-eye daisy is a good flower for you. It helps you get to the center of your uncertainty and sort it out. This will support the decisions you make. When you make decisions only from your intellect, you may overlook or mistrust your inner awareness. Although your decision may appear rational, it may not be for your highest good.

Ox-eye daisy teaches you the balance between intellect and intuition. Integrate your inner knowing with your intellect. Gain wisdom, understanding, and clarity as you explore your inner awareness. Enjoy the bright, cheerful nature of ox-eye daisy. Let it lift your spirits.

Tender offshoots of ox-eye daisy are quite tasty and can be eaten in salads. Roots and young leaves can be eaten steamed or cooked. Parts of the plant are also known as a tonic and antispasmodic in the treatment of chest problems, bronchial catarrhs, coughs, asthma, and nervous excitability.

Bees have a magnetic attraction to the daisy family. Along with ox-eye daisy's aromatic fragrance, nectar is found in the yellow center or the "eye" of the daisy that attracts other kinds of pollinators too, such as ants, moths, and beetles.

Ox-eye daisy's flower essence water smells strong and sweet. It offers a full, pleasant, and strong taste. One may experience more energy and become more insightful when taking this essence.

✦ Affirmation ✦

> I honor and trust my inner awareness in helping me make decisions and life choices.

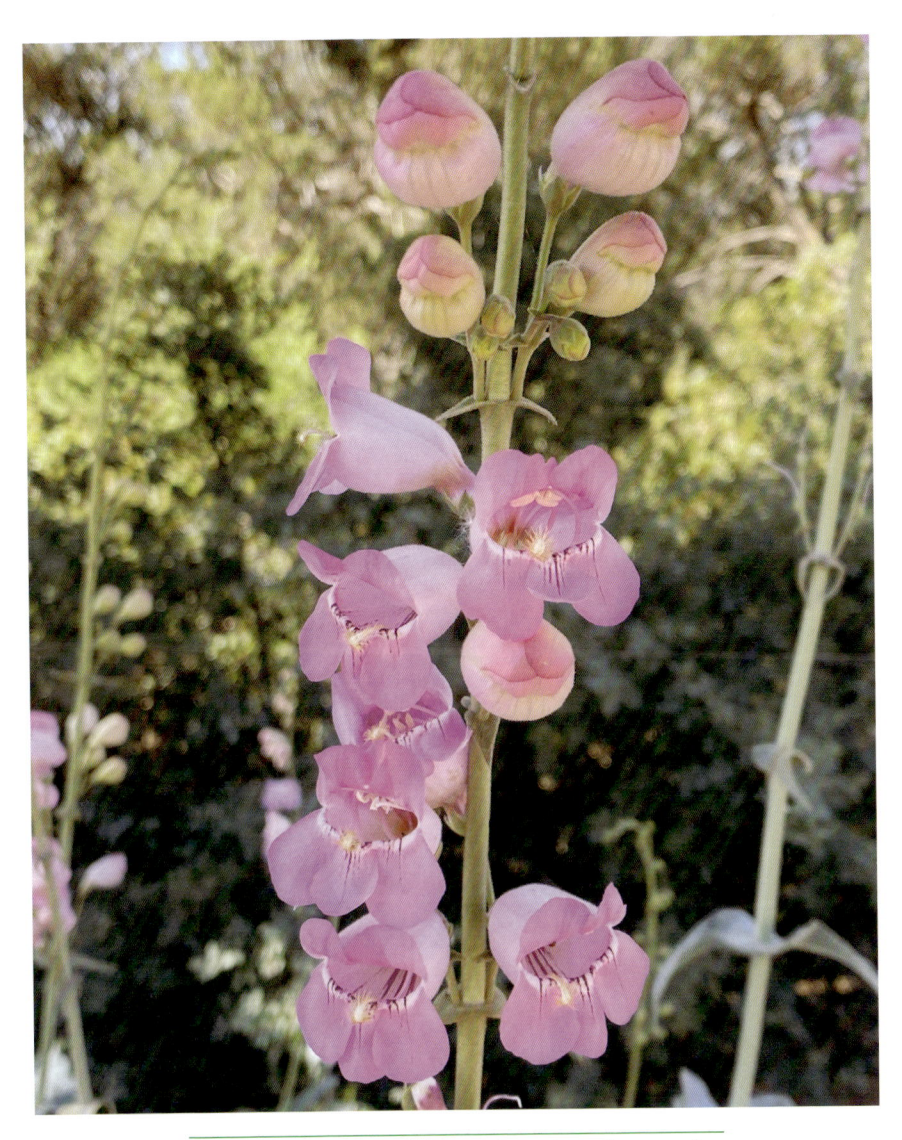

Palmer's penstemon blooms its voice of expression

PALMER'S PENSTEMON
(Penstemon palmeri)

Primary quality: truthful communication
Energy impact/chakra correspondence: third, fourth, fifth, and sixth chakras

Voice of the Flower

To speak from the heart is the gift I offer you. Inside my soft, pinkish-lavender chambers is my inner essence, filled with the sweet taste of nectar. Imagine what my nectar tastes like. Allow it to fill your heart, mind, and soul.

Feel the warmth of my soft pink glow in your heart. Imagine being inside my open mouth–shaped flower petals. Bring my scent and my presence into your energy field. I will help you recognize and explore your own inner essence. Let my glowing nature and compassion fill your heart. Your heart is the bridge to the essence of your soul.

Stir your senses with the messages you receive and feel in your heart. Connect with your inner essence—your nectar—which you hold in your heart. Give yourself a voice to speak your truths from your heart.

Bring the glow and compassion that I share with you as you step outside my chamber and into the opening of my petals. Be aware of any sounds you make and how you make them. Listen to the words you say and how you say them. Express yourself from your heart. Notice how the world around you responds when you do.

Insight

Palmer's penstemon calls to you to look truthfully at the ways you express yourself. Maybe in some way you communicate reactively, from the mind or the emotions.

Palmer's penstemon's bright pink flowers have a tubular shape with two upper petals flared backward and three lower petals flared downward. The open flower resembles a large mouth. Lavender-colored variegated lines on the lower petals guide bees to the nectar inside its short tube. Four fertile, anther-bearing stamens emerge from the roof of the mouth. A sterile fifth stamen has replaced its anther with a dense cluster of yellow fuzzy hairs. It zooms out from the center of the flower's mouth like a tongue. The young buds have a line through their middle that separates the upper and lower petals, resembling a tight jawline.

Palmer's penstemon inspires you to experiment with new ways of speaking and communicating in a heartfelt and honest way that voices your true feelings and thoughts. Listen to the words and tones you express. Notice how they sound and feel to you. Open your heart and discover how others respond to you when you do.

Practice clarity in your voice. Look into a mirror and share your feelings and voice with yourself. Listen closely to your tone and where your words are coming from. Feel the connection you have with your heart. Make any sounds you want to express. Feel them deeply in your heart. Experience the freedom of expressing your truths from your heart.

There are over 250 species of penstemons native to North America. Native Americans use the leaves to make a poultice for the skin and as a wash to treat eye problems. A tea is made to treat constipation, bronchitis, kidney problems, and whooping cough.

Palmer's penstemon's flowers appear cupped and open-mouthed, shaped to allow a variety of insects such as butterflies, bees, and moths to partake of their sweet nectar.

Palmer's penstemon flower essence water carries a sweet, full fragrance, even more so than the flower itself. To the contrary, its taste is strong and slightly bitter.

✦ *Affirmation* ✦

I speak my truth from deep within my heart.

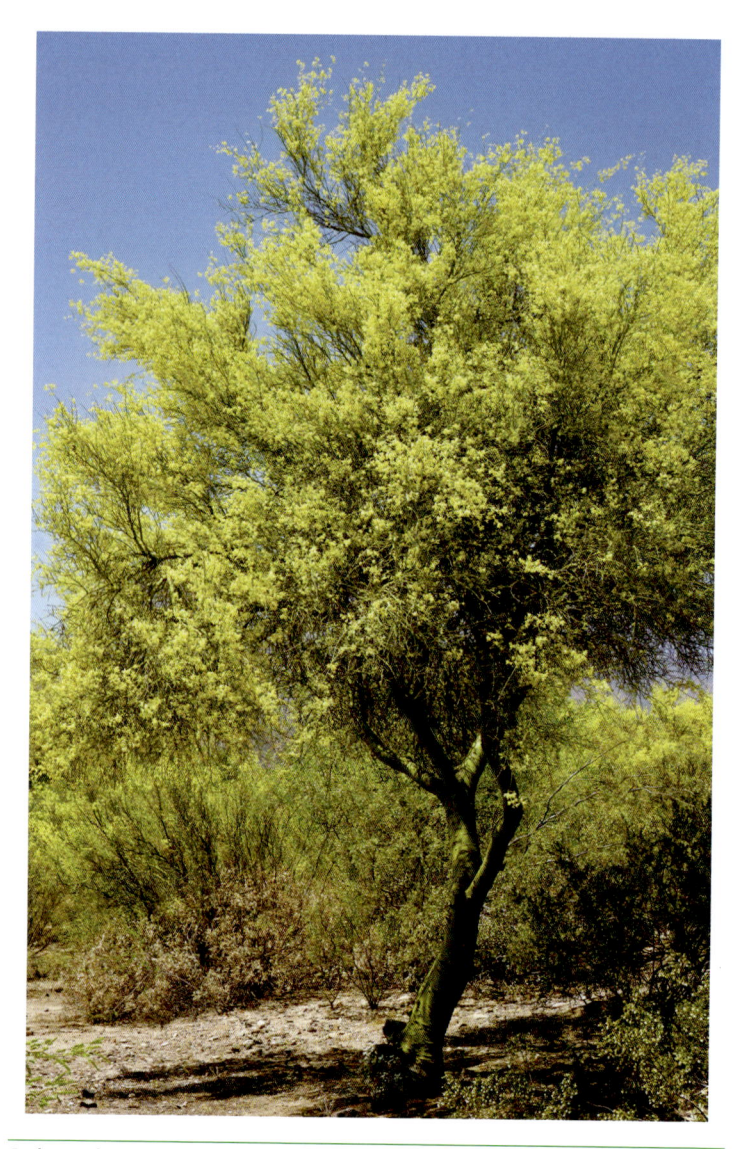

Paloverde tree offers its revealing green presence on the desert floor

PALOVERDE
(Cercidium floridum)

Primary quality: feeling rooted
Energy impact/chakra correspondence: first, second, and third chakras

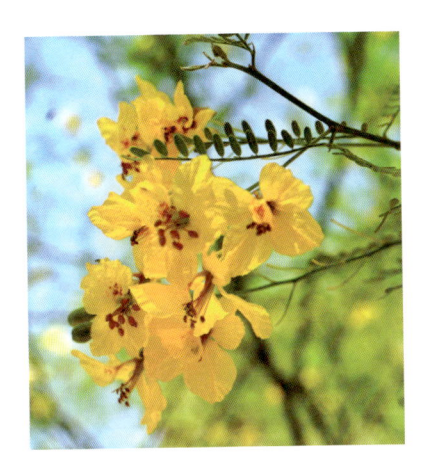

Paloverde flowers expose their stunning beauty

Voice of the Flower

It's a glorious sight to see me in full bloom. I offer the gift of beauty and inspiration in the desert landscape. Imagine being in the Desert Southwest, sitting on the ground, face-to-face with my blue-green trunk. Look at my bark and examine it closely with your eyes and then with your hands. With your hands, follow the smooth lines on my trunk and bark.

Visualize my tree roots extending below you and building a bridge that connects to the base of your spine. Feel what it's like to be connected to the earth and my roots. Notice that my roots are connected with other paloverdes that grow nearby. The larger and scalier roots are older, and the tender young shoots are beginning to grow new trees.

Feel into the powerful connection with my roots and the earth in which they ground. Now look above. See my many bright yellow blossoms with hints of reddish orange. Feel my presence on the desert floor. My gift is to remind you to ground yourself. Explore your inner depths and embrace the higher wisdom that already exists in you.

It is my soil, my sacred ground, that I bring to your awareness as your own inner sanctuary. Authentic wisdom is not based on outside conditions or what others tell you. It is a wisdom that comes from within. Plant the seeds of wisdom in your choices and in all your relations. Discover the value of making wise choices in life from a place of being grounded and rooted. Sometimes one's decisions may draw unwanted consequences. Based on a deeper connection with yourself, experience the inherent wisdom of a lesson learned. If you truly made a connection, the outcome will be supported and aligned with who you authentically are. As you walk in harmony on the Earth, reenact your role as a co-creator to sustain Earth life. This is the foundation of grace in the world and the wisdom from which it arises.

Insight

Paloverde leads you on a pathway of healing that wants you to connect with and relate to the Earth, with yourself as a provider and a resource.

Paloverde's bright yellow five-petaled flowers with a hint of orange offer a sweet fragrance and flavor. Their message is about learning ways to heal yourself while being rooted. Make amends with yourself and with whomever else you need to forgive.

Paloverde helps you ground and connect with the wisdom and gifts that the Earth provides. Align yourself with nature and her elements. Feel into the root of who you are. Tap into your natural inherent wisdom. Take time to consider the big picture. Be aware of the consequences of the choices you make. Become aligned with who you really are and live by your authentic nature. Walk in harmony on the Earth. Find ways to sustain her, yourself, your family, and all your relations.

Native Americans ground the seeds of paloverde as a food source to make flour; birds and other wildlife also eat the seeds. Some animals eat the branches and pods.

Numerous kinds of pollinators are drawn to the beautiful display of paloverde flowers, including especially bees and butterflies. The flowers support the desert ecosystem with their nectar in the Southwest.

Paloverde offers a very full, sweet, earthy, herbaceous scent. It's flower essence water turns light yellow and the flowers open wide in the water. The essence offers a full feeling of being rooted, with a tingling sensation that runs through the body. Its flower essence tastes sweet and tangy, with a vegetable flavor.

✦ **Affirmation** ✦

> I sink deep into my roots that ground me and experience the depth of who I am.

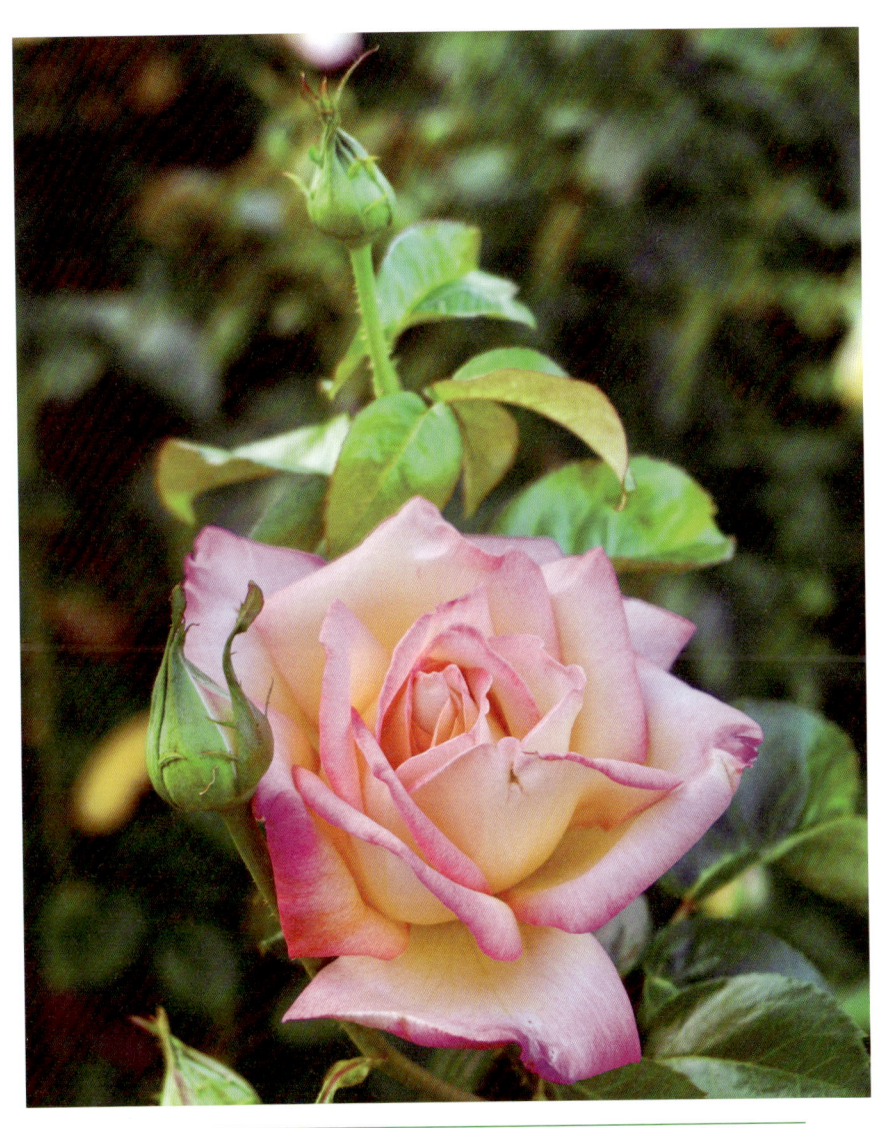

Peace rose blossom fills your senses with a sweet, delicate fragrance

PEACE ROSE
(Rosa "Peace")

Primary quality: serene peace
Energy impact/chakra correspondence: first, fourth, and seventh chakras

Voice of the Flower

Imagine yourself as a lush peace rose bush. Visualize my prickly thorns spreading out on long stems. Choose a thorn and identify that thorn in your life now. Look the thorn over carefully. In what way does the thorn prevent you from blossoming into a flower? How does it make you feel and think? Are you ready to let the thorn in your thoughts and feelings go? If so, tell the thorn that you no longer want it in your life. Thank it for how it has helped you and how you have grown from it. Say goodbye to the thorn. Allow it to fall where it wants to fall.

With all the thorns in your life, your pains and sorrows, my gentle and endearing presence has always been there.

My ivory-pink rosebud offers a peaceful and pleasant fragrance. Visualize being inside my soft, tightly closed petals as I begin my blossoming journey. Breathe my rose-scented fragrance into your heart. Watch as my bud slowly begins to unfold its petals. Feel your heart open wider as my rose petals gently emerge. Allow the petals to take their time. Let your heart open with the flower. Feel the warmth of love and peace for yourself in your heart.

My flower, like an angel, offers you the gifts of beauty, love, and serene peace. Allow yourself to emerge as a peace rose, inspired by love. Set your heart free.

Insight

Peace rose draws you to the awareness of what you feel in your heart. The gentle fragrance and color of peace rose sweeps through your heart, increasing your capacity for love. An opportunity is created for you to find peace within your heart-mind-body, no longer to be held back by life's thorns. Nothing remains the same, nor is it like it was. The flowers bloom according to the season. We, too, bloom in relation to our life cycles. Sometimes there are only a few blossoms on one rosebush, and other times there are many more.

Peace rose's flower gives you the courage and faith to face the thorns in your life. Accept life's cycles and open your heart to receive love. Make peace with yourself. Peace rose gives you an opportunity to help you come to terms with loving yourself. Share that love with others.

The rose family began its long European history in Greece. The rose became known as "the gift of the angels" due to its safe, soothing, and healing nontoxic qualities. Rosewater became popular for cooking and drinking. In the sixteenth century, an essential oil called *attar* (or *otto*) was prepared from rose petals. Peace rose petals are common in potpourris and offer a soothing aroma associated with love and femininity.

Bumblebees and yellow jackets collect pollen and nectar from the sweet fragrance of the peace rose and from roses in general.

Peace rose flowers are more aromatic in the plant's flower essence water—very pleasant, with a distinctly roselike fragrance. The essence's heartwarming taste is similar to its scent and offers a peaceful feeling throughout the body.

✦ *Affirmation* ✦

I allow love and serene peace within.

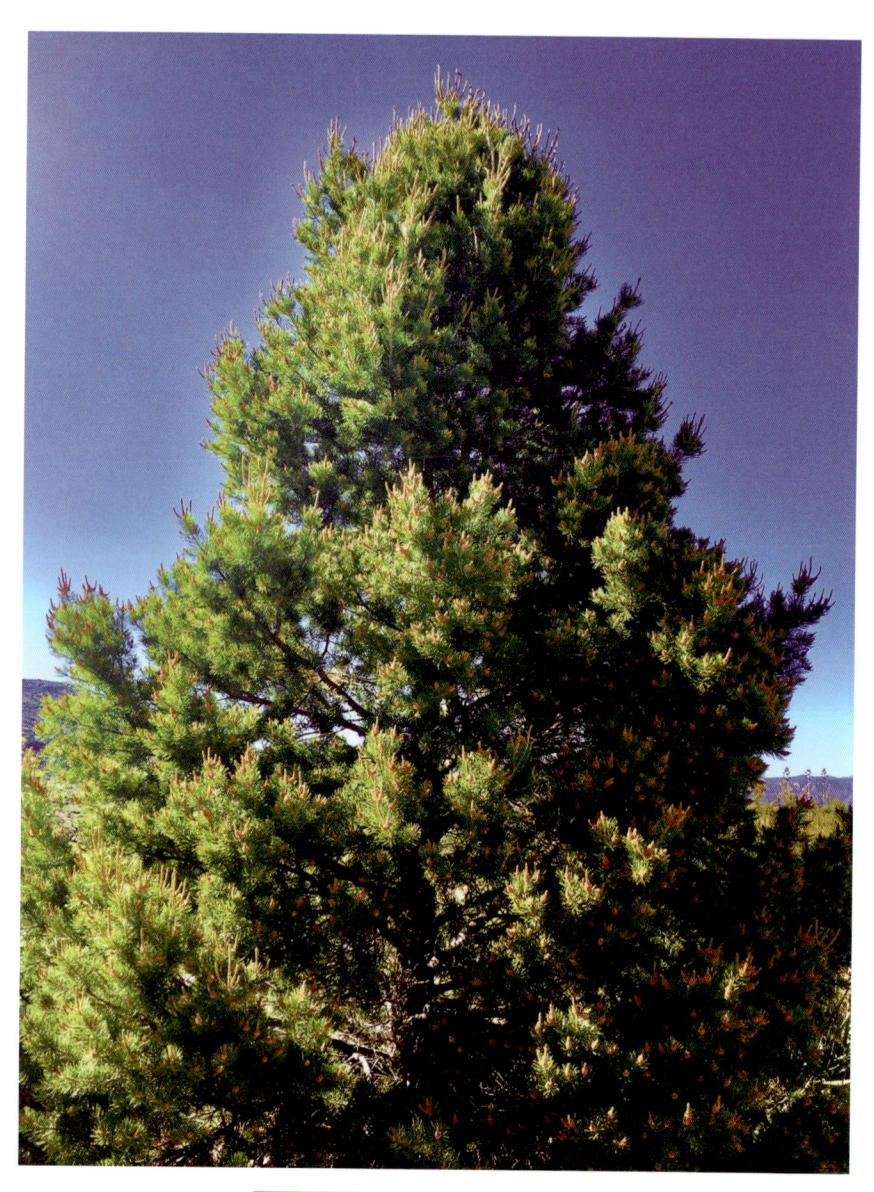

Pinyon tree displays its endurance

PINYON
(Pinus edulis)

Primary quality: trusting in patience
Energy impact/chakra correspondence: first, fourth, and sixth

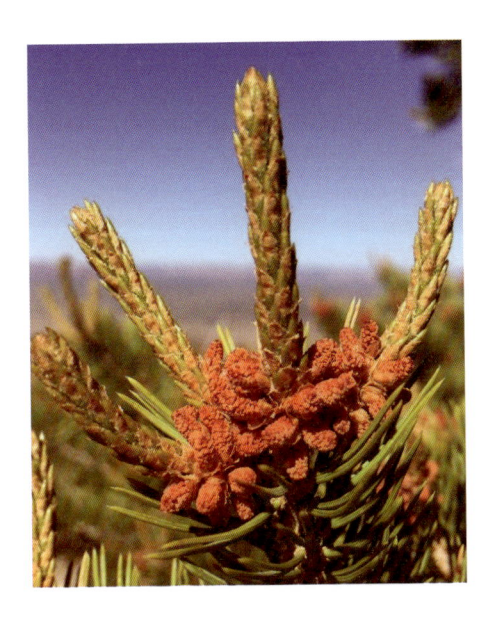

Pinyon catkins evolve into pine cones

Voice of the Flower (Catkin)

I stand firm, in fortitude. I am graceful, yet persistent and enduring. My needles are light and delicate, yet spiny and strong. Listen to my branches and needles as I dance with the wind. I provide an appreciation for simplicity, endurance, and trust.

The scent and taste of my needles and resin is fresh, cleansing, and rejuvenating. If you bite into one of my needles you may at first experience a bitter taste. It may remind you of any bitterness you may be feeling. Inside the center of my needle there is a strong taste of pine without the bitterness. It's like discovering a powerful essence inside of you that reveals something about your true nature that you haven't felt before.

I am a teacher of great patience and perseverance. I honor the process of steady growth and slow maturation. I offer you patience in your personal growth, without shame, guilt, or time constraints. Love who you are and develop a new sense of self.

Trust the new foundation you are building. Be strong and enduring. Come to terms with yourself and make dependable choices. Be patient with yourself. I offer you a newfound freedom. Bear the fruits of trusting your enduring patience.

Insight

Pinyon (or piñon) reminds you to take time for yourself. The conelets on the pinyon tree take twenty-six months to mature, a reflection of the pinyon's patience and perseverance. The slow but steady growth of the tree and its delicious pine nuts show you the importance of being patient and persevering in your own life. You, too, can bear your fruits through your steadfast endurance and patience. Breathe in the scent of pinyon's resin and pine needles; its refreshing and cleansing presence invites you in.

Pinyon provides cleansing, purification, and rejuvenation. It is traditionally used in prayers or ceremonies dealing with the death of a person or to release an old part of yourself that no longer serves you.

The pinyon nut, called a *pine nut*, contains twenty amino acids that make a complete protein. Pine nuts can be eaten raw, roasted, boiled, or ground into a flour. Pinyon pitch can be used as a dressing to treat open wounds. The smoke from burning the tree's gum can be inhaled to treat head colds and earache. The inner bark of the pinyon can be boiled slowly to make a tea, and then sweetened with honey to make an expectorant. Incense can be made with the resin to clear negative energy. Pinyon makes a wonderful healing salve for infections and skin irritations. An essential oil is made both from the pinyon needles and from the cones. Incense is made from the resin. Pinyon's scent offers a powerful clearing of energy and a grounding connection to your body and the Earth.

Pollination of the pinyon pine is via the wind rather than by insect pollinators.

Pinyon's flower essence water offers a revitalizing piney scent. It tastes just like its pine scent, but even more refreshing, smooth, and soothing—as is the feeling it gives you when you drink it.

✦ *Affirmation* ✦

I am patient with myself. I trust my journey.

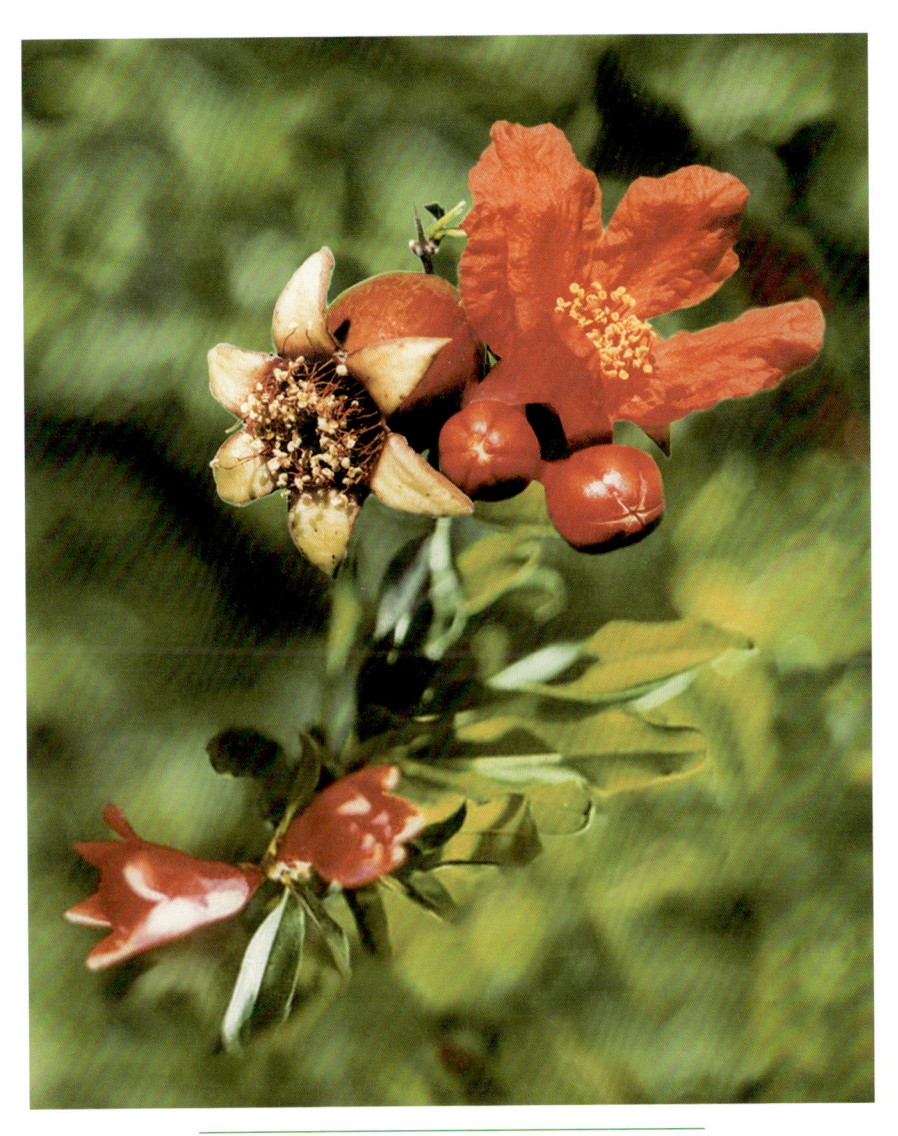

Pomegranate flower radiates its exotic vibrancy

POMEGRANATE
(Punica granatum)

Primary quality: passion
Energy impact/chakra correspondence: first, second, and third chakras

Voice of the Flower

My showy, orangish-red flowers emerge at the end of my young branches. My fragrant flower has five to seven rounded, waxy, wrinkly, papery petals. A group of prolific yellow stamens appear at the center of my flower. My fruit is protected by my plump, rose-to-red-colored skin. When my watery fruit is ripe, it bursts forth, the juicy taste of my sensual fruit and ruby-red seeds with their dripping red flesh offer you a glimpse of my exotic nature. I am a powerful symbol of female fertility, emotion, and sexuality. My signatures represent a place within you where life-promoting energy is awakened.

Come enter my flaming orange petals and embrace the darkness where your innate wisdom lies. Allow me to stir your deepest passions, joy, and creativity. Awaken your vital life force. Celebrate the fullness of your sensuality. Discover the depths of your primal feminine self. Receive the fruits of your abundance and beauty, and honor them within yourself. Draw on your resources. Treasure these gifts as you delight in your freedom. Express your passion for life and the joy of living.

I will help you get in touch with the power of your emotions and the energetic imprint you carry in your emotional being. Connect with yourself through your own emotional realms. Feel a new sense of trust in who you are. Feel the essence of my vitality and pulsating energy.

Awaken to new steps that stir your passion in the dance of life.

Insight

Pomegranate is here to teach you about your inner wisdom, beauty, and power.

Bring your attention to what you are feeling. Notice the force within you that builds your emotional drive. Become aware of your feelings and where they came from. What stirs your passion?

Pomegranate has long been known as an ancient symbol of fertility due to its striking reddish-orange color and its juicy fruit. Fertility is the opportunity to plant new seeds. Imagine the sensation a farmer may feel driving their tractor and tilling fertile soil to plant new seeds. Take in the earthy smells of the plowed earth. Notice the dark, wet richness each row shows as it is turned over.

Imagine the fertile flesh of pomegranate. Recognize the fertility of the foundation within yourself. Stir your inner soil to receive new seeds. Whatever your seeds may be, let them germinate and burst forth. Experience all the gems within you. Abundance comes in many forms, as does passion.

In Greek mythology, the goddess Persephone was said to have eaten six seeds of a pomegranate after she fell into Hades, the underworld. As a symbol of union, the pomegranate bound her to Pluto, god of the underworld, for six months, from fall to spring (each seed representing one month). Despite her descent to Pluto's hidden kingdom, the image of Persephone eating the pomegranate seeds symbolizes a birthing period and her return to the light. The underworld helped her discover her hidden wisdom, beauty, and power, and allowed her to confront her fears in the darkest moments of her life. In the spring, Persephone was free and emerged with the newly found gifts she had given herself.

Fertilize your seeds of growth. Let them ripen and burst forth in their fullness. Be the power of your passion!

The medicinal history of pomegranate dates back to the Roman naturalist and philosopher Pliny, in the first century AD. The root and bark have been used since ancient times to expel worms from the intestinal tract; they have been found to be most beneficial in cases of tapeworm infection. If you bite into the rind of a pomegranate, you will experience its astringent nature. The powdered fruit rind is used as an astringent and has also been used to treat dysentery, diarrhea, excessive perspiration, intermittent fever, and as a gargle for sore throats. In modern times pomegranate has been hailed for its antioxidant properties.

Pomegranate's single flowers are pollinated primarily by bees.

Pomegranate's flower essence water emits a gentle, subtly sweet, fruitful fragrance. The flower essence tastes slightly sweet, delicate, and fruity, and it lingers at the back of the tongue. You may feel its energetic power in your sacral region.

✦ Affirmation ✦

I lovingly nurture the seeds within me;
I am the power of my passion.

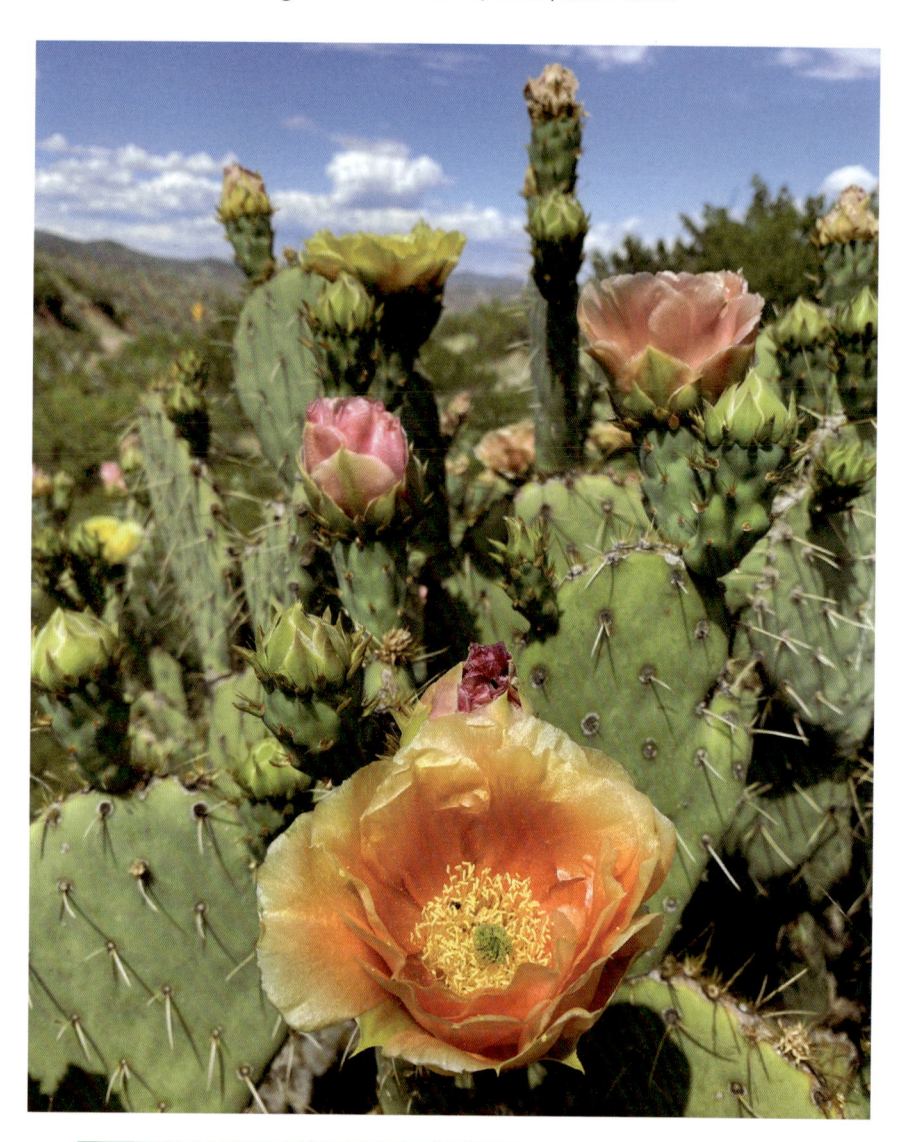

Blooming prickly pear cacti's emerging beauty among the desert flora

PRICKLY PEAR CACTUS
(Opuntia engelmanni)

Primary quality: the strength to be me
Energy impact/chakra correspondence: first, second, and third chakras

Voice of the Flower

I am a survivor of many habitats, from deserts to mountains, and a plant of many uses. When you first look at me you may not realize what I am made of and how my healing properties can help you. You may be attracted to my shiny, thick pads and my showy, yellow to yellowish-orange, waxy flowers. However, my spiny stems and leaf hairs may scare you away. In the center of my flower you will see one firm pistil with a lobed stigma in a garden of yellow stamens nestled around it.

Join me in nurturing a grounding energy within you. Build your self-confidence and independence, and appreciate your uniqueness. Experience the free spirit of my nature from a place of security, strength, and protection. You, too, can create this energy for yourself.

Feel the power of my presence. Allow life to unfold naturally. I am much more than how I appear. Likewise, you, too, may go unnoticed by others, but within the core of you is the inner flesh of who you authentically are. This only belongs to you.

Insight

Prickly pear guides you on a journey of arousing your primal sense within. Prickly pear has the ability to regenerate itself in sandy soil through its pads and seeds, thereby establishing a root system that can survive in diverse habitats.

Prickly pear pads or flattened stems grow rapidly and multiply in production. The pads symbolize the different parts of who you are. As prickly pear exists in different environments, it adds new experiences and builds new pads. Each pad strengthens the core of the plant. This represents the different parts within you that bring strength and stability into the core of your being. It's the pads, or life experiences, that strengthen the core of who you are. Trust how you navigate your life experiences. There may be times in life when you feel you don't know who you are. We develop thorns on each pad to protect us until we have grown into who we really want to become.

The plant's flower represents how you nurture yourself. Have you grown beyond the thorns? Do you allow people to see and experience who you really are? Removing your thorns brings you into the heart of what's inside of you—your inner treasures.

The raw inner flesh of the prickly pear's pads hold healing properties that can be used for poultices, cuts, bites, stings, and burns. The juicy, purple-colored, bulbous fruits burst forth with sweetness and tiny edible seeds and they can be juiced or made into jams, jellies, wines, and simple syrups. They are also very delicious and offer a delightful magenta color in margaritas! Rhonda's aunt, Marilyn Schirch, made a tasty prickly pear jam, among many other desert jams that she created and sold with Rhonda's uncle Reldon in their Desert Kettle gift store in Fountain Hills, Arizona.

As a survivor in nature's harsher landscapes, prickly pear offers many other wonderful healing gifts. There are many varieties in the prickly pear tribe. If you do choose to eat the flesh, be mindful of which variety is safe to eat and which is not.

One of the most valuable plants of the Southwest is prickly pear. Its dark purple, deep red fruits are known for treating diabetes, high cholesterol, obesity, and hangovers, as well as for their antiviral and anti-inflammatory properties. The raw flesh of prickly pear pads should be cooked or roasted to offset the cold temperature within the pad. The tender pads, known as *nopalitos*, are commonly eaten in salads and are very popular in the Southwest. The inner flesh of the pads is used as a poultice for wounds, cuts, abrasions, burns, and even venomous bites and stings that include rattlesnakes, scorpions, and various insects. Please use prickly pear with caution and know which species are safe to consume and which are not.

The fruity nectar of prickly pear cactus flowers entices pollinators such as various species of bees and hummingbirds. The Desert Southwest in general also attracts hawkmoth and bat pollination to sustain its ecosystem.

The scent of prickly pear offers a uniquely fruity, cool, earthy scent. Its flower essence water taste is also earthy and mildly sweet.

✦ Affirmation ✦

I allow my life to evolve naturally.
I am grounded and secure in who I am.

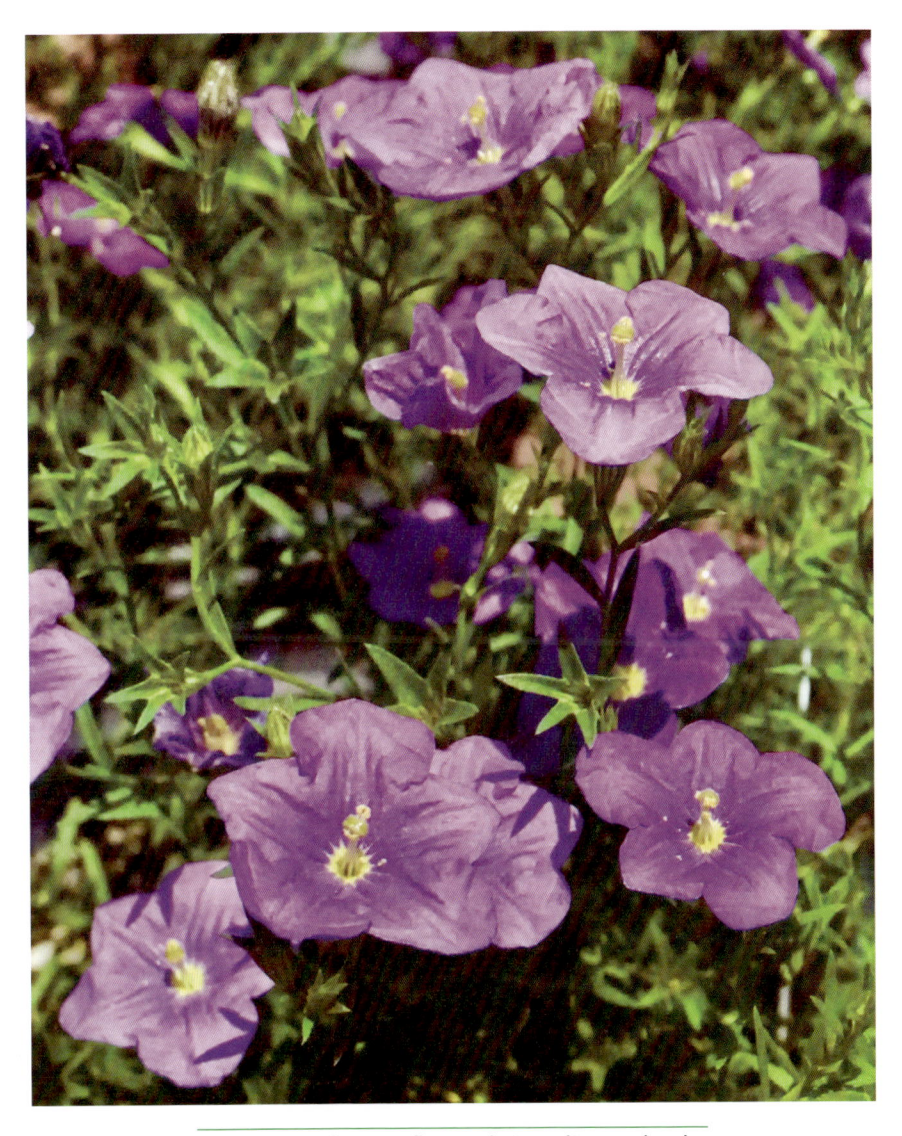

Purple robe flowers flaunt their radiant splendor

PURPLE ROBE
(Nierembergia scoparia)

Primary quality: awakening vision
Energy impact/chakra correspondence:
third and sixth chakras

Voice of the Flower

My deep purple flower bursts into a star-shaped pattern from within the center of my petals. My firm, thick, yellow style—part of my female structure—displays a cluster of yellow stamens that evolve out of the center of the star. I am a prolific plant that grows low to the ground and is widely spread. I produce an abundance of flowers that are only one inch wide. The structure of my plant is light, delicate, and flexible. My cupped flowers appear tender, although my petals are quite strong. I do not fade in even the brightest sun. I offer you a sense of strength and persistence to awaken, grow, and spread your inner light.

I am a plant of beauty and simplicity. I bring you gifts of abundance.

Despite my fullness, I am very humble. The small yellow eye in my center is a gift of abundance to awaken and expand your vision, insights, and understanding.

My inner star-shaped pattern provides inspiration and illumination. I offer you the ability to trust the depths of your own nature. Stir your awakening vision.

My message to you is to show you that you have unlimited opportunities. Supply is the law of expansion and fruition. The universe supplies us with infinite resources, from within ourselves to outside of ourselves.

Take a moment to go within and find your inner silence. Let my flower's energy deepen your awareness and awaken your vision. Become aware of the supply of your own resources within. Allow your inner resources to give you a new sense of purpose, insight, and wisdom. Take in my spirit of splendor and awaken your vision with boundless treasures.

Insight

Purple robe offers you a pathway of healing where the feeling of lack in your life is replaced with the feeling of plenty. Purple robe is a prolific, widely spread-out plant that produces an abundance of flowers. The finely textured foliage evolves on multiple stems, with stiff linear leaves about a half inch long.

Purple robe demonstrates its quality of abundance by the way it grows and reproduces. The purple cupped flowers appear delicate, although the petals are actually quite strong and pronounced. This plant's signature suggests the sense of strength and persistence needed to grow and spread, and a gentle approach in doing so.

The rich purple color of the flower with its lemony-yellow center is characteristic of the brow energy center, the sixth chakra. It gives you a sense of purpose, spiritual insight, and wisdom. Experience the abundance of purple robe. Deepen your awareness of the abundance already within you.

Native to Argentina, purple robe is a widely spreading plant that can be used for ground cover and makes an attractive addition in flower arrangements and wreaths.

Purple robe's cup-shaped flower is a magnet for pollinators and especially for hummingbirds and bees. Its vibrant purple color is a wondrous attraction in pollinator gardens.

Purple robe flower essence water offers a full and sweet fragrance that tastes strong and sweet, soothing and powerful. The taste is warming, and it gives you a feeling of expansion in the way that you can have a clearer vision.

✦ *Affirmation* ✦

> There is an unlimited supply of what I need in my life.
> I expand and awaken my vision to create it.

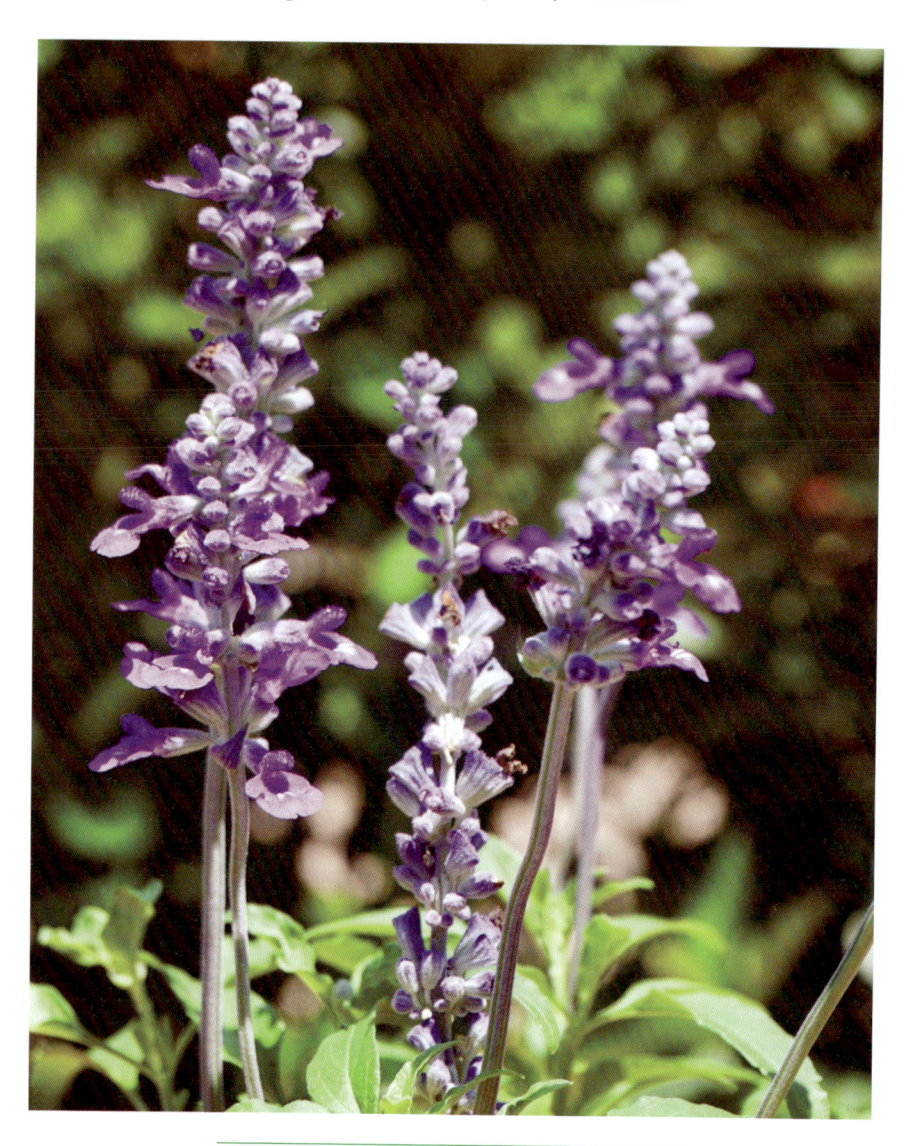

Sage flowers suggest their tasteful elegance

SAGE
(Salvia officinalis)

Primary quality: inner wisdom
Energy impact/chakra correspondence: first, third, fourth, fifth, and seventh chakras

Voice of the Flower

My violet to purple and bluish flower blossoms form whorls along my stem. My aromatic flowers are deep-throated and two-lipped, either straight or arched. They look like an open mouth with lips and tongue. They appear spurlike. The fuzzy base of my calyx is bell-shaped. The opening of my flower looks like a gateway. Two white streaks appear at the front of my mouth or lower lip. A white color emerges from the center of my opening and comes into sight like a tongue. There is a tiny ring of hairs on the inside of each of my flowers. Stamens with purple anthers emerge from the flower's center. My soft sepal looks like a five-pointed cup that gently holds the flower.

Step inside my cool chambers and hear my sacred voice. I offer you guidance on a path toward wholeness. I assist you in exploring your inner wisdom. Become conscious of how you integrate your higher purpose in life with your daily patterns of living.

Connect with your inner wisdom in the way you live your life.

Listen to my sounds. Take in my refreshing breath. Experience cleansing of your body, soul, and mind. I invite you to come fully into your divine presence with your own voice and song through sounds, speech, touch, and senses.

May you feel whole through this connection with yourself. Allow your inner wisdom to bring coherence into your life.

Insight

Sage helps you to become aware of the sounds you make and the words you choose. Notice and feel the sensations inside your throat. Breathe deeply into the sensations and slowly exhale. Experience how these sensations stir your inner realms and the wisdom that comes as a result.

The violet-purplish color of sage corresponds to the brow energy center, or sixth chakra, which serves as a visionary or guide. This signature opens us to see beyond our ordinary vision. It helps us connect with our own true Self and our inner realms.

Come to an understanding of the ways that you integrate your inner wisdom with practical applications of daily living. Sage offers spiritual inspiration and visionary guidance. It is useful in times of transition and life-cycle changes. Hear sage beckon you on your journey. Listen to your inner voice as you go deeper into your exploration of inner wisdom.

Sage flowers offer a slightly spicy and somewhat minty, refreshing aroma. The flower essence is refreshing and cooling. It has a slightly tingling and cool energy felt from the throat to the brow.

Herbalists today use *Salvia officinalis* to treat a variety of conditions such as sore throat, tonsillitis, mouth irritations and sores, sexual debility, hot flashes, irregular menses and menopause, colds, coughs, and diarrhea. Sage is also used to promote hair growth and improve memory. Sage essential oil is known for its cleansing properties and uplifting spirit, along with a variety of other healing properties.

A broad range of pollinators that include bees, butterflies, and hummingbirds are drawn to sage's aromatic properties.

Sage's flower essence water offers a slightly spicy, minty, refreshing aroma. Its taste is similar and is cooling to the mouth and throat.

✦ *Affirmation* ✦

I awaken the gift of my wisdom.

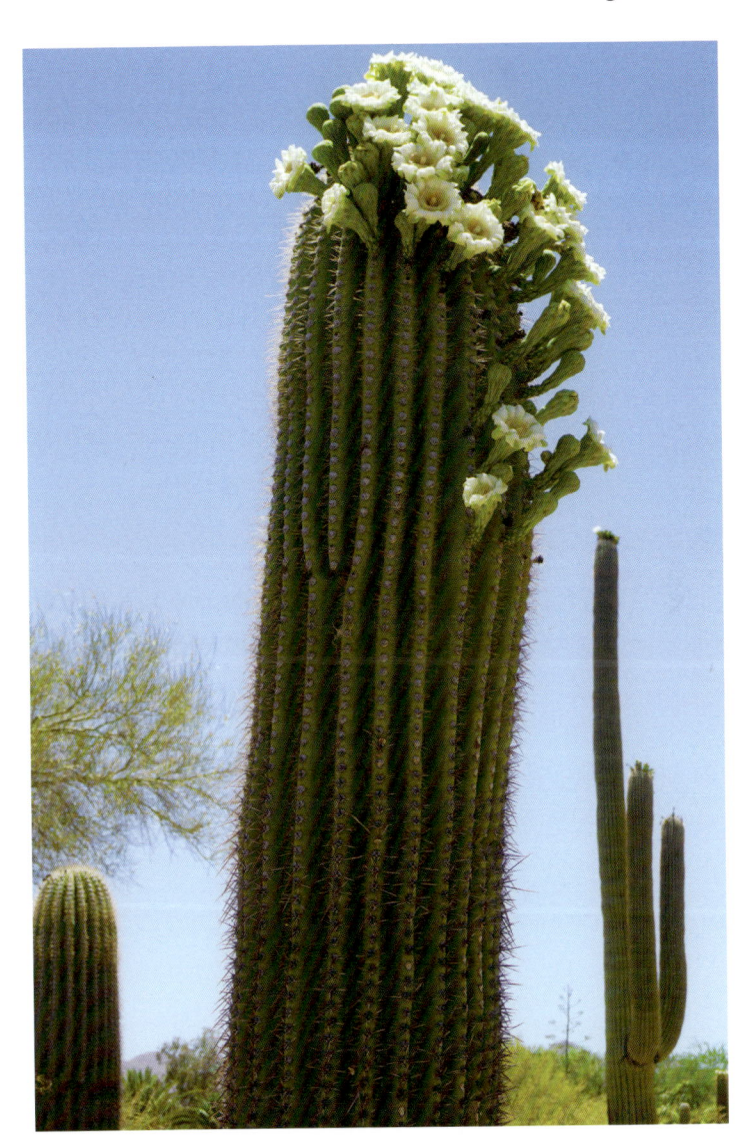

Saguaro cacti stunningly adorn the Sonoran desert

SAGUARO
(Carnegiea gigantea)

Primary quality: protector
Energy impact/chakra correspondence: first, fourth, and seventh chakras

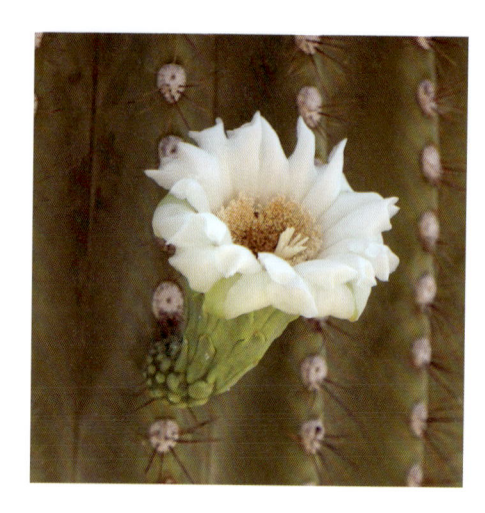

Saguaro flower invites you into its heavenly, sweet scent

Voice of the Flower

Imagine you are walking along a Sonoran desert trail, ascending gracefully to a mesa. You are drawn to a distant ridge on the edge of the mesa. As you begin to approach the ridge, feel the thermal winds rising in the current of hot air above you. Notice my family of mature saguaros that beckon to you. You find yourself standing in the center of our circle. Feel your strength stirring inside of you. Feel the shield of protection offered by our towering presences.

Listen to the inner silence of the desert.

I have a profound ability to endure and grow at a slow and steady pace. When it rains, I soak up water and store it in my body to build up reserves for hot desert days.

I feel protected inside my slow-growing bud as my flower petals leisurely unfurl. As each of my individual petals builds their strength and security, they open up to a soft, billowy crown. My creamy-white flower petals are waxy and soft. I carry a heavenly sweet scent that arouses the sweet nectar of life.

My patient flowers and my slow growth guide you to be equally patient with yourself as you grow stronger on your journey. Feel secure in the protection you already hold within you. Imagine a warm glow that fills you with anticipation. Be patient and enduring on your journey. Feel a soft, cuddly, white blanket wrapped around you. Allow the tapestry of your own flower to unfold.

Insight

Saguaro teaches you how to persevere and trust that you are protected. Saguaro helps you to feel rooted and balanced. It awakens and stimulates each sacred energy center, from root to crown. Saguaro helps you to restore, stretch, and expand.

Saguaros grow in large communities scattered throughout the Sonoran Desert. Their presence suggests protection. They appear as overseers or guardians of the desert due to their size. They are the largest cacti in the world, averaging thirty to fifty feet in height, although they're known to grow even taller. Their diameter is about two and a half feet, and they weigh up to nine tons. Their green trunk is characterized by columns with twelve to thirty prominent ribs that branch out from the trunk as they grow older, forming branches or "arms" as large as twenty inches in diameter. It takes 50–65 years for a saguaro to grow its first branch. Saguaros have an uncanny ability to create a variety of human and animal shapes out of their fleshy arms.

Saguaros grow at a slow, steady pace and can live up to two hundred years or longer. During its first year, a saguaro grows only about a half inch tall. When it is about nine years old, it stands at only six inches. It takes nearly fifteen years to reach one foot. When it has grown about eight feet in height, the first flowers begin to bloom.

Saguaro's creamy-white flowers bloom only once, during late spring or early summer. The flowers offer a sense of crowning expansion. They begin at nighttime and stay open during part of the next day. Once the saguaro has grown its first branch, it becomes a host to nearly 100 or more flower blooms on a branch. Once the first branch has emerged, other branches develop quickly. Although individually short-bloomed, flowers continue to appear on the saguaros' branches throughout the period of their flowering season, inviting pollinators to support their flourishing reproduction.

The succulent, deep red fruit of saguaro emerges from the base of the flower as the flower's life span comes to an end, generally just before monsoon season. An average mature saguaro produces about 150 sweet and red-fleshed fruits per year, which "contain dark red pulp laden with an average of more than 4,000 seeds and are contained by a rind that remains green on the exterior until maturity when it turns a reddish pink."[10] The magic of this special fruit is indicative of the mystery of saguaro in all the many ways that it grows and appears. Saguaro teaches you that it is the fruit of your endurance and hard work that allows the flower within you to blossom.

Experience your consciousness expanding as you understand the deeper purpose in your life. Embrace the choices you make. Thrive in the protectiveness of this powerful desert giant. Feel its presence within you.

The saguaro has had many uses for Native Americans of central and southwestern Arizona for centuries. The Hohokam and the Tohono O'Odham (the "desert people") would dislodges the fruit from the high branches with pieces of saguaro ribs tied together. The syrup, yams, fruit, wine, and flour made from the seeds sustained them during the hot summer months.

Dried saguaro fruit is a special delicacy that tastes slightly sweet and nutlike. The wooden ribs of dead saguaros have been used to make roofs, shelters, fences, hiking sticks, and more. There is so much to learn and explore about this sacred plant, and there aren't enough words to describe how important saguaro and the entire cacti family is to the evolution of plant growth, their stamina and perseverance, and the many gifts they bring to the ecosystem of the Sonoran desert.

Saguaro flowers' pollination is birthed into the nighttime by bats, hawkmoths, and other insects. Daytime pollinators include doves, woodpeckers, orioles, and bees.

The flower essence water of saguaro offers a strong, powerful, fruity, and nectarlike fragrance. Its taste is very similar and smooth. Its compelling presence offers an energy shield and a feeling of the ability to survive whatever your present state or condition is within you and all around you.

✦ Affirmation ✦

I create a shield of protective energy all around me.
I am secure and defended.

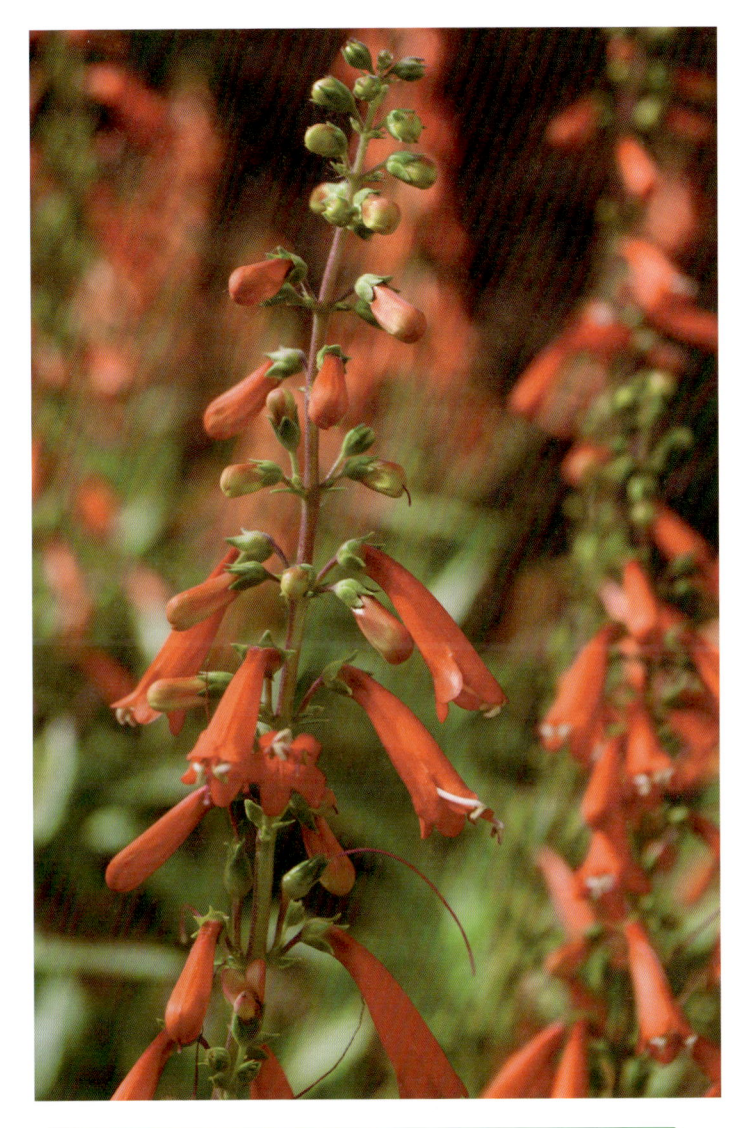

Scarlet penstemon flowers show off their scarlet red vitality

SCARLET PENSTEMON
(Penstemon barbatus)

Primary quality: self-confidence
Energy impact/chakra correspondence: first, second, third, and fifth chakras

Voice of the Flower

My radiant scarlet flowers lean toward the earth. I rise in pairs from my upper leaf axils. Deep inside my long, narrow tube is my sweet nectar. It stirs a strong and courageous intention in you to go deep inside to find it. Once the nectar is found, its sweet taste brings comfort. Hummingbirds especially thrive on my nectar.

The scarlet color of my flower relates to the root energy center, the first chakra, where you came from and who you are at the very core of your being. My reddish-orange color invites creativity, emotion, and sensation. These colors offer my signature of courage, vitality, and strength.

My unique tubular flower opening appears as an upper lip with two tiny "teeth" that project forward. My lower lip bends downward and back with a "beard" of long yellow hairs that dangle toward the earth.

I offer you a sense of having the self-confidence and voice to step into your power, to release something old in order to receive something new.

My message to you is to step into your strength. Awaken all the self-confidence you have. Accept life's challenges as opportunities to strengthen your faith in yourself. Fortify your courage and self-confidence to take the next step forward.

Seek your inner guidance and find the strength and self-confidence to go deep within. Take a sip of your sweet nectar and allow yourself to be vulnerable to love and to give love. Be soft and nurturing with yourself. It takes courage and a willingness to take risks in order to follow your higher life path. And it takes even more courage to face life's setbacks and to trust that you are being provided for.

Insight

Scarlet penstemon brings awareness to your self-confidence. The flower faces downward as an expression of surrender and grounding. Its long, narrow tube contains sweet nectar deep inside.

Scarlet penstemon offers you the strength and energy to go deep into yourself. It tells you to explore the ways in which you have given away your power. You may have allowed other people or situations to override your self-confidence.

You are being asked to be conscious of others in your life and how you respond to them. Insecure people tend to feed off of others' insecurities. If there is a person in your life who is critical and who projects that out to you, notice the negative energy you feel inside when you are put down. This adds to your insecurity. Most likely that person feels powerful by making you feel insecure. This allows them to feel more secure about themselves. This type of person gains security by exploiting others' insecurities.

Step into your strength and courage. Go deep within. Find your inner nectar and the essence of your being. Once the nectar is found, let its sweet taste comfort and nurture you. Trust in yourself and who you are.

There are over 250 species of penstemons native to North America. Native Americans used the leaves to make a poultice for the skin and as an eyewash to treat eye problems. A tea made from leaves treats constipation, bronchitis, kidney problems, and whooping cough.

Scarlet penstemon's flower essence water is slightly pungent and slightly sweet. Similar to its odor, the essence is sweeter and fuller.

✦ *Affirmation* ✦

I claim my power. I trust my self-confidence and the inner essence of my being.

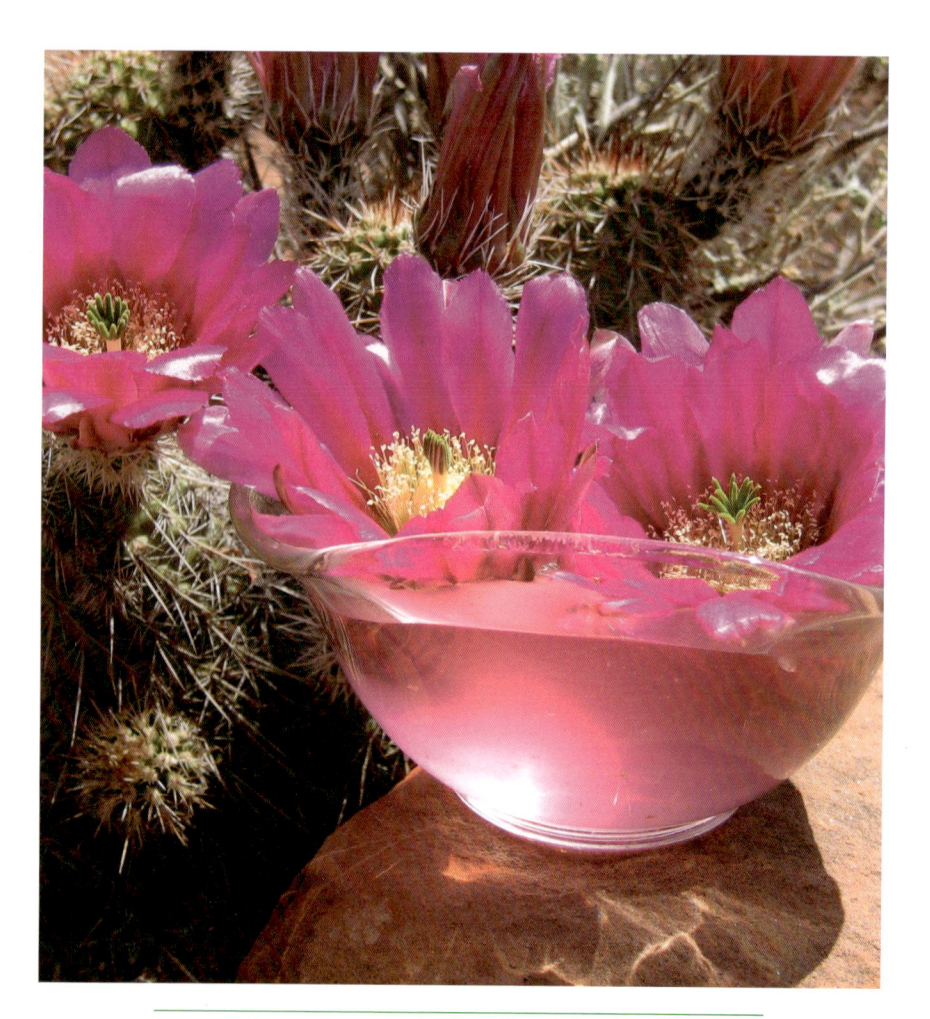

Immersed strawberry hedgehog flowers' sensual presence creates a natural pink hue in the flower essence water

STRAWBERRY HEDGEHOG
(Echinocereus engelmannii)

Primary quality: sensual pleasures
Energy impact/chakra correspondence: first, third, and fourth chakras

Voice of the Flower

I have great passion for living. I appreciate and love the joys life has to offer me. The secret of enjoying life's magnificent pleasures is to open your heart and tap into your ecstatic nature. The desire realms within your heart are the key to your passion for joy and pleasure.

My cucumberlike organ or stem is very delicate. It is covered with a thick, waxy layer that helps me hold water that my roots absorb. My needles provide protection. My flower emerges from the sustenance offered by my stem. I awaken within you the sacred energy that rises up the spine, spiraling to the heart, and out the top of your head.

My deep magenta, cup-shaped flower is sensual, soft, and elastic. A style encircled by golden-yellow pollen, with a receptive stigma, rises from the top of my ovary. My inner petals are deep and rich in color. My outer petals are a softer pink. Dozens of soft, airy, lemon-yellow stamens spread out in a circle inside the center of my flower. My sweetly fragrant flowers bloom for several days. They attract bees and beetles due to their abundance of pollen.

Enjoy life as a celebration of discovery. Become absorbed in my passion. Give yourself permission to be completely and unconditionally receptive to the celebration of your own creative passion and sensual pleasures.

Insight

Strawberry hedgehog helps you look at the ways in which you experience different pleasures in your life. This plant awakens and stirs your senses. Its passion runs deep. Feel the excitement of its vibrant beauty. Strawberry hedgehog's instinct is strong when it comes to the senses—feel this sensuous vibration as you look at its photo.

Awaken to the senses that give you pleasure. Include all of your senses—taste, smell, touch, sound, sight, as well as your intuitive power within. Often we lose sight of our senses or forget that each one has their own joy and fulfillment. Connect with your individual senses. Give them a voice. That's what gives pleasure to your senses. Listen to your heart. Notice how it feels when you connect with your senses.

The miraculous power of this beautiful, sensuous flower emerges through a cluster of spine-bearing tubercles that join together to surround and protect it. With a burst of passion, the strawberry hedgehog flower embodies freedom. It blooms despite the challenging environment of the desert.

The passionate magenta petals of the flower are strong, yet yielding and gentle. Strawberry hedgehog helps you cultivate a relationship with yourself and with others. Experience your desire to awaken your senses in a bigger way. Enjoy the sensual nature of this flower. Open yourself up to love and compassion. Appreciate yourself and all that is good in your life.

Strawberry hedgehog is a long-living succulent, a survival plant of the desert and a treasure to the Desert Southwest's ecosystem. Its shallow and wide fibrous roots grow close to the earth's surface and they absorb rainwater to support the plant. After the flowers are pollinated, they mature into brightly colored fuchsia fruits with tiny black seeds. The strawberry-tasting fruits offer food to wildlife such as rodents, coyotes, javelinas, and birds.

The inner flesh of strawberry hedgehog's stem can be used as a poultice for sunburn, bites, stings, open wounds, cuts, and abrasions. It also lowers blood sugar and can treat earache.

A variety of bees and flies are attracted to the abundantly sweet nectar of strawberry hedgehog, carrying the pollen amidst the desert flora.

The scent of strawberry hedgehog flower essence water is roselike, subtle, and soft. Its taste is similar, although fuller. The flower essence water color turns into a soft pink, glowing hue.

✦ Affirmation ✦

I awaken all my senses and live a passionate life.

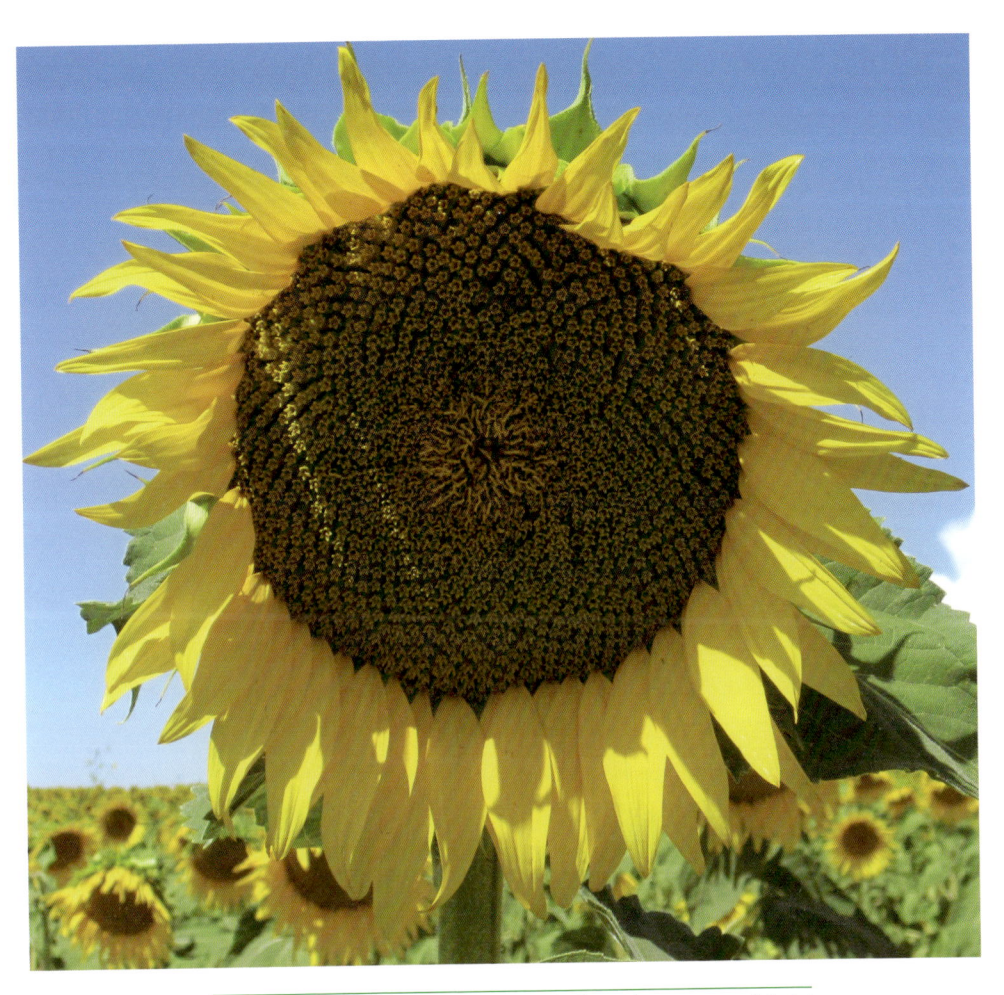

Sunflower head beckons you to follow the power of light

SUNFLOWER
(Helianthus annuus)

Primary quality: empowering radiance
Energy impact/chakra correspondence: third chakra (solar plexus)

Voice of the Flower

As the sun rises in the east, I awake refreshed. My flower head faces the sun to greet the new day. The center of my disk appears as an open eye. It is encircled by brilliant ray flowers. These fertile flowers are composed of small tubular blooms without petals that ripen into seeds. My seed head forms a dazzling geometric circle pattern.

In the center of my flower's disk I feel an opening. The warmth and light of the sun slowly invite my golden-yellow petals to stretch further outward. Throughout the day, I follow the sun. I bask in the sun's rays. I let its light into me.

My deep root system is far-reaching. It gives me the ability to draw out trace minerals that may not be found in the uppermost topsoil. My root system absorbs water from the soil. It is believed to open pathways in the soil that allow the natural warmth of the sun to pass through.

My stalk is covered with coarse hairs and is sturdy and tall. My showy, broad leaves alternate along the stem. My presence offers you a feeling of being in your power—a feeling of strength and endurance.

I attract sunlight all day long. Even my round, golden-yellow head is symbolic of the sun. I represent the fire of life, the will. Like me, I invite you to follow the sun and let my radiant light come through in you.

Turn toward me and follow the brilliance of my golden-yellow light. I awaken you to your own source of love and power. Discover your deepest sense of purpose, what you came into this life to accomplish. Trust that you will fertilize the seeds of your life purpose. Lovingly nurture your seeds. Empower your growth.

Feel light entering the soles of your feet. Let it move up your legs to your belly. Feel warmth from deep within you and all around you. Allow wisdom and strength to embellish you, to take you in, and to hold you in that place. Experience a deep sense of your own empowering radiance.

Insight

Sunflower guides you to follow the light and power of the sun. Let its radiance shine on you wherever you turn. Bring your awareness to those aspects of yourself that give you a sense of purpose, joy, and optimism. Notice your thoughts and feelings.

Sunflower restores youth and innocence, fun and play, liveliness and pleasure. Bring life to the child within you. Allow the positive nature of sunflower to stir your ability to focus on the light aspects of life. Imagine that all day long you can bring light into your root system. Empower your inner radiance.

Feel the warmth of the sun shining down on you. Give thanks for its expansive energy. Allow the life-giving power of the sun and its representative plant, the sunflower, to awaken the seeds of expansive energy within you. Be renewed by your own radiance and light. Let your personal power shine from deep within your roots and outward toward the sun. Create loving thoughts and feelings from the awareness of how it feels to empower all that you are.

The sunflower is believed to have originated in Peru, where the sun-worshiping Incas wore headdresses of the flower and adorned their temples with flowers wrought in gold. Aztec sun priestesses also adorned themselves with sunflowers and gold jewelry with sunflower emblems. The sunflower has for thousands of years been known as a symbol of the sun.

Sunflower was cultivated over three thousand years ago by Native American peoples, and archaeologists also found sunflower seeds in clay containers made at about that same time. Sunflower seeds are rich in vitamins and minerals, and sunflower oil offers a low-saturated fat content.

There are many traditional uses for sunflower, including sunflower soap, snares and arrows, flutes, flour, cereal, mush, breads, soups, oil, and dyes. Medicinally, sunflower root can be used to treat snakebite, rheumatism, and inflammation, and the stem juice can be used to clean cuts and wounds. An infusion of the pith stalk can be used as an eyewash and to treat cases of sore, inflamed eyes. Sunflower is a multitasking plant; all parts of it can be used, and it has too many uses to name here.

Numerous honeybees and many species of native wild bees are attracted to sunflowers and they are the plant's main pollinators.

Sunflower's odor is strong and musty, yet its flower essence is light and airy. It's one of the few flowers where the essence water turns a distinct shade of golden yellow.

✦ Affirmation ✦

> I empower the radiance that glows within me.
> I create loving thoughts and circumstances
> from a place of joy, wisdom, and strength.

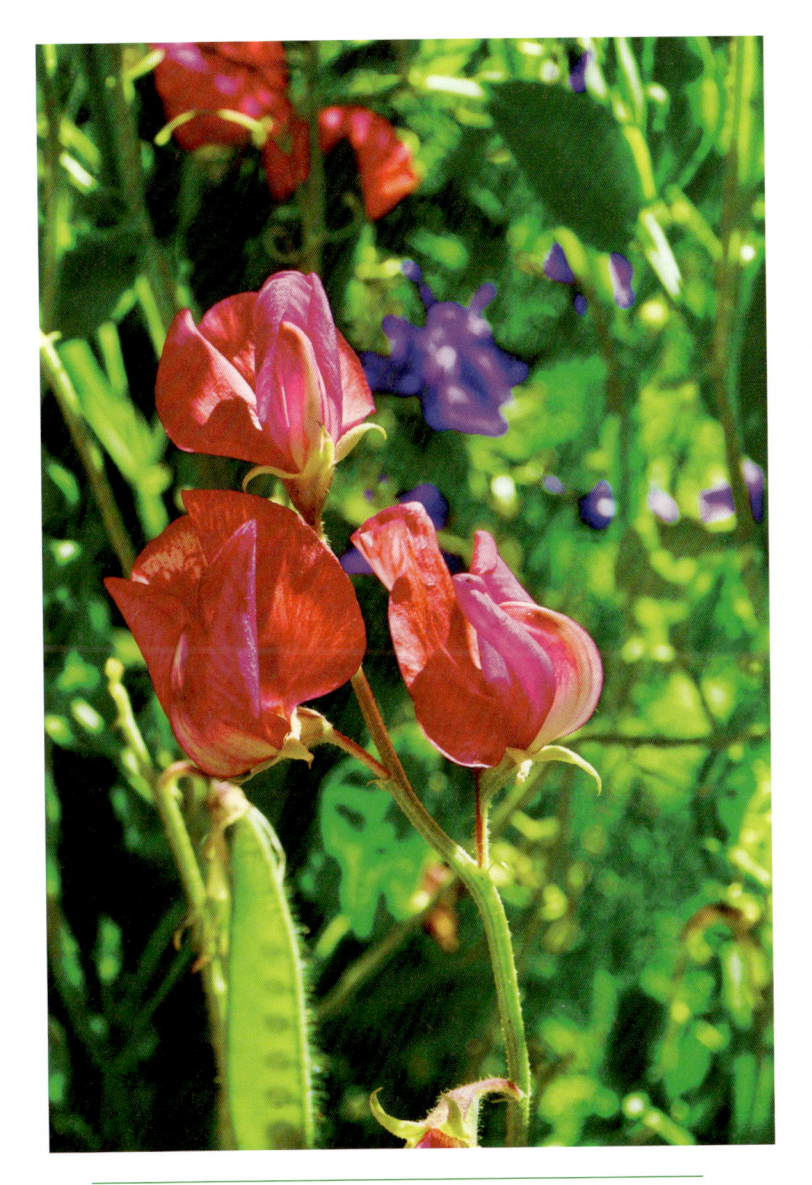

Sweet pea flowers in the moment with their lush presence

SWEET PEA
(Lathyrus latifolius)

Primary quality: inner security
Energy impact/chakra correspondence: fourth chakra

Voice of the Flower

Within my tender folds I offer you a place of security and protection. In this place, feel my great compassion and taste my sweet essence.

My broad, hood-shaped petal represents protection. Imagine a child sitting with a hood or cap covering her head. Inside the hood, the child feels safe, calm, and secure. My two side petals resemble wings that indicate freedom. My two folding lower petals offer protection and security.

My soft beauty and gentle nature are a reminder of the gentleness and compassion needed to raise a child. Bring your attention to your inner child. The essence of my flower is slightly sweet and light, reinforcing my sweet and gentle nature. It also offers a quiet and soothing presence.

My tendrils attach and twine around other flowers or structures to help me thrive. I am nurtured and supported by their presence.

I give you the strength to love yourself unconditionally and to nurture yourself as you change and grow. Honor yourself and embrace your personal growth as you walk your life journey. Slow down. Find your own footholds. Take time to establish your support system. Discover what brings you security from within. Find your own trellis of strength that sustains you. Climb into the protection I offer in my flower. Nurture yourself in the secure knowledge of who you are.

Insight

Sweet pea awakens your inner child. It offers a soft, gentle beauty. Its presence gives a feeling of compassion, security and protection.

Open your heart to the child within you. Imagine nurturing yourself as you would nurture a child.

A support structure is needed to encourage the security for sweet pea to climb. The vines require a truss on which to grow. A child, or your inner child, also needs secure footholds in order to gain confidence and security.

Often, we as adults forget to honor our child within. We may look for security externally. But it's the inner child that knows what security really is. So often in life we look to other people or things to help us feel secure. Listen to your inner child. What is she saying to you? Stir your childlike nature within. Do things you liked to do when you were younger. What did you do for yourself as a child to feel secure? What can you do now for yourself to feel secure? What footholds in life will create the support your inner child needs to feel secure?

Father Cupani, a Sicilian priest, gave sweat pea seeds from his monastery garden to a schoolmaster in London, England. These seeds are reputed to be the ancestors of all the common sweet peas found in our gardens, greenhouses, and natural settings. There are hundreds of varieties of sweet peas that vary in color, petal shape, and fragrance.

Sweet pea flowers offer a beautiful visual presence to the garden buffet in addition to enriching its biodiversity. They invite pollinators such as butterflies, bees, moths, flies, and beetles who treasure their nectar.

The scent of sweet pea is sweetly fragrant and relaxing, just like its flower essence tastes, and so is the sensation the essence offers when drinking it.

✦ *Affirmation* ✦

I establish an inner structure of support.
I feel secure in who I am.

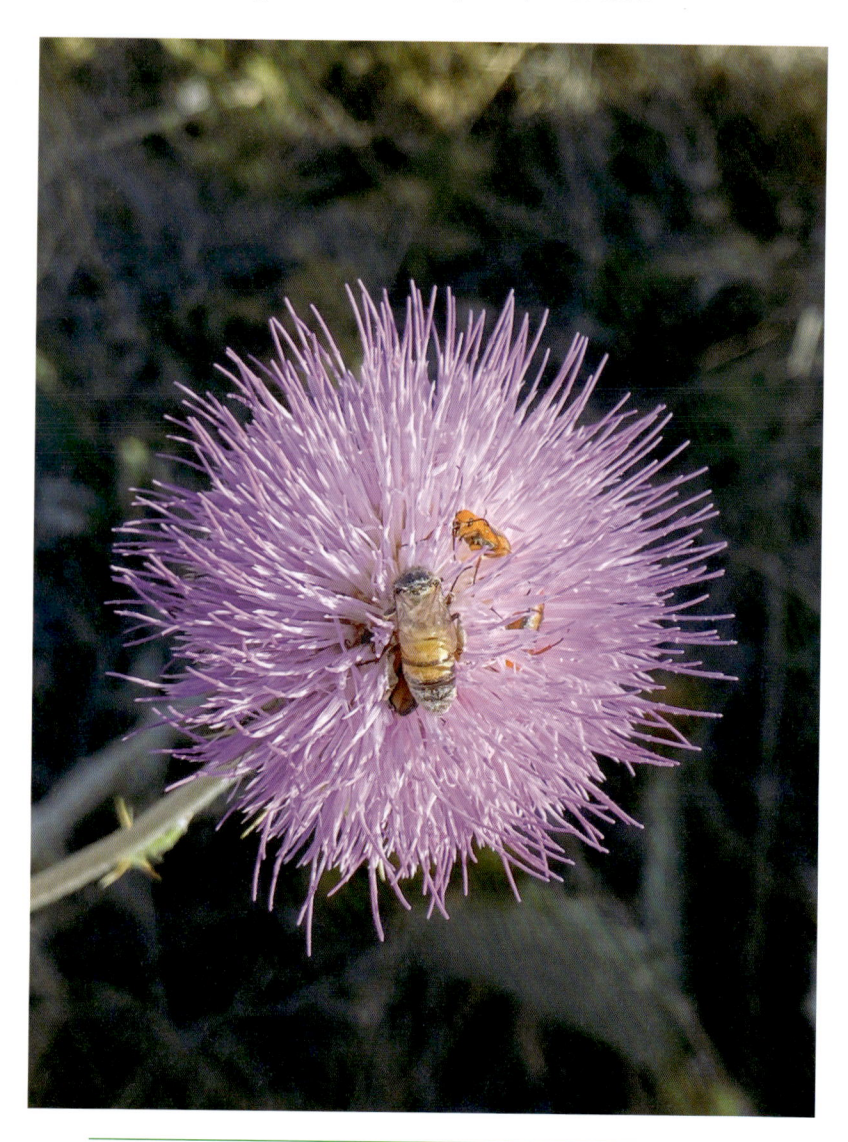

Thistle flower presents its encircling soft array of purple delight

THISTLE
(Cirsium mexicanum)

Primary quality: feeling centered
Energy impact/chakra correspondence: fourth, sixth, and seventh chakras

Voice of the Flower

My spiny stems and prickly leaves are rough, edgy, and thorny. They offer me protection. Inside my stem lies a sweet juice. From my stem emerges my soft and delicate flower.

My purple flower head is composed of a soft array of tender, stringy spines that emerge from my center. They form a round, plush, lavender circle. Midway inside the circle, my lavender spines become white, with tiny white tips. The very center of my flower is filled with soft, deep pink and lavender tips on short lavender spines. These short spines offer a symmetrical center within the circle. They hold a protective energy within my flower.

Energy flows within me and all around my center. My flower head expresses the essence of that shape. It forms a nearly perfect circle around the center. There's nothing that forces it into that shape in nature. It holds its own in the form of a circle with a constant swirl of energy.

It is the center of my sacred circle that holds the power of union between inner and outer, hard and soft, light and dark, sweet and bitter. It reflects the magic within you to discover your power at the center of your being. See yourself standing in the center of a circle. Experience the power of circular energy in motion all around you. Step into that flow of energy.

When you connect with your center, a natural balance of energy and power radiates from your heart. Imagine my flower caressing you and your heart. Feel a gentle sensation all around you. Breathe light and love into the center of your heart.

Insight

Thistle encourages you to search for balance in your life. It assists you to soften your character or to protect yourself in those situations where you need to maintain clear boundaries.

The thorns and roughness that grow on thistle's stem and leaves reflect back to us our own bristly characteristics—characteristics to work with in order to capture our own beauty and sweetness from deep within. Thistle teaches balance and helps us to get in touch with our center.

Experience that place within you where darkness meets light. Support the feeling of being centered and balanced. This allows your heart center to open. Radiate a creative force of energy and power. Feel this energy within and around your heart and spiraling outward.

There at least seventeen species of thistle in the American Southwest, and numerous other species in other parts of the United States, Europe, and Asia. Thistle infusions can be used as a tonic, astringent, and diuretic. They are known to treat stomach conditions, fever, diarrhea, dysentery, skin eruptions, ulcers, and poison ivy.

Native American peoples ate the roots of the New Mexico thistle raw, boiled, or roasted. These thistles make good emergency food. They are easy to identify and grow abundantly. Thistle flower buds picked at the immature stage can also be eaten raw or steamed and dipped in lemon butter, tasting similar to artichoke hearts.

Bees, butterflies, and moths are the chief pollinators of thistle in the Southwest flora.

The odor of thistle flower essence water is pleasantly sweet, offering a mild, lavenderlike aroma. However, its taste is slightly bitter. This is another example of thistle's ability to bring opposites together to create balance.

Affirmation

Energy flows within me and all around my center.

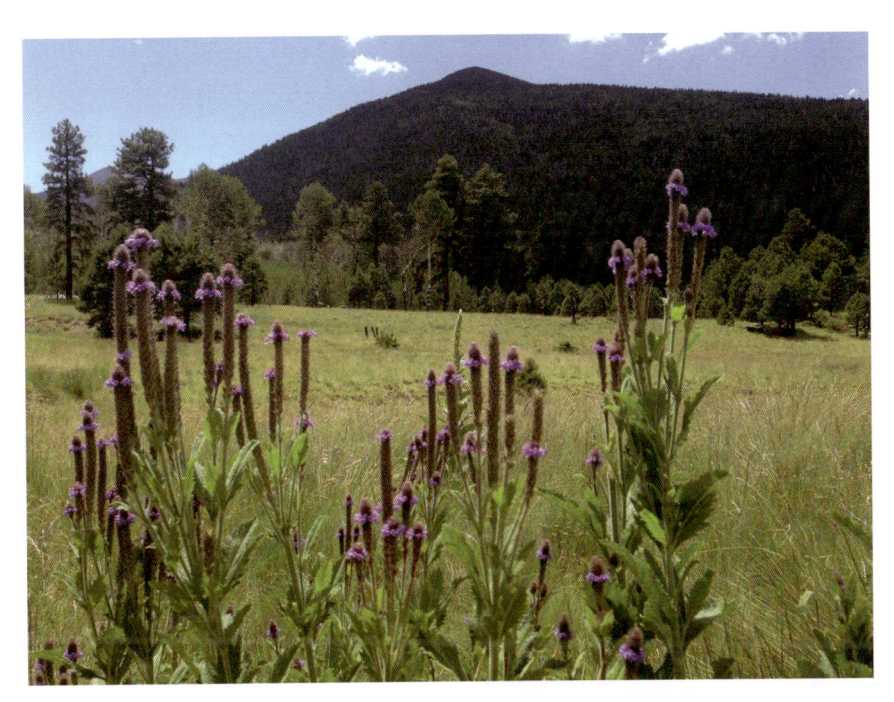

Vervain plants emerge to help you follow your dreams

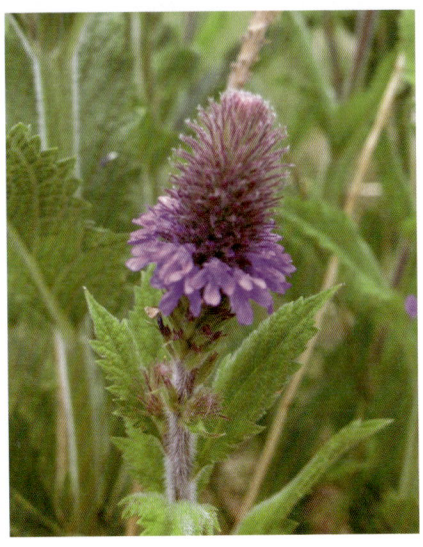

Vervain flower reaches to new heights

VERVAIN
(Verbena macdougalii)

Primary quality: inspiring direction
Energy impact/chakra correspondence: sixth and seventh chakras

Voice of the Flower

My strong, thick, square stem is sticky and composed of many layers. It is hairy all around. Branching stems arise from my spreading roots. My dark green, lance-shaped, mintlike leaves are widely spread and grow in opposite pairs. My prominently veined leaves are prickly yet fuzzy, and my entire plant has a slightly bitter smell.

My lush purple flowers first open at the bottom of my long, erect spike. They form a ring around the spike and appear to progress up the spike. As each circle of flowers moves upward along my stem, I remain open to the journey of every moment as it reveals itself to me.

Seed pods appear below and flower buds appear above my ring of flowers. My tiny singular flower has five petals or lobes. Three petals bend downward and two bend upward. The center of each of my tiny flowers is whitish-yellow and star-shaped.

As my roots sink deeper into the earth, my spiral grows higher toward the sky. I feel hope and joy that I am on a higher path. Imagine being in the center of the circle of my flowers as they move upward along the stem. Be open to your journey. Feel your feet as roots sinking deeper into the earth. Visualize your body spiraling like my stem. Hold yourself in that space. Release any tensions you may be carrying. Let your inspirations guide your journey. Allow life to unfold and become aware of your dreamtime.

I inspire you to hold your vision. Enjoy your journey, moment by moment. Reach for your destiny. Experience my light shining forth like brilliant stars lighting your way.

Insight

Vervain supports you to gain clarity in your direction. The formation of the spike and the ring of flowers progressing upward signifies a sense of crowning achievement.

Vervain gives you insight and perspective to see what lies ahead. It encourages you to remain relaxed, grounded, and focused while you take each step along the way.

The tiny star shape in the center of the tiny flowers symbolizes an upward direction, as if encouraging you to reach for the stars. Stay open and receptive to a new, positive direction.

The organizational structure of vervain offers a uniform appearance in its spiraling spikes. Its ring of flowers and layers along the stem suggest simplicity and moderation. This represents vervain's ability to see ahead and to strive for an upward direction. Vervain's spreading roots and its sturdy branching stems symbolize the plant's ability to remain grounded and connected to the earth.

Let your inspiration guide your journey, moment by moment. Allow life to unfold naturally as your endeavors reap the rewards of your crowning achievement.

The genus *Verbena* is referred to as "holy bough," and vervain is known as "the enchanter's plant." It has been associated with mysticism and magic for centuries. Known as the "herb of Venus," vervain was also used in love potions and lucky charms. In seventeenth-century England, herbalist Nicholas Culpeper used vervain to treat "pain in the secret parts."

Today, vervain has multiple medicinal uses—as a sedative, mild tranquilizer, diaphoretic, emetic, diuretic, bitter tonic, and antispasmodic. Vervain eases conditions such as nervous tension, depression, insomnia, and headache. A salve made from vervain leaves is used to treat sprains, deep bruises, and muscle tension.

Vervain offers a unique exquisiteness in the mountainous landscape or in the fall garden, enticing pollinators such as hummingbirds, bees, and butterflies.

Vervain flower essence's scent is subtle and somewhat bitter. It tastes full, pleasant, soft, and slightly sweet, unlike its smell. You may feel a warming, tingling sensation when you drink a vervain flower essence. You may want to take it at bedtime to help you in your dreamtime.

✦ *Affirmation* ✦

I reach for my own brilliant stars to guide me on my journey. As I follow my dreamtime, I am inspired to be all that I am.

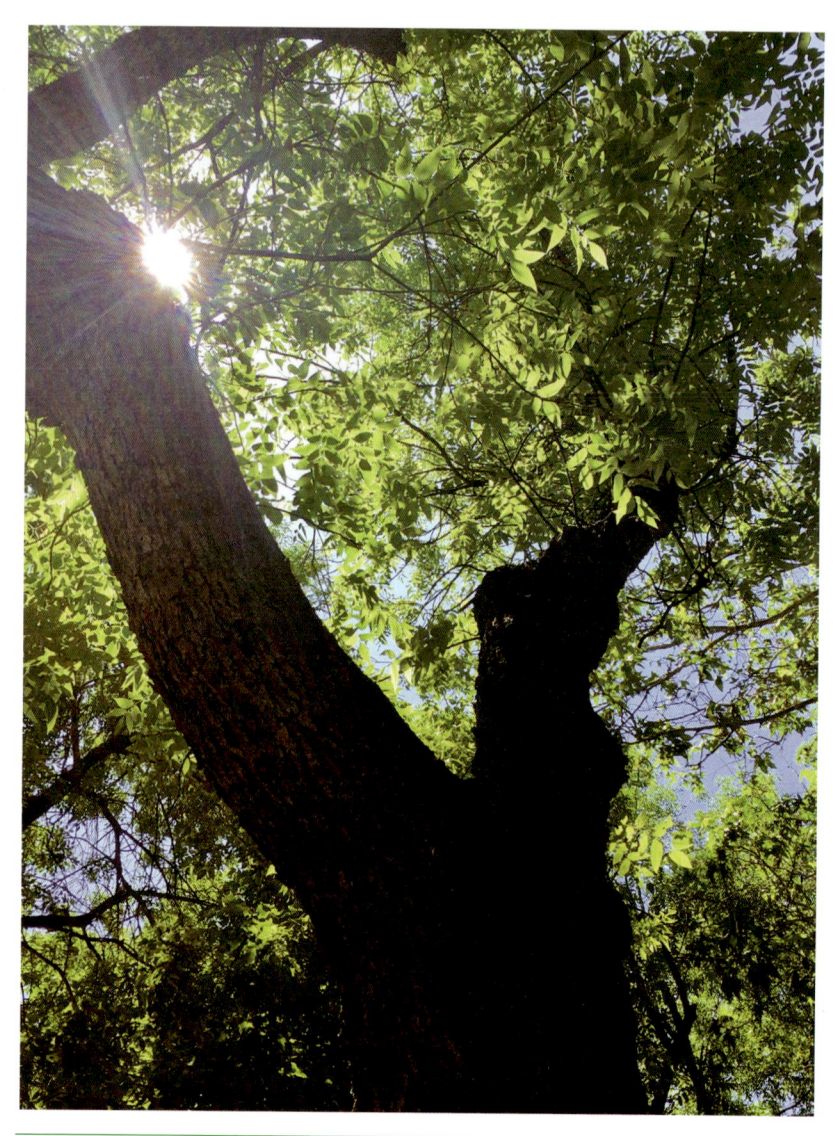

Walnut tree encourages standing strong on your journey as you begin anew

WALNUT
(Juglans major)

Primary quality: new beginnings
Energy impact/chakra correspondence: first, second, third, and seventh chakras

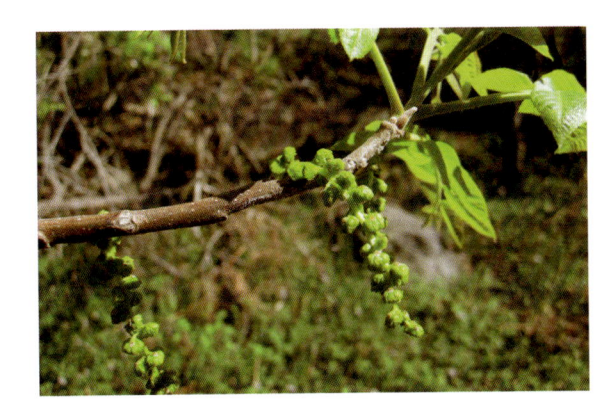

Walnut catkins are plush and firm, vibrant and tenacious

Voice of the Flower (Catkin)

Step away from the outside world . . . it's just you and me. Make yourself comfortable under my canopy of support and protection. If for any reason you feel vulnerable next to my distinctive presence, I encourage you to explore all that I am. Notice the deep, fertile soil below me from which I grow. My roots extend up to fifty feet or more away from my trunk, yet they are no more than three to seven feet deep.

My grayish-brown bark becomes rough and rugged as I mature. I have deep, scaly ridges that run vertically up and down my trunk. My leaves are pinnate and grow in pairs of leaflets. They are coarsely toothed and lance-shaped, aromatic, and spicy. I am one of the first trees to lose leaves in the fall and the last to leaf out in the spring.

Press your nose against my gnarled trunk and take in the subtle scent of my being. I secrete a natural herbicide known as juglone, which is harmful and growth-stunting to many other plants and prevents them from growing close around me, including even my own offspring. All my parts—leaves, roots, husks, fruit, bark, and nuts—contain juglone, which protects me from unwanted invaders yet is safe for humans.

Let your eyes focus on my trunk and then gaze up at my branches. Notice my catkins and flowers hanging from a stem, displaying a sense of position and strategy, knowing their place. My catkins are plush, firm, and taste bitter. They offer a sense of vibrancy and tenacity to stay true to yourself, to learn from your journey and to trust it is beginning anew.

Visualize my outer green husk as a protective covering for my walnut, my fruit. My walnut kernels find security within their shells, which are blanketed by this green outer husk. With its place in the center, two halves joined as one, my walnut kernel resembles a human brain and also a human heart.

When my walnuts fall from my branches, they will not flourish if there is too much juglone in the soil. The ones that bounce away from me have a much better chance of survival than those that fall directly into the soil below my canopy.

I offer you encouragement to move forward in your life, to explore and trust the depths of your life's experiences. Sometimes it takes stepping away from yourself and whatever situation you may be facing to gain a fresh perspective so you can see where you really want to be. Try moving outside of your inner circle to be inspired by new thoughts and new realities. Allow them to unfold naturally.

Hold the presence of my protection within you as you go forth into the outside world. Make way for new beginnings.

Insight

Harvest time for walnuts occurs during the month of August. The thin green outer hull covering the nut, which is about the size of a baseball, but softer like a softball, starts to crack open and exposes the hard, brown shell protecting the nut. The actual walnut kernel found inside the woody shell consists of two ridged, light brown lobes, which give the appearance of a human brain—hence walnut's association with the brain and intellectualism. The lobes are covered with a papery thin skin, and the two lobes are attached in the center.

The outer green husk as a covering for the walnut offers the signature of a head—it resembles the external membrane of the skull, the pericranium, and corresponds to the ability to know how to protect oneself from the outside world to prevent unnecessary hardships. It teaches you to learn how to adapt to and endure hardships if and when they do occur, and to step into new places when you feel shielded and protected.

The smooth woody shell around the kernel further underscores walnut's signature, that of a human skull, while offering yet another layer of protection for the actual kernel inside. This signature is of a shield that protects you while allowing you to explore your innermost depths, so that you feel supported to move forward.

Juglone, the fungicidal and antibacterial compound found in walnut trees, presents a signature of strength, endurance, and protection, as juglone wards off predators, pests, and other invasive plant life. This refers to your ability to live consciously while warding off any dangers that inhibit your vitality.

When the walnuts fall from the tree, those that bounce away from the tree stand a much better chance of surviving than those that fall on the ground directly under the parent tree, which is infused with juglone. This is a signature of how you as an adult support your inner child to trust and move forward in life, allowing you to find a new direction. Know that your roots are supported and protected. The new walnut sprouts need to separate themselves from the existing host energy in order to create a new mode of survival and to begin anew.

As you stretch forward and choose new directions to build new beginnings, feel the guidance and support that walnut offers you. Trust that your strength and endurance will protect you on your journey.

Walnut leaves and bark are astringent and antiseptic. A tea can be made to treat diarrhea, dysentery, asthma, the sinuses, excessive menstruation, and parasites. Walnut is an excellent source of iodine, which supports the thyroid gland. Walnuts and walnut oil are flavorful and nutritious. They are also a significant food source for wild animals. The wood of walnut trees is strong, very hard, and strikingly beautiful.

Walnut trees are wind-pollinated. Walnut catkins carry a tender, aromatic, uplifting, and subtly spicy yet slightly bitter aroma. The essence water tastes similar and is also very earthy. The essence invites you to ground new beginnings you're bringing into your life.

✦ Affirmation ✦

> I trust that the core of my inner strength carries me through my life's journey. I walk in new directions to create new beginnings.

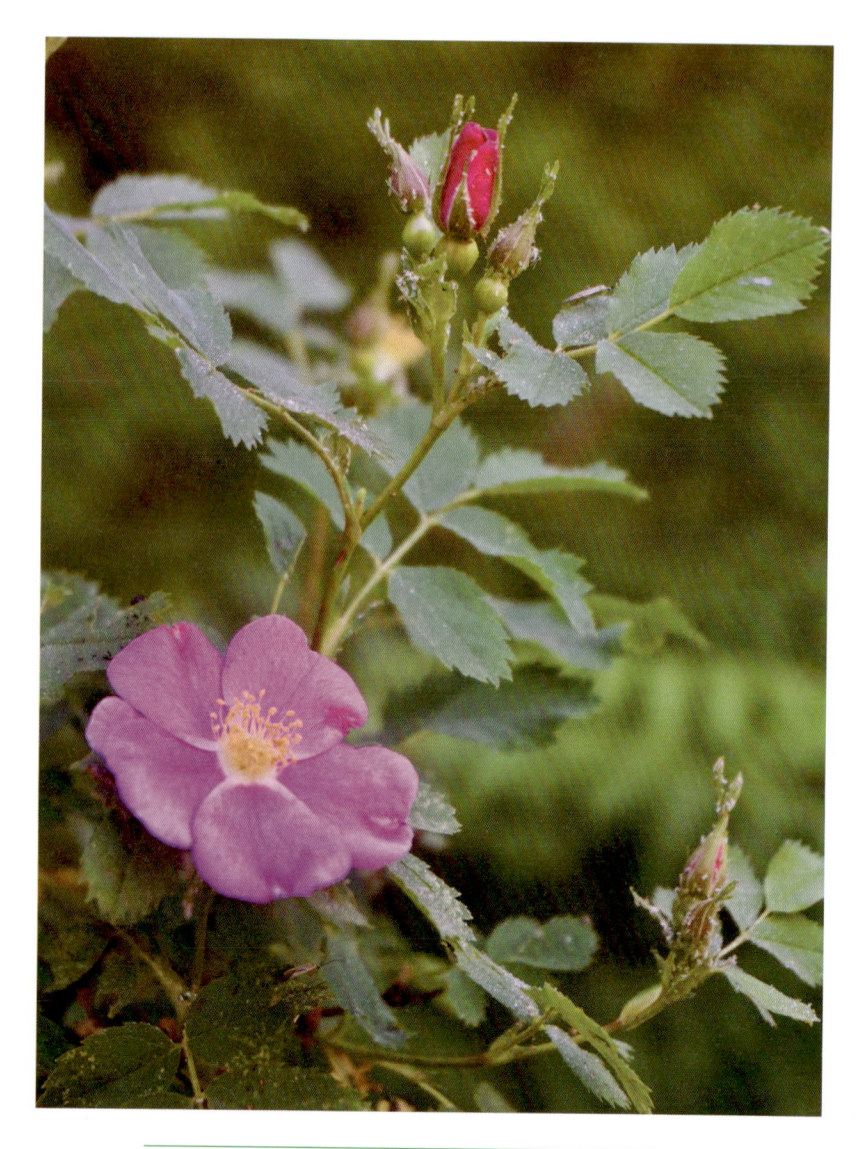

Wild rose blossoms lusciously flourish along the stem, exuding their growth and soft pink hues

WILD ROSE
(Rosa acicularis)

Primary quality: heart awakening
Energy impact/chakra correspondence: third and fourth chakras

Voice of the Flower

My flower carries a gentle rose fragrance that is sweeter than most other roses. I have five beautiful pink, wavy petals with a clump of yellow stamens that emerge from my center. My stems are brownish in color, with hooked thorns. My leaves alternate with five to nine toothed leaflets. My fleshy, rounded, ruby-colored rose hips birth an abundance of seeds. Harvest my tiny jewels and receive my inner medicinal treasures.

I have long been known as a powerful symbol of love, beauty, and adoration. The Greek goddess of love, Aphrodite, is often shown with a crown of roses around her head.

Imagine lying on a velvety pink blanket charged with my silky wild rose petals. Wrap my blanket of love around yourself. With eyes closed, hold a flower in the palm of your hand. Bring my flower to your nose and smell its sweet fragrance. Now bring me to your lips and gently kiss me. Place my flower on your heart. See a soft pink glow all around you. Let my fragrance stir you deep within your heart and all around you. Take in my tender, loving presence.

I invite you to awaken your heart and receive the love that is already within you. May you find an opening within your heart to love the gift of being alive. Embrace each opportunity to face your challenges and your pain.

Give yourself over to love. Nurture your heart. Feel your blood flowing from your heart and throughout your body.

Your heart is your greatest teacher. I am the love within you.

Awaken the love in your heart.

Insight

Wild rose awakens you to your heart energy. It calls you to discover your powers of love and compassion. Listen to your heart as you live your life.

Wild rose embodies abundance and growth, love and beauty. It reminds us of the power of our emotions and thoughts, sometimes stuck among the thorns. Soften your thorns and allow a new journey to unfold, a journey of being pure love.

Take time to feel your pain and your love. Let your pain—represented by the rose's thorns—find its way to untangling itself. See yourself unwinding the pain. It's the mind and the unprocessed emotions that keep pain alive in you, that keep those old thoughts and hurts constantly running in the background.

When you love deeply, your pain and the love you're feeling get mixed up together.

May you open the doorway of your heart so that the power of love can pour through you. Trust in love. Plant the seeds of love in your heart's soil. Nurture all the ways you love yourself. Give yourself permission to love yourself first, before anything or anyone else. Nourish your heart, mind, body, and soul. Be love.

Native American peoples gathered the wild rose for ornaments and for medicinal use. Young men picked wild roses for their brides. Wooden needles from the rose bush were used for leatherwork. Rose petals were used with bear grease to treat mouth sores, and they made a rose powder to treat fever, sore, and blisters.

Wild rosebuds and rose hips can be made into a pleasant tea to treat diarrhea and to expel kidney stones. The petals offer an added flavor to medicines in the form of a syrup and have been used in tonics and gargles to treat catarrh, sore throat, mouth sores, and stomach problems. The petals, diluted in water, make a safe eyewash that acts as a mild astringent. Roses in general can be made into a simple syrup for teas and drinks. Rose flowers and stems can also be used in facial toner to decongest blocked pores and draw out dead skin cells.

Insect pollinators are attracted to the pollen and protein-rich golden yellow stamens in the wild rose. These include many bees, hoverflies, and wasps.

Wild rose flower essence water carries a soft, subtle, rosey fragrance. Its flower essence is also especially soft and roselike, tastes soothing, and offers a quiet, easygoing peacefulness thoughout the body.

✦ Affirmation ✦

I begin this day in love and live in love all day long.

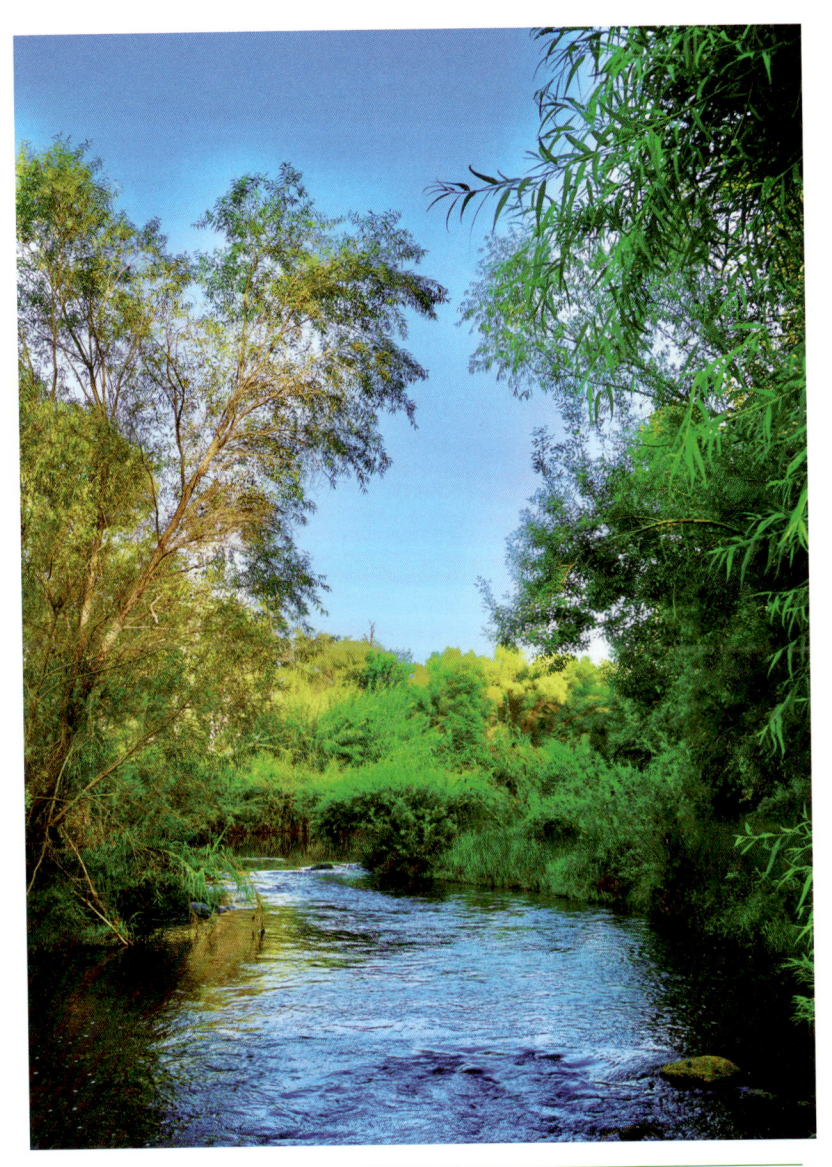

Willow trees whose roots hold strong, letting the flow of water move on

WILLOW
(Salix gooddingii)

Primary quality: compassion
Energy impact/chakra correspondence: fourth and seventh chakras

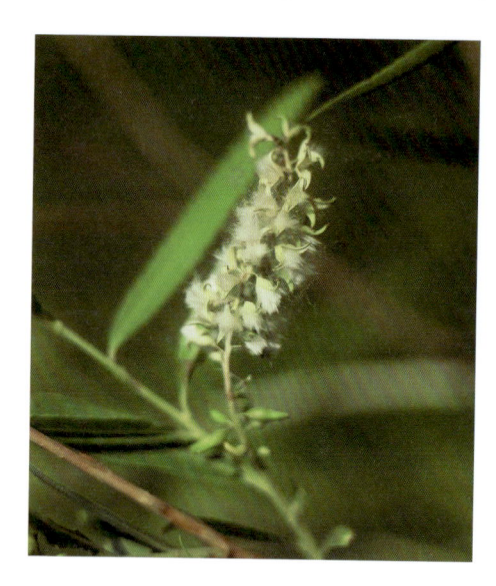

Willow catkin's white cottony seed buds sway in the wind

Voice of the Flower (Catkin)

I protect the waters that flow around me. I am nurtured by these waters as my roots sink deep into the earth. My deep root system holds the soil and stops streambed erosion. When the creek or stream rises, I hold the soil together to keep it from being washed away.

I offer you the inner strength needed to help recognize the erosion of your spirit. Feel my compassionate presence as you spend time with me.

I am trustworthy and flexible. My wispy branches bend and sway gracefully in the wind. My smaller branches are limber and flexible, like reeds sweeping in the slightest breeze. See my shiny green and curved leaves quake. My catkin flowers with their white, cottony seed buds shimmer in the sun. My entire being is a dance in the wind, giving and receiving, bending and yielding. I stir the energy of freedom and compassion from within.

I invite you to open your heart. Join me in my dance of freedom and compassion. Bring your burdens to me. Free yourself of the past.

My strength is to help you recognize what burdens you are carrying. Find out who and what you need to forgive. I will help you reveal your compassion.

Be flexible along with me. Get to know me through my compassion and willingness to stretch and bend. My invitation to you is to imagine being me, growing along a stream. Overhead you hear the flapping of wings from a pair of mallard ducks. Upstream you hear the trickling flow of nearby waters. Slowly breathe in and breathe out.

Feel the rustling of the wind flowing through your branches, which are your arms. Slowly move your arms, neck, and head from side to side.

Next, take a step with one foot and allow your whole body to bend and sway. Feel the energy stirring in your body. Let your movements be guided by your intuition. Experience all that you are in the freedom of your dance.

Insight

Willow provides an opportunity to look at the ways you move with the ebb and flow of change in your life. To encourage change and to make peace with the past, step away from identifying with any suffering you have endured. If you feel pain or hurt from someone else's actions, you are being asked to face the situation and deal with your feelings. Let go of comparing your pain with the pain of others. Your resolve is based on the compassion of forgiveness.

If you harbor bitterness in your heart, that bitterness will become a burden. Choosing to forgive is choosing to let go of the burden. Free yourself of the past. Get to a place where you are ready to stop identifying with your suffering. Acknowledge what it is you are ready to forgive. And forgive yourself for holding onto pain. Feel compassion for yourself first.

Willow teaches you to be flexible in your approach to life. Move with the ebb and flow of life's wisdom and grace. Let the compassionate nature of willow open your heart. Bask in the peace that forgiveness brings. Revel in the growth and excitement of your spirit rising. Shine in your heart's radiance. Feel the warmth in your heart that forgiveness brings.

There are many species of willow, so it can be difficult to identify some species due to variations and cross-breeding. Willows grow abundantly along streams and washes. A tea made of willow leaves will relieve nausea and a nervous stomach. A tea made from willow bark treats headache, fever, and inflammation. *Salix* and associated plants rich in salicin are used as an analgesic and antirheumatic to relieve muscle pains, arthritis, and toothache.

Native American peoples used willow branches as poles for tipis and to build sweat lodges. Willow leaves were fed to livestock as fodder. The down of some types of willow that comes from the tree's white feathery catkins was made into stockings. Basket makers have used the plant shoots to make sturdy baskets, and the resilient wood is also used to make handles and fences. Today, willow branches are still commonly used to make sweat lodges, especially in the Southwestern United States, and they provide the structure for hoop weaving and dream catchers as willows are known for their flexibility and strength.

Some willow trees have an especially well-known connection between male catkins, which provide nectar and pollen, and the tree, which attracts a variety of bees and butterflies.

Willow catkin essence water offers a very fragrant, earthy green, spicy aroma. Its taste is potent, cooling, somewhat bitter and strong, providing a sense of flow yet also a feeling of being rooted in the body.

✦ Affirmation ✦

> I dance in the freedom of my compassion to forgive.

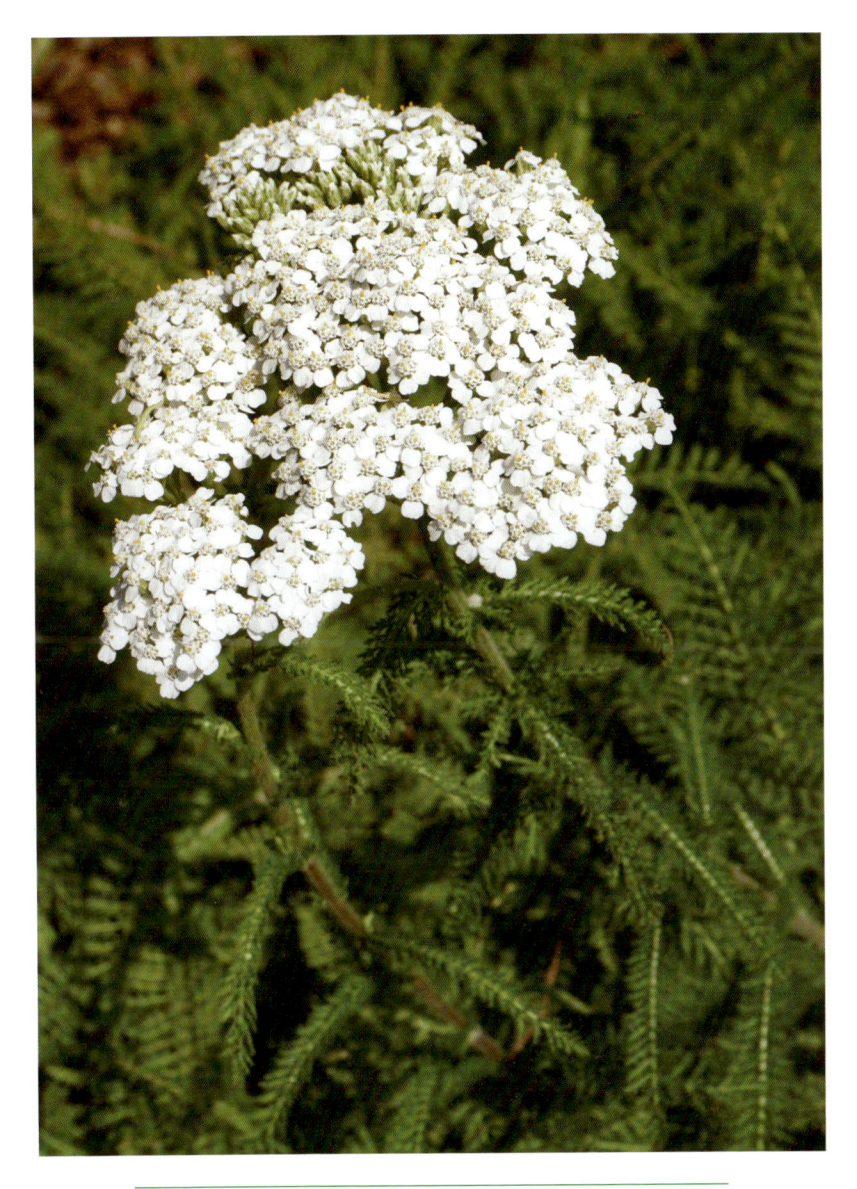

Yarrow flowers shield you in their protective energy field

YARROW
(Achillea millefolium)

Primary quality: energy protection
Energy impact/chakra correspondence: seventh chakra

Voice of the Flower

I am a thriving plant with creeping underground roots. My roots spread quickly to nurture large colonies. My pale green, slender stem is finely hairy and hollow. My slightly woolly, grayish, ferny green leaves are feathery and light. They are narrow and swordlike, yet lacy in appearance and highly aromatic. They give off a spicy, earthy odor that continues after being dried. My tiny seeds are flat and tear-shaped.

My tiny flowers are bone white in color and daisylike, and bloom in flat-topped clusters along my stem. They also form additional clusters toward the top. Sometimes they appear slightly pinkish. My tiny disk florets are composed of five petals, five tiny stamens, and five pale yellow anthers. My pollen is a soft orange. Breathe in my flower's pungent woody scent.

I offer you an energy shield to protect you from feeling drained by others or by life's circumstances. When you feel energetically depleted, you are given a choice to guard against unwanted influences. Create security within yourself. Find ways to feel safe and free. You have the choice to protect the ways in which you expend your energy. Empower yourself. Form a shield of protection within you and all around you.

Embrace the glow of my bone-white petals. Feel energized and protected by their warmth. Experience the power of my protection. Protect the energy that you give out. Empower yourself for healing to take place.

Insight

Yarrow is a way-shower in the ways that you may be giving your energy away. It brings to your awareness how you may be expending your energy in a way that leaves you with no reserves.

Yarrow has a powerful ability to thrive and heal. Yarrow may come to you at this time of healing to remind you to avoid overextending your energy where it concerns others. Save some energy for yourself, it says.

One of yarrow's characteristics is its feathery, lacy, saw-toothed leaves. They point to the plant's ability as a woundwort remedy that treats cuts, burns, and blood and inflammatory conditions.

The flowers' lacy appearance and bone-white color brings to mind our bones and blood. When you feel "cut to the bone," yarrow supports a safe place for healing. Yarrow's tough and nurturing underground root system is symbolic of the yarrow-type person who feels a need to be tough and strong.

Yarrow's strong scent, volatile oils, and bitter qualities also make a statement about its healing powers. Yarrow promotes cleansing. It helps us release toxic build-up, stagnation, and tension at all levels of our being.

When you have experienced the pain of feeling reduced and cut to the bone, the essence of yarrow shows you how the scar of your pain is imprinted on you. As your healing takes place over time, the pain gradually fades, yet the imprint may linger, leaving a scar that can either remind you of the pain or the growth that the pain has taught you.

Take in all that you can from the presence of yarrow. Let the energy of its protection surround you and fill you with an inner light.

Yarrow pollen on fossils in Neanderthal burial caves indicate that the plant's history of human use dates back sixty thousand years. Some three thousand years ago, the Greeks used yarrow in the Trojan Wars, and the Greek hero Achilles is said to have staunched the bleeding of wounded soldiers with yarrow leaves. Yarrow's reputation as a woundwort remedy continued through the American Civil War. Yarrow has also had a reputation for being a magical herb and was included in the Saxon amulets for protection. Yarrow leaves are used externally to treat burns, skin rashes, bruises, cuts, wounds, and to reduce swellings and ease rheumatic joints. Native Americans drank yarrow leaves and flowers in a tea for spiritual guidance and to treat an overall run-down feeling, as well as for conditions such as internal bleeding, fevers, and indigestion. Yarrow offers a wealth of medicinal healing well worth to learn about.

Yarrow, both wild and in gardens around the world, grows abundantly and attracts a multitude of various species of bees and gossamer-winged butterflies as their foremost pollinators.

Yarrow flower essence water smells fresh, strong, slightly pungent, and earthy green. It tastes cool, refreshing, and is smooth, bittersweet, and astringent.

✦ *Affirmation* ✦

I empower what energy means to me and and how I use it. I create an inner shield of light that glows within me and all around me.

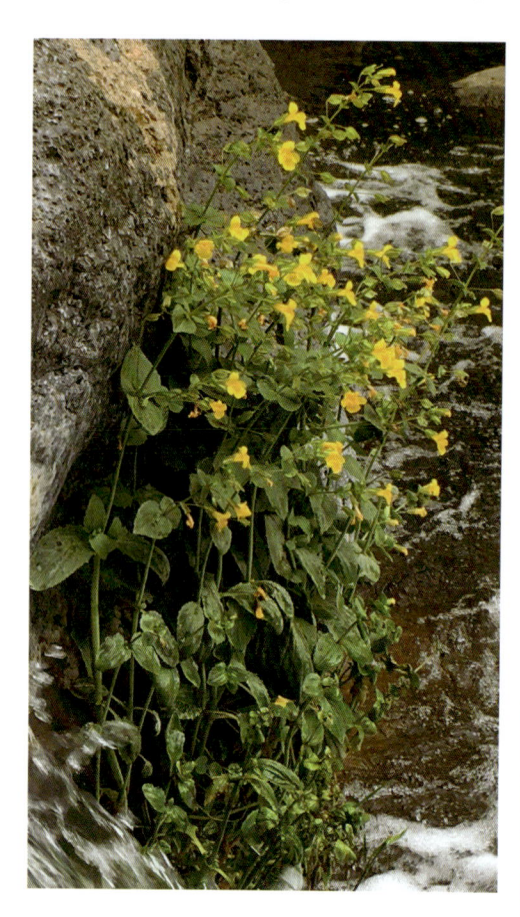

Yellow monkeyflower plants teach us to trust the flow of life

Yellow monkeyflower blossom helps you to let go of fear and step into trust

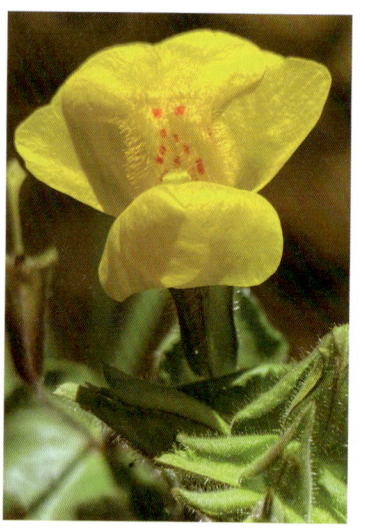

YELLOW MONKEYFLOWER
(Mimulus guttatus)

Primary quality: trust the flow
Energy impact/chakra correspondence: first, second, third, and fifth chakras

Voice of the Flower

My yellow flower with its red spots and mouthlike shape looks a monkey's face. This is how I got my name. My upper lip has two broad lobes that join to form a tunnel, and they point upward. My lower lip has three broad lobes, and they point downward. Both my calyx and corolla have reddish-orange spots. Larger spots can be seen toward the outside of my flower and smaller spots toward the inside. Two pairs of threadlike stamens with yellow anthers emerge from my center.

My root is easily pulled and develops from fallen stems where they contact the soil. My smooth, hollow, bending stems root at the nodes and develop clumps on cliffs and along rocks in wet places. My dark green, oval, sticky leaves have toothed margins and grow in opposites.

The steady flow of the waters I live in strengthens my roots as they search deeper for their foothold into the earth below. I feel a profound fear that my roots will lose hold when the water's force becomes swifter and stronger. I am afraid that its current may sweep me away, yet something inside of me knows that I can relax and go with the water's flow. With trust and confidence, I let go of my fear.

I allow the current of the water to move through me and all around me. I move with this flow. As I do, I let go of my fears and trust my newfound freedom. I give you this opportunity to allow yourself to move forward with the currents of life. Let go of your fears and embrace what is to come. Trust the flow of life.

Insight

Yellow monkeyflower helps you recognize your fears. You may in some way be hiding your fears from yourself and thus your true expression of self. Are you feeling trapped by life's setbacks and situations?

Yellow monkeyflower grows in or near flowing waters. Water represents the emotions, moods, and our sacral energy. This plant prefers moving waters, symbolizing how you flow or move in your emotional field. Its leaves are sticky, moist, and viscous. Yellow monkeyflower encourages you to move with the flow of life and to release whatever is making you feel stuck.

Yellow monkeyflower's reddish-orange spots get smaller as they go deeper inside the flower's tunnel, eventually disappearing. This represents what it takes for you to trust your journey of going deep within so that you can gather your courage and strength.

Yellow monkeyflower's petals express a mouthlike opening. The funnel part of the petals appear as a throat that opens into a mouth. This is the plant's way of helping you identify your fear of finding your voice. This fear might be related to not being heard. When you do share your truth, you may not be validated for your true feelings.

The sticky, viscous leaves of yellow monkeyflower are a reminder to let go of sticky relationships or situations you may find yourself in, and the fear that you may hold inside as a result of feeling stuck.

Yellow monkeyflower is a gentle kindred spirit who reminds you to trust and believe in yourself. It is here to feed your strength, to support you to express your uncertainties without fear. Flow with the natural currents in life that feed your soul. Take in confidence and trust that which yellow monkeyflower shares with you. Release your fears and enjoy your journey. Swim in the waters of your newfound freedom!

Yellow monkeyflower roots are traditionally used as an astringent. The sticky leaves taste somewhat buttery and were included in the diet of Native Americans, who also crushed the raw leaves and stems to use as a poultice to treat rope burns and wounds. The fresh plants can be eaten raw in salads. The leaves and stems make for an herbal steambath or a poultice to treat aches and pains.

A variety of butterflies, bees, flies, birds including hummingbirds, and moths are the major pollinators of yellow monkeyflowers.

Yellow monkeyflower carries a warm, musky odor. Its flower essence taste is smooth and mellow. When drinking yellow monkeyflower essence, the authors have experienced a noticeable tingling on the palate and the back of the tongue before swallowing.

✦ **Affirmation** ✦

I face my fears with strength and confidence.
I trust my life's flow and lovingly embrace my freedom.

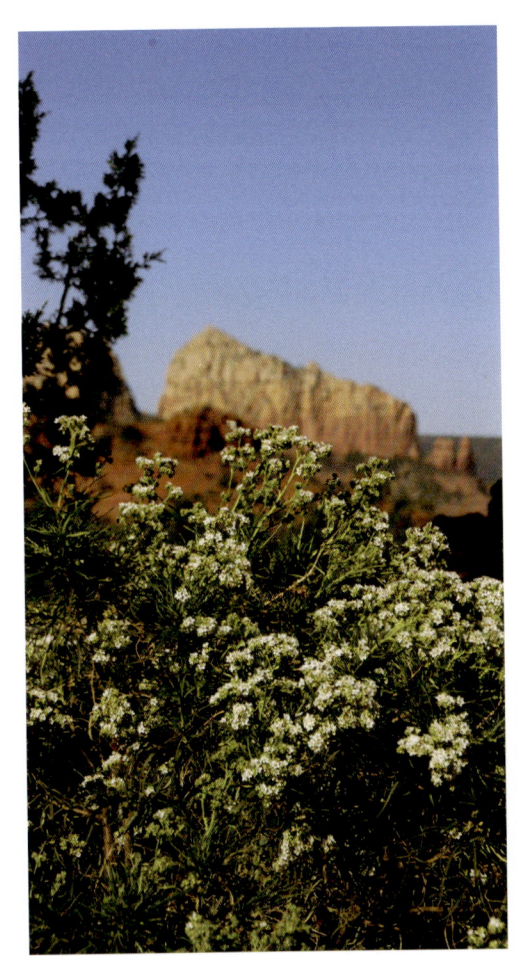

Yerba santa bush's sweet aroma guides you to connect with your higher self

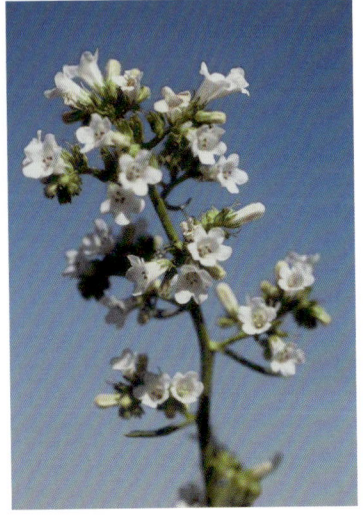

Yerba santa flowers offer cleansing and purification

YERBA SANTA
(Eriodictyon angustifolium)

Primary quality: self-discovery
Energy impact/chakra correspondence: seventh chakra

Voice of the Flower

My name, yerba santa, means "holy herb." I am recognized for my cleansing properties.

I am a woody bush that grows from two to six feet tall. My leaves have lanceolate and slightly notched edges. My outer leaves are sticky, smooth, and resinous. My lower, slightly woolly leaves are a dull green. They have a marked central vein with numerous small, elegant veins. They have a unique scent, similar to licorice—sweet-smelling and powerfully spicy.

My flowers are white and funnel-shaped. They grow in loose terminal clusters at the end of my stems and have five tiny petals and five tiny stamens with five dark yellow anthers. Breathe in my sweet, resinous aroma. My flower essence water tastes very strong and resinous. Taking in my essence water invites a warm, cleansing, gentle sensation throughout your body.

My invitation to you is to step inside my beautiful funnel-shaped flower. Breathe in my pleasant aroma. Touch my soft, delicate petals. Visualize my flower as an aide to help you reach into the depths of your inner world. In this place, what comes to your awareness? What is it in your inner world that calls for your attention? I offer cleansing and purification in your deepest places as you delve into discovering who you are. Talk to that part of you that needs your attention. Ask what you can do for it and how you can nurture it. Give it a voice. Let me guide you on your path of self-discovery. Cleanse yourself of whatever it is that causes you discomfort.

Feel renewed with the healing power of my light-filled radiance. Hold the power of my sacredness deep inside of you. When you feel ready, step outside my flower petals. Keep the inner light within you alive. Let this renewal inspire you to enjoy your path of self-discovery.

Insight

Yerba santa offers new ways to renew yourself by going deep within and taking time to explore who you truly are.

The sticky, astringent, mucilaginous, resinous qualities of yerba santa leaves strongly indicate the plant's use for treating chest colds, bronchitis, asthma, and more. If you look closely at the underside of the leaves, you can see tiny veins that look like bronchioles. This characteristic suggests the plant's practical and medicinal uses. It also demonstrates the powerful cleansing effect that yerba santa has on both the inner and outer body.

Yerba santa is a wonderful healer and teacher that helps you sort out your inner layers of confusion and pain. It helps you to reach into the depths of your inner world to discover pathways of healing that bring you cleansing and solace. Yerba santa guides you to follow through with your outer tasks as you meet your inner needs.

Yerba santa's signature as a woundwort remedy is indicated by the leaf's shape, which resembles a knife or swordlike instrument. This signature demonstrates the plant's natural ability to serve as a Band-Aid that can hold both sides of a cut together. There are two different sides of the leaf: the outer leaf, which is smooth and shiny, relating to the skin; and the underside leaf, which is dull and veiny, relating to the veins. We are shown the duality of healing what is on the inside and what is on the outside.

Yerba santa, "holy herb," was adopted by Spanish colonizers, who learned of the plant from Native Americans. The fresh or dried leaves of yerba santa can be boiled or made into a tea to expel phlegm, restore the liver, clear the urinary tract, and treat chest colds, sore throats, bronchitis, head congestion, asthma, and more. Yerba santa also has a reputation as a woundwort remedy. Due to this plant's rich history it is worth mentioning that it brings to your awareness your relationship with your own inner sanctuary. This awareness will help you navigate out of old internal conditions to discover what it is that will lead you to your own psychological healing.

Yerba santa flowers attract butterflies as their primary pollinator.

Yerba santa's flower essence water smells slightly sweet and refreshing. It tastes subtly of fennel or licorice, especially if leaves are included in the essence. Its taste is strong, powerful, and resinous. When drinking it, you might feel a warm tingling sensation and an opening in your heart that travels to your crown chakra that is gentle yet persuasive.

✦ *Affirmation* ✦

I explore the depths of my inner world.
I discover a newfound renewal.

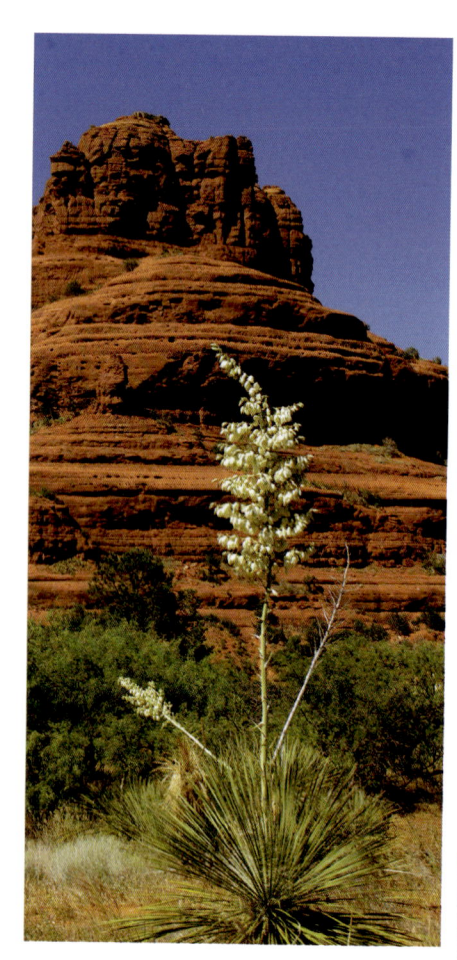

Yucca plant flourishes to achieve new heights

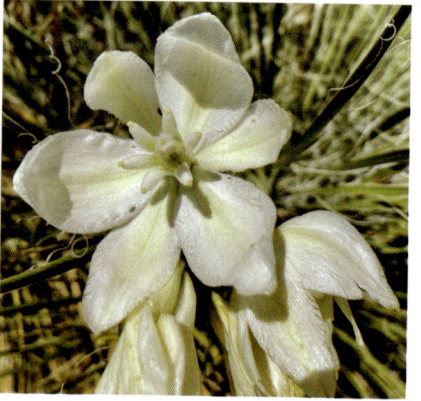

Yucca flowers reveal their soft and creamy inner aura

YUCCA (SOAPTREE)
(Yucca elata)

Primary quality: focus
Energy impact/chakra correspondence: seventh chakra

Voice of the Flower

I stand with great endurance as my roots burrow deep into the earth. My sturdy stalk reaches to meet the sky above. The high saponin content of my roots helps me flourish in the desert terrain. I am protected all around my base with spiny-tipped and fibrous leaves. My narrow leaves rise in a rosette from a central stem.

I am a very useful plant. My leaves can be used to make cordage and baskets, among other things. Many parts of me are cleansing. The taste of my flowers is divine. You may notice that they are creamy-colored, with a slight pink hue around them and rising in clusters toward the top of my stalk.

My flowers have a soft, subtle, sweet, yet bitter smell. My flower petals are thick and rubbery. They grow alternately, upright, and close together along the stem. Each flower has six petals and is bell-shaped in the daylight and star-shaped at night or when placed in a bowl of water. My clustered flowers glow in the moonlight and look like a softly burning candle.

Six fuzzy, creamy-white stamens with yellow anthers are protected inside my flower. The pistil is somewhat thick and crunchy. It tastes like a raw green vegetable. My flower is followed by a symmetrical, three-celled, cylindrical seed capsule and a large, succulent fruit. My entire flower tastes good.

I bloom even in the dark of the night. I offer you my shining light to help you stay focused on your life's dreams and your life purpose.

Take in my gentle, light-filled energy. Let me shed light on your journey. I share with you my strength and endurance. Join me in discovering your destiny. Stay focused on your life's path.

Insight

Yucca is calling you to focus on your direction and how you invest your energy.

Yucca is a night-blooming plant. The flower essence is best made at night under a full moon. The flowers open in the water and appear like a six-pointed star. This important signature represents the light this plant offers, even in the darkness. Like a shining star, yucca shines its light to help you see where you're going so you can stay focused on your journey.

Yucca offers great strength, endurance, and grounding energy. The plant's sprout grows upright. When it reaches maturity, yucca stands tall and rises like a spear to meet the sky. Its high saponin content from roots to flowers gives yucca the ability to thrive on its own resources. Yucca reflects a powerful cleansing effect. Its medicinal qualities are diverse and have multiple uses.

Yucca helps you stay centered and focused on your life's direction. Tap into the enormous power of yucca. Feel its fullness. Be empowered to take actions that will help you move forward in life. Let the light of yucca shine on you and guide you on your path.

The yucca was depicted in several petroglyphs in prehistoric times by the Pueblo in Boca Negra Canyon in New Mexico. Native peoples of the Southwest ate the flowers, buds, and young stalks, which are rich in vitamin C. The saponin-rich yucca root is known since ancient times for its use in cleansing and was made into a shampoo by the traditional peoples of the Southwest to stimulate hair growth and prevent dandruff. It was also used as a soap for cleansing before ceremonies and dances. A root poultice or salve can be made to treat skin disorders, skin eruptions, sprains, breaks, and rheumatism. A tea made from the root treats pain such as arthritis, and is still used today as a laxative. An infusion of the tea is known to treat urethral and prostate inflammation. Yuccas have a multitude of other natural healing properties.

The yucca plant and the yucca moth depend upon each other for survival; they cannot live without each other. It is one of the most amazing relationships that exists between an insect and the plant that it pollinates. Rhonda experienced this phenomenon of nature with farmer and floral designer Kate Watters on Perkinsville Road near Jerome, Arizona, during a magical moment of understanding this interdependent relationship.

Yucca flower essence water emits a deep, full, sweet fragrance. Just like its scent, the yucca essence tastes thick, full, rich, potent, and sweet. It sends warmth throughout the body, from the feet to the crown.

✦ *Affirmation* ✦

I am focused on my journey. I move forward in my life.

Notes

INTRODUCTION.
SYNCHRONICITY AND INTERCONNECTEDNESS

1. "Thoughtforms and Synchronity—Assume the Impossible," YouTube, Nov. 23, 2021.
2. Wood, *Seven Herbs*, 101.
3. Wood, 108.

CHAPTER 1.
THE LANGUAGE OF PLANT ENERGY

1. Sánchez, *Breaking Ground*, 6.
2. Buhner, *Plant Intelligence*, 31.
3. Popham, *Evolutionary Herbalism*, 165.
4. Wood, *Magical Staff*, 15.
5. Hahnemann, *Organon*, 9–10.
6. Gladstar, Facebook post on October 4, 2023.
7. Childre and Martin, *Heart Math*, 9.
8. Buhner, *Secret Teachings*, 111–12.
9. HeartMath, "What Is Heart Coherence?"
10. McKusick, *Electric Body*, xxvii.
11. Buhner, *Secret Teachings*, 159.

CHAPTER 2.
PLANTS' SENSORY INPUT

1. Chamovitz, *What a Plant Knows*, 24.
2. Chamovitz, 29.
3. Mancuso and Viola, *Brilliant Green*, 57.
4. Mancuso and Viola, 67.
5. Mancuso and Viola, 76–77.
6. "Tel Aviv scientists record sounds emitted from plants under stress," YouTube, April 3, 2023.
7. Yang, "Plants can talk."
8. Micalizio, "Can Plants Hear?"
9. "Tel Aviv scientists record sounds emitted from plants under stress," YouTube, April 3, 2023.

CHAPTER 3.
DYNAMICS OF THE BIOFIELD

1. Trivedi et al., "Effect of a biofield treatment."
2. Wood, *Book of Herbal Wisdom*, 23.

CHAPTER 4.
FLOWER ESSENCES: UNSEEN GIFTS OF NATURE

1. Wood, *Holistic Medicine*, 46.

CHAPTER 5.
PATHWAYS UNITING BODY, MIND, AND SPIRIT: THE CHAKRAS

1. Winston and Maimes, *Adaptogens*, 291.

CHAPTER 7.
AN INVITATION TO A PLANT JOURNEY: WELCOME A NEW DOORWAY INTO YOUR LIFE

1. Graves, *White Goddess*, 171.

THE GUIDING VOICE OF FLOWERS, TREES, AND PLANTS: ASPEN TO YUCCA

1. Nabnan and Pinera, *Agave Spirits*, 61.
2. Moore, *Medicinal Plants of the Desert and Canyon West*, 28.
3. Bigfoot, *Useful Wild Western Plants*, 12–13.
4. Moore, *Medicinal Plants of the Desert and Canyon West*, 28.
5. Moore, *Medicinal Plants of the Desert and Canyon West*, 67–68.
6. Ross, *Smoke Plants*, 115.
7. Urtecho, "What's in your Watershed: Manzanitas."
8. Moore, *Medicinal Plants of the Desert and Canyon West*, 73–75.
9. Ross, *Smoke Plants*, 116.
10. Yetman et al., *The Saguaro Cactus*, 64.

Bibliography

Andrews, Ted. *The Healer's Manual: A Beginner's Guide to Vibrational Therapies.* St. Paul, MN: Llewellyn Publishing, 1996.

Bach, Edward. *The Collected Writings of Edward Bach.* Bath, England: Ashgrove Press, 1998.

———, and F. J. Wheeler, M.D. *The Bach Flower Remedies.* Keats Publishing, 1979.

Beitman, Bernard, and Richard Grossinger. "Thoughtforms and Synchronicity—Assume the Impossible." *Connecting with Coincidence* podcast episode 229, YouTube, November 23, 2021.

Bergner, Paul. *Medical Herbalism: Materia Medica and Pharmacy.* Boulder, CO: North American Institute of Medical Herbalism, 2001.

Bigfoot, Peter. *Useful Wild Western Plants* (self-published class material, no date).

Boericke, William. *Boericke's Homeopathic Materia Medica and Repertory.* New Delhi, India: B. Jain, 1995.

Bowers, Janice. *100 Desert Wildflowers of the Southwest.* Tucson, AZ: Western National Parks Association, 1987.

———. *100 Roadside Wildflowers of Southwest Woodlands.* Tucson, AZ: Western National Parks Association, 1989.

———. *Shrubs and Trees of the Southwest Deserts.* Tucson, AZ: Western National Parks Association, 1993.

Brennan, Barbara Ann. *Hands of Light: A Guide to Healing through the Human Energy Field.* New York: Bantam Books, 1988.

British Institute of Homeopathy Diploma Coursework. Surrey, England: Homeopathic Studies Ltd., 1996.

Bruyere, Rosalyn L. *Wheels of Light: Chakras, Auras, and the Healing Energy of the Body.* New York: Fireside Publishing, 1994.

Buhner, Stephen Harrod. *Sacred Plant Medicine: The Wisdom in Native American Herbalism.* Boulder, CO: Roberts Rinehart Publishers, 1996.

———. *The Secret Teachings of Plants: The Intelligence of the Heart in the Direct Perception of Nature.* Rochester, VT: Bear and Company, 2004.

———. *Plant Intelligence and the Imaginal Realm: Beyond the Doors of Perception into the Dreaming of Earth.* Rochester, VT: Bear and Company, 2014.

Chamovitz, Daniel. *What a Plant Knows: A Field Guide to the Senses.* New York: Farrar, Straus and Giroux, 2017.

Childre, Doc, and Howard Martin. *The Heart Math Solution: The Institute of HeartMath's Revolutionary Program for Engaging the Power of the Heart's Intelligence.* New York: HarperCollins Publishers, 1999.

Clarke, John Henry, M.D. *A Dictionary of Practical Materia Medica.* New Delhi, India: B. Jain, 1994.

Cook, Trevor. *Homeopathic Medicine Today: A Modern Course of Study.* New Canaan, CT: Keats Publishing, 1989.

Darwin, Charles, and Francis Darwin. *The Power of Movement in Plants.* Cosimo Classics, 1880.

Dodge, Natt D. *Flowers of the Southwest Deserts.* Tucson, AZ: Southwest Parks and Monuments Association, 1992.

Elmore, Francis H. *Shrubs and Trees of the Southwest Uplands.* Tucson, AZ: Southwest Parks and Monuments Association, 1976.

Elpel, Thomas J. *Botany in a Day: Thomas J. Elpel's Herbal Field Guide to Plant Families.* Pony, MT. Hops Press, 2000.

Epple, Anne Orth. *A Field Guide to the Plants of Arizona.* Helena, MT: Falcon Press, 1995.

Epstein, Ron. *Making and Using Flower Essences.* Los Angeles, CA: self-published, 1986.

Evans, Mark. *A Guide to Herbal Remedies.* Essex, England: C. W. Daniel Co., 1990.

Gaumond, Andrew. "Hollyhock Flower Meaning, Popular Types, and Uses." Petal Republic website, April 7, 2021.

Gerber, Richard. *Vibrational Medicine: New Choices for Healing Ourselves.* Santa Fe, NM: Bear and Company, 1988.

Gimbel, Theo, D.C.E. *Healing Through Color.* Essex, England: C. W. Daniel Co., 1980.

Gladstar, Rosemary. *Rosemary Gladstar's Family Herbal: A Guide to Living Life with Energy, Health, and Vitality.* North Adams, MA: Storey Publishing, 2001.

Graves, Robert. *The White Goddess*. New York: Farrar, Straus and Giroux, 1997.

Gunther, Bernard. *Energy Ecstasy and Your Seven Vital Chakras*. Van Nuys, CA: Newcastle Publishing Co., 1983.

Gurudas. *Gem Elixirs and Vibrational Healing, Vol. 1*. Boulder, CO: Cassandra Press, 1985.

———. *The Spiritual Properties of Herbs*. San Rafael, CA: Cassandra Press, 1988.

Khait, I., O. Lewin-Epstein, R. Sharon, et al. "Sounds Emitted by Plants Under Stress Are Airborne and Informative." *Cell* 186, no. 7 (2023): 1328–36.

Hahnemann, Samuel. *Organon of Medicine*, 6th ed. New Delhi, India: Homeopathic Publications, 1921.

Hall, Manly P. *Paracelsus*. Los Angeles, CA: Philosophical Research Society, 1964.

Harrington, H. D. *How to Identify Plants*. Denver, CO: Sage Books, 1957.

Harris, James G., and Melinda Woolf Harris. *Plant Identification Terminology: An Illustrated Glossary*. Spring Lake, UT: Spring Lake Publishing, 2013.

HeartMath Institute. "What is Heart Coherence?" HeartMath website, Sept. 13, 2022.

———. "Why Heart Coherence Matters." HeartMath website, Oct. 12, 2022.

Heaven, Ross, and Howard G. Charing. *Plant Spirit Shamanism: Traditional Techniques for Healing the Soul*. Rochester, VT: Inner Traditions, 2006.

Heline, Corinne. *Color and Music in the New Age*. Marina del Rey, CA.: DeVorss and Co., 1985.

———. *Healing and Regeneration through Color*. Marina del Rey, CA: DeVorss and Company, 1983.

Hoffmann, David. *The Herbal Handbook: A User's Guide to Medical Herbalism*. Rochester, VT: Healing Arts Press, 1998.

———. *The Holistic Herbal*. New York: HarperCollins Publishers, 1983.

Holmes, Peter. *The Energetics of Western Herbs: A Material Medica Integrating Western and Chinese Herbal Therapeutics*. Vols. 1 and 2. Boulder, CO: Artemis Press, 1989.

Hutchens, Alma R. *Indian Herbalogy of North America: The Definitive Guide to Native Medicinal Plants and Their Uses*. Boston: Shambhala Publications, 1973.

Judith, Anodea. *Wheels of Life: A User's Guide to the Chakra System*. St. Paul, MN: Llewellyn Publications, 1988.

Judith, Anodea, and Selene Vega. *The Sevenfold Journey: Reclaiming Mind, Body, and Spirit through the Chakras*. Freedom, CA: Crossing Press, 1993.

Kane, Charles. *Medicinal Plants of the American Southwest*. Lincoln Town Press, 2006.

Kent, J. T. *Kent's Repertory*. New Delhi, India: B. Jain, 1988.

Kruger, Anna. *An Illustrated Guide to Herbs: Their Medicine and Magic*. Surrey, England: Dragon's World Ltd., 1993.

Lagos, Leah. *Heart, Breath, Mind: Train Your Heart to Conquer Stress and Achieve Success*. Audiobook. New York: Houghton Mifflin Harcourt, 2020.

Lanner, Harriette. *The Pinyon Pine: A Natural and Cultural History*. Reno, NV: University of Nevada Press, 1981.

Leadbeater, C. W. *The Chakras*. Wheaton, IL: Theosophical Publishing House, 1987.

———. *Man Visible and Invisible*. Wheaton, IL: Theosophical Publishing House, 1977.

Llewelyn, C. J. *Chakras and the Vagus Nerve: Tap into the Healing Combination of Subtle Energy and Your Nervous System*. Woodbury, MN: Llewellyn, 2023.

Lommen, Ursula K. E. *Essential Oils Reference Manual*. Maple Plain, MN: Una Publishing, 1994.

Magley, Beverly. *Arizona Wildflowers: A Children's Field Guide to the State's Most Common Flowers*. Billings, MT: Falcon Press, 1991.

Maier, Kat, and Rosemary Gladstar. *Energetic Herbalism: A Guide to Sacred Plant Traditions Integrating the Elements of Vitalism, Ayurveda, and Chinese Medicine*. Chelsea, VT: Chelsea Green Publishing, 2021.

Mancuso, Stefano, and Alexandria Viola. *Brilliant Green: The Surprising History and Science of Plant Intelligence*. Washington, DC: Island Press, 2018.

Mansfield, Peter, and Shaun Williams. *Flower Remedies: An Introduction to over 200 International Flower Remedies, Their Benefits and Uses*. Boston: Charles E. Tuttle, 1995.

McKusick, Eileen Day. *Electric Body, Electric Health: Using the Electromagnetism Within (and Around) You to Rewire, Recharge, and Raise Your Voltage*. Audiobook. New York: Macmillan, 2021.

———. *Tuning the Human Biofield: Healing with Vibrational Sound Therapy*. Rochester, VT: Healing Arts Press, 2014.

Meadows, Kenneth. *The Medicine Way: How to Live the Teachings of the Native American Medicine Wheel*. Edison, NJ: Castle Books, 1997.

Micalizio, Caryl-Sue. "Can Plants Hear?" *National Geographic* online (education blog), May 24, 2017.

Moore, Michael. *Medicinal Plants of the Desert and Canyon West.* Santa Fe, NM: Museum of New Mexico Press, 1989.

———. *Medicinal Plants of the Mountain West.* Santa Fe, NM: Museum of New Mexico Press, 1979.

Myss, Caroline, Ph.D. *Energy Anatomy: The Science of Personal Power, Spirituality, and Health.* Boulder, CO: Sounds True, 1996.

Nabnan, Gary Paul, and David Suro Pinera. *Agave Spirits: The Past, Present, and Future of Mezcals.* New York, NY: W. W. Norton, 2024.

PallasDowney, Rhonda. *Aromatherapy and Essential Oils.* Ogden, UT: Woodland Publishing, 2010.

———. *The Complete Book of Flower Essences: 48 Natural and Beautiful Ways to Heal Yourself and Your Life.* San Rafael, CA: New World Library, 2002.

———. *The Healing Power of Flowers: Bridging Herbalism, Homeopathy, Flower Essences, and the Human Energy System.* Ogden UT: Woodland Publishing, 2007.

———. *Voices of Flowers: Learning to Use the Essence of Flowers to Heal Ourselves.* San Fransisco, CA: Red Wheel/Weiser, 2006.

Panos, Maesimund, and Jane Heimlich. *Homeopathic Medicine at Home: Natural Remedies for Everyday Ailments and Minor Injuries.* Los Angeles, CA: Jeremy Tarcher, 1980.

Pollan, Michael. *The Botany of Desire: A Plant's-Eye View of the World.* New York: Random House, 2001.

Popham, Sajah. *Evolutionary Herbalism: Science, Spirituality, and Medicine from the Heart of Nature.* Berkeley, CA: North Atlantic Books, 2019.

Ritchason, Jack. *The Little Herb Encyclopedia: The Handbook of Nature's Remedies for a Healthier Life.* Orem, UT: Biworld Publishers, 1982.

Ross, Mairi. *Smoke Plants of North America: A Journey of Discovery.* Jerome, AZ: MultiCultural Educational Publishing Co., 2002.

Saint-Exupery, Antoine de. *The Little Prince.* New York: Reynal and Hitchcock, 1943.

Sánchez, JoAnna Castigliego. *Breaking Ground.* Self-published curriculum studies, 2016.

———. *Seed Sowing.* Self-published curriculum studies, 2013.

Scheffer, Mechthild. *Bach Flower Therapy: Theory and Practice.* Rochester, VT: Healing Arts Press, 1988.

Schneck, Marcus. *Cacti.* Avenel, NJ: Crescent Books, 1992.

Trivedi, Mahendra, Gopal Nayak, and Nandini Altekar. "Effect of a Biofield

Treatment on Plant Growth and Adaptation." *Journal of Environment and Health Science* 1, no. 2 (2015). 1–9.

Urtecho, Paula. "What's in Your Watershed: Manzanitas." The Watershed Project website, Jan. 13, 2021.

Weiner, Michael. *Weiner's Herbal: The Guide to Herb Medicine.* Briar Cliff Manor, NY: Stein and Day, 1982.

———. *Earth Medicine, Earth Food: The Classic Guide to the Herbal Remedies and Wild Plants of the North American Indians.* New York: Ballantine Books, 1990.

Winston, David, and Steven Maimes. *Adaptogens: Herbs for Strength, Stamina, and Stress Relief.* Rochester, VT: Healing Arts Press, 2007.

Wood, Matthew. *The Book of Herbal Wisdom: Using Plants as Medicines.* Berkeley, CA: North Atlantic Books, 1997.

———. *Holistic Medicine and the Extracellular Matrix: The Science of Healing at the Cellular Level.* Rochester, VT: Healing Arts Press, 2021.

———. *The Magical Staff: The Vitalist Tradition in Western Medicine.* Berkeley, CA: North Atlantic Books, 1992.

———. *Seven Herbs: Plants as Teachers.* Berkeley, CA: North Atlantic Books, 1987.

———. *Vitalism: The History of Herbalism, Homeopathy, and Flower Essences.* Berkeley, CA: North Atlantic Books, 2005.

Yang, Allie. "Plants Can Talk. Yes, Really. Here's How." *National Geographic* online, April 12, 2023.

Yetman, David, Alberto Búrquez, Kevin Hultine, and Michael Sanderson. *The Saguaro Cactus: A Natural History.* Tucson: The University of Arizona Press, 2020.

Additional website references:
americansouthwest.net
honey-plants.com
gardenfundamentals.com
nrcs.usda.gov

Index

abundance, 233–35
adrenal glands, 52, 54
air element, 40, 58, 65, 77–78, 88
animals, flower essences for, 46, 47
archetypes, 1
archeus (vital force), 18
aspen, 18, 101–3
aster, 24, 62, 104–6
aural communication, 27–29

Bach, Edward, 38–40
balance
  and centering, 257
  of the chakras, 50
  chamomile for, 36
  in the endocrine system, 52
  flower essences for, 38, 41
  and the heart, 59
  honeysuckle for, 173–75
  as taught by plants, ix, 16
beauty, inner, 140–42
beginnings, new, 262–65
Beitman, M.D., Bernard, 2
beliefs, new, 197–99
bells of Ireland, 107–9

biofield, the, 31–34, 42
black cohosh, 3
black-eyed Susan, 110–12
blanketflower, 113–15
bliss and the seventh chakra, 63–65, 83–84
blue flag iris, 116–18
bouncing bet, 119–21
boundaries, 205, 257
brain, heart and, 21
Breaking Ground, 16
breath
  in heart/brain connection, 21
  in plant journeys, 91, 93
  in the universal energy field, 23
Brilliant Green: The Surprising History and Science of Plant Intelligence, 27, 28
Buhner, Stephen Harrod, 18, 22, 23

calendula, 46, 57, 122–24
California poppy, 125–27
centering, 256–58
century plant, 15, 32, 128–30

Index

chakras
  Chakra Spread, 80–84
  colors of, 50–52, 80
  and the endocrine system, 52–53
  fifth/throat/voice, 60–61, 81, 83
  first/physical/root, 54–55, 81–82
  fourth/heart, 58–59, 81, 82–83
  opening of, 64
  plant communication with, 50
  and plant readings, 69
  second/emotional/spleen, 55–56, 81, 82
  seventh/crown/bliss, 63–65, 81, 83–84
  sixth/brow/third eye/insight, 61–63, 81, 83
  third/personal power/solar plexus, 57–58, 81, 82
  and the vagus nerve, 54
chamomile, 36, 46, 131–33
Chamovitz, Daniel, 25, 27
chaparral, 57, 134–36
children, flower essences for, 45–47
chi/prana/Spirit, 18
choices, inner wisdom for, 212–14
circadian clocks, 25–26
circle of life, 169–72
cleansing, 133, 179–82
cliff rose, 137–39
colors of the chakras, 50–52
columbine (yellow), 140–42
comfrey, 143–45
communication, 60–61, 215–17
compassion, 269–72
confidence, 139, 243–45
Connecting with Coincidence, 2
consciousness
  of the chakras, 58
  connecting with higher, 63–64

conscious/unconscious connection, 1
divine consciousness, 22, 74
and human-plant connection, 15
merging energy with, 65
crabapple, 146–49
creativity, 59, 176–78, 206–8
crimson monkeyflower, 56, 150–52
cryptochromes, 25

Darwin, Charles, 30
decisions, inner wisdom for, 212–14
desert larkspur, 153–55
desert marigold, 156–58
desert willow, 59, 159–61
digestive system, 53, 54
divine, the, 79–80, 89
doctrine of signatures, 6, 15, 16, 35–37, 90–91

earth element, 40, 54, 65, 72–73, 79, 89
ease, experience of, 156–58
eastern direction, 77–78, 88
echinacea, 162–64
electromagnetic field, 22, 23, 31, 32
emotions
  balancing, 38, 41
  calendula for, 123
  California poppy for, 125–26
  chamomile for, 36, 131–33
  of children, 46, 47
  emotional power, 150–52
  energy of, 23
  healed via flower essences, 42
  heart coherence and, 23
  onion for, 37
  in plant readings, 68
  and red/orange/yellow flowers, 51
  and the second chakra, 53, 55–56, 82
  understanding of personal, 5, 8

unwinding painful, 267
water and, 78
empowerment, 250–52
endocrine system, 52–54
energy
  of the chakras, 50, 51
  children's sensitivity to, 45
  of color, 51
  energetic protection, 273–75
  of flower essences, 39–42
  of grief, 94
  in group plant readings, 69
  held/obstructed in the body, 52, 54
  of the life force, 16–19, 55
  merged with consciousness, 65
  of the plant biofield, 31–34
  plant energy readings, 67–70
  quintessential, 77
  and telepathic communication, 61
  unique expression of, 40
  universal field of, 22–24, 64
  See also plant energy medicine; vibrational healing
entanglement, 4, 5, 267
enthusiasm, 113–15
ether element, 60
evening primrose, 165–68

fertility, 228–29
fire element, 40, 57, 65, 78, 88
Five Elements Circle of Life Spread, 70, 76–80
flower colors, 51–52
flower/plant essences
  for animals, 47–48
  for children, 45–47
  how to make, 39, 42–43, 87–93
  in plant readings, 67, 68
  and quintessence, 77

safety of, 44
subtle medicine of, 5–6
use of, 45–48
vibrational healing by, 40–42
Flower Spread, 70, 71–74
focus, 282–84
forgiveness, 59
four elements, 40
fragrance/scent, 26–27
freedom, 114
frustration, 4, 5

Gaia, 24, 71
giving, 73
Gladstar, Rosemary, x–xi, xiii, 7, 20
Grandfather Oak, 93–95
Grandmother Manzanita, 85–93
gratitude prayer, 88, 93
grief, 37, 94, 209–11
Grossinger, Richard, 2–3
grounding
  by black cohosh, 5
  feeling rooted, 218–20
  in the Flower Spread, 71
  in plant journeys, 90
  strength for, 203–5
growth, personal, 59, 75, 76

habits/patterns
  cleansing of emotional, 126, 127
  and the doctrine of signatures, 35
  flower essences for new, 40
  juniper for cleansing of, 180–81
  new beliefs, 197–99
  release of old, 10, 41, 56, 58, 59, 74, 181, 207
  Seed Spread for changing, 74
  understanding of, 5, 8
harmony, 43, 50, 131–33

healing
  acknowledging need for, 75
  and Chakra Spread flowers, 80
  and doctrine of signatures, 35
  and endocrine balance, 52
  and the five elements, 77
  via flower essences, 40, 42–43, 45, 46, 47
  of grief, 94, 209–11
  and the human energy field, 23
  of the inner child, 107–9, 254–55
  via the life force, 18–19
  via plant meditations, 66–67
  via plant readings, 69
  power of plants for, 7
Healing Power of Flowers: Bridging Herbalism, Homeopathy, Flower Essences, and the Human Energy System, The, 43
hearing/sound, 27–29, 50
heart, the
  awakening of, 266–68
  connecting with wisdom of, 20–24
  expression from, 60
  as the fourth chakra, 53, 58–59
  heart coherence, 23
  manzanita and, 186–89
  open, 146–49
  seeing with, 50
  trust in, 148, 149, 188
HeartMath Institute, 23
herbalism, 16, 17, 31
Hildegard of Bingen, 100
Hippocrates, 14, 18
hollyhock, 169–72
homeopathy, 19, 35, 38
honeysuckle, 173–75
humans
  ancient cultural knowledge of, 14

  biofields of, 31
  as interconnected, 1–2
  life force of, 17–18, 19
  relationship with nature, 33
  sustainable lives of, 2, 33

identity, personal
  and the second chakra, 56
  strength to be authentic self, 230–32
  trusting, 231, 234, 245
Indian paintbrush, 55, 176–78
inner child, 107–9, 251, 254–55, 265
insight, 61–63, 68, 104, 105
instinctual wisdom, 17, 108
intention, in plant readings, 68, 69
interconnection
  in the biofield, 31
  human-plant connection, 15, 32, 38
  and the life force, 20
  synchronicity and, 1–3
  as universal, 9, 100
intimacy, 200–202
invisible, trusting the, 190–93

journaling with plants, 68, 70, 92
journeys
  and the first chakra, 54–55
  inspired direction for, 261
  journeying with plants, 7, 9–10, 85–95
  journey of life, 9
  via plant readings, 69
  of the soul, 135
  as true Self, 58
juniper, 60, 179–82

kundalini energy, 120

Index

larkspur, 60, 153–55
life
  circle of life, 169–72
  ecological interrelatedness of, 33
  energy of, 16–19, 22–23, 45
  finding purpose in, 57, 183–85
  flexibility with experiences of, 156–58
  flow of, 276–78
  guiding choices in, 71, 73
  journey of, 9, 43
  moving forward in, 264, 265
  passion/enthusiasm for, 114
  universal field of, 22–23
light, response to, 25
listening to flowers/plants, ix, 10, 68, 100
lotus flower, 64
love
  awakening of, 266–68
  blissful union, 119–21
  and the heart, 22, 53, 58–59
  love potions, 142, 261
  nurturing of, 159–61
  as our birthright, 10
  self-love, 139
lupine, 62, 183–85

Maier, Kat, 31
Mancuso, Stefano, 27
manzanita, 59, 85–95, 186–89
marriage, sacred inner, 120
McKusick, Eileen, 23
meditating with plants, 7, 66–67
memory, 30
mental patterns, 52, 54
mesquite, 190–93
Mexican hat, 194–96
Milgram, Dave, 5
mind, quieting the, 67

monkeyflower, 6, 46, 56, 150–52, 276–78
morning glory, 197–99
Mother Earth, 24, 71
mullein, 200–202

National Geographic, 28
nature, 33, 35
nervous system, 18, 21, 52–54
new beliefs, 197–99
northern direction, 79, 89

oak, 55, 86, 203–5
O'Connor, Sandi, 7, 57
ocotillo, 56, 206–8
olfactory communication, 26–27
oneness, 83–84
onion, 37, 209–11
ox-eye daisy, 212–14

pain
  freeing, 194–96
  healing from, 281
  and heart awakening beyond, 267
PallasDowney, Curt, xiv, 33, 41, 95
PallasDowney, Rhonda, 3, 8, 32, 86, 95
Palmer's penstemon, 60, 215–17
paloverde, 55, 218–20
pancreas, 53, 57
passion
  and enthusiasm for life, 113–15
  and love/sexual love, 119–21
  pomegranate and power of, 227–29
  and sensual pleasure, 247
patience, 224–26
peacefulness, 122–24, 221–23
peace rose, 221–23
penstemon, 60, 215–17, 243–45
perseverance, 116–18

personal power, 57–58
photosynthesis, 25
pineal gland, 53, 63
pinyon pine, 224–26
pituitary gland, 53, 61
plant energy medicine
    ancient understanding of, 14
    and doctrine of signatures, 15, 16, 35, 37
    in flower essences, 39–42
    life force energy and, 16–19
    medicine spreads, 70–84
    and merging with plant spirit, 34
    plant readings for, 67–70
    resonance/power of, 14–15
plants
    biofields of, 31–34
    doctrine of signatures, 6, 15, 16, 35–37
    electromagnetic field of, 22
    flower colors, 51
    healing power of, 9, 14–15
    heart-plant connection, 23–24
    as inherent to life, ix
    instinctual wisdom of, 17
    journeying with, 7, 9–10, 85–95
    language of, 14–16
    life force of, 18
    lifelong relationship with, x
    meditations with, 66–67
    merging with spirit of, 34, 70
    quintessence of, 77
    readings with, 67–70
    response to light, 25
    sensory inputs from/for, 25–30
    wisdom of, x, 9, 16, 17, 31, 34, 67, 71, 94, 95, 100
pleasure, 246–48
pomegranate, 56, 227–29

Popham, Sajah, 18
power
    emotional power, 150–52
    of passion, 229
    personal, and the first chakra, 57–58
Power of Movement in Plants, The, 30
prana/chi/Spirit, 18
prickly pear cactus, 230–32
protection
    aspen for, 102
    bells of Ireland for, 108
    California poppy for, 126
    juniper for, 181
    mullein for, 201
    ocotillo for, 207–8
    prickly pear cactus for, 231
    saguaro for, 240–41
    sweet pea for, 254
    trusting in, 241
    walnut for, 264–65
    yarrow for, 37, 273
purple robe, 233–35
purpose in life, 57, 73, 183–85, 250

quintessence/divine center, 79–80, 89

radiance, 250–52
reception, 73
red root, 95
relationships with plants
    and learning their language, 16
    lifelong, x
    means of intimacy in, 32, 34, 100
    and merged biofields, 31
    via plant journeys, 85–95
    via plant readings, 67–70
renewal, 74, 76, 179–82, 281
reproductive glands, 52–53, 55
Rescue Remedy, 40

resonance, 14–15, 22, 24, 42
rhythm, gentle, 101, 103
rose
   cliff rose, 137–39
   peace rose, 221–23
   wild rose, 266–68

sadness, 37, 94
sage, 62, 236–38
saguaro, 33, 63, 239–42
Sánchez, JoAnna Castigliego, 16, 35
scarlet penstemon, 243–45
scent/smell, 26–27
security, inner, 253–55
seeds, 17–18, 65, 94, 250
Seed Spread, 70, 74–76
Self, higher/true
   black-eyed Susan for, 110–12
   blossoming of, 71
   blue flag iris and, 118
   bouncing bet and, 120
   and the chakras, 58, 63
   connecting to all levels of, 16, 80
   crimson monkeyflower and, 151
   echinacea and, 163
   flower essences for, 43
   and the heart, 23, 59
   Mexican hat and, 195
   ox-eye daisy and, 213
   as the quintessence/center, 79–80, 89
   sage and, 237
   See also soul, the
self-acceptance, 137–39
self-confidence, 139, 243–45
self-discovery, 279–81
self-expression, 153–55
self-worth, 165–68, 202
sensory inputs from/for plants, 25–30

sensuality, 246–48
Seven Herbs: Plants as Teachers (Wood), 6, 7
sexuality, 55, 56
snakeroot, 4
soil quality, 27
solar plexus, 57–58, 123
soul, the
   aligned with nature, 5, 33–34
   communication from, 61
   emotions and, 56
   and flower essence healing, 41–42
   heart as bridge to, 22, 59
   journey of, 135
   as the quintessence/center, 79–80
   stepping into deepest, 10
   See also Self, higher/true
sound, 27–29, 50, 103
southern direction, 78, 88
Spirit/chi/prana, 18
spiritual traditions, 1
strawberry hedgehog, 246–48
strength, 203–5, 230–32
stress, 52, 55
sunflower, 18, 57, 249–52
support, 143–45
sustainable living, 2, 33
sweet pea, 253–55
synchronicity, 1–3

taste, 27
teachers, plants as, 9, 34
telepathy, 61
thistle, 256–58
thymus gland, 53, 58
thyroid gland, 53, 60
touch, 30
transformation, 128

trust
  of contradictions, 174
  in darkness, 111, 167
  in flow of life, 277–78
  in the heart, 148, 149, 188
  of inner strength, 166, 201, 265
  in the invisible, 190–93
  in love, 268
  and patience, 225, 226
  in rhythms of life, 102–3, 147, 276
  in your insight, 105
  in your instincts, 108
  of your journey, 126, 185, 263, 278
  in your senses, 167
truthfulness, 215–17

unconscious/conscious
    interconnection, 1
universal energy field, 22–23

vagus nerve, 52–54
vervain, 259–61
vibrational healing
  and doctrine of signatures, 6
  and electromagnetic energy, 23
  by flower essences, 40–42
  and the heart, 22
  and the human energy field, 23
  human-plant-universal, 24
  and the life force, 16–19, 22–23
  via merging with plant biofield, 31–34
  and plant journeys, 87, 88
  and plant readings, 67
  of plants, 7
  and resonance, 14–15

Viola, Alessandra, 27
vision, awakening of personal, 233–35
vitality, 162–64
voice, 53, 60–61, 103
Voices of Flowers, 9, 10

walnut, 262–65
water element, 40, 55, 65, 78–79, 88
western direction, 78–79, 88
wholeness, life in, 9
wild rose, 47, 59, 266–68
willow, 159–61, 269–72
wisdom
  ancient herbal, 14
  awakening to plant, 10
  awakening to your, 10, 236–38
  divine, 74
  of the heart, 20–24
  inner, 212–14
  interconnection and dawning of, 2
  of plants, x, 16, 17, 31, 34, 67, 71, 91, 94, 95, 100
  and the sixth chakra, 61–62
  trusting your inner knowing, 213, 214, 245
Wood, Matthew, xiii, 5, 6, 7, 9, 25, 35, 39

yarrow, 36–37, 273–75
yellow monkeyflower, 6, 276–78
yerba santa, 6–7, 63, 279–81
yoga, 54
yucca, 18, 63, 282–84

About the Authors

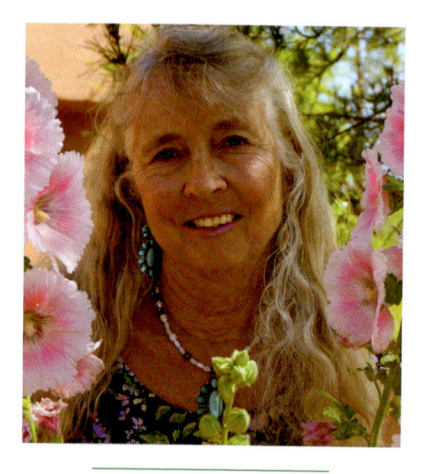

Rhonda PallasDowney
(photo by Curt PallasDowney)

Rhonda PallasDowney received a certificate of Herbal Medicine and the Wisdom of Nature with Matthew Wood/Sunnyfield Herb Farm in 1999. She has a Diploma in Homeopathy from the British Institute of Homeopathy, UK, and she is a flower essence practitioner. Rhonda has an M.A. in Education from Ohio State University and more than twenty-five years of experience in education and social services, with a dedication to the field of developmental disabilities and mental health.

Along with her work in social services, Rhonda founded Living Flower Essences and the Center for Plant Studies and Healing Arts, both of which were her driving force in the natural health and products industry as a product formulator and manager.

Rhonda's understanding of whole plant medicine and whole person healing as associated with the human energy system known as the chakras continues to drive her passion for plants and flowers, nature, health, and wellness. Her fascination with the doctrine of signatures of plants and their folklore ignited her delving deeper into plant communication, plants' sensory perception, and the psychology of plants as shown in the language of flowers.

Rhonda—as a plant whisperer, intuitive teacher, and plant and spiritual medicine guide—is an instrument for illuminating whole person healing with whole plant medicine. She inspires those who are on a path of personal transformation and growth to open new portals of awareness within themselves. Her desire is to share all that she's learned about the gifts of plants, how they communicate, and how they live as energetic beings, and to combine and share these gifts through teaching others.

Rhonda is the author of *The Healing Power of Flowers: Bridging Herbalism, Homeopathy, Flower Essences, and the Human Energy System* and *Voices of Flowers: Learning to Use the Essence of Flowers to Heal Ourselves*. She also has a CD called *Voices of Flowers: 7 Flowers & Chakra Meditation Sound Bath* and a DVD called *A Journey Into Plants & Flowers*, which was featured in the 2014 Sedona Film Festival and selected by the 2022 International Herb Symposium.

Rhonda is a mother and grandmother and resides in Cottonwood, Arizona, with her husband, Curt.

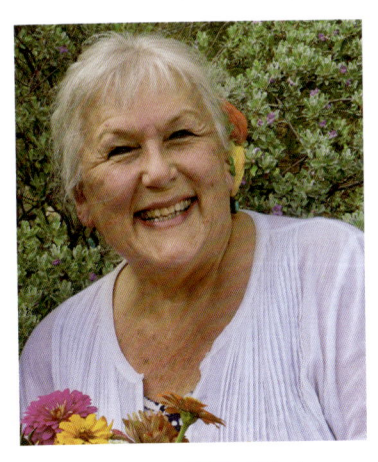

Sandi O'Connor
(photo by Curt PallasDowney)

Sandi O'Connor has worked for more than thirty years in social services, specializing in the field of developmental disabilities. Studying, exploring, and practicing herbalism in her daily life, she met and worked with Rhonda and was inspired to further pursue her interests in herbalism. She became a flower essence practitioner and also a plant medicine guide. Sandi's expertise is in the symbols and myths of flowers and plants and how they correspond to peoples' patterns and behaviors.

Sandi is a lover of plants, animals, and nature. Delving into the symbols and myths of flowers has stirred her passion for the doctrine of signatures and the language of flowers. Sandi is a naturally gifted person and plant whisperer who helps others connect in a deeper way to themselves and to the plant kingdom.

Sandi resides in Clarkdale, Arizona.

A beautiful friendship and a shared passion between Rhonda and Sandi has resulted in collaboration on many projects.

Contact the authors at the Center for Plant Studies and Healing Arts (centerforplantstudies.com, info@centerpsha.com, or on Instagram @pallasdowney).